The Health of Native Americans

The Health of Native Americans

Toward a Biocultural Epidemiology

T. Kue Young

Department of Community Health Sciences
University of Manitoba, Winnipeg, Canada

New York   Oxford

OXFORD UNIVERSITY PRESS

1994

Oxford University Press

Oxford   New York   Toronto
Delhi   Bombay   Calcutta   Madras   Karachi
Kuala Lumpur   Singapore   Hong Kong   Tokyo
Nairobi   Dar es Salaam   Cape Town
Melbourne   Auckland   Madrid

and associated companies in
Berlin   Ibadan

Published by Oxford University Press, Inc.,
198 Madison Avenue, New York, New York 10016

Oxford is a registered trademark of Oxford University Press

Library of Congress Cataloging-in-Publication Data
Young, T. Kue.
The health of Native Americans: toward a biocultural epidemiology/by T. Kue Young.
p. cm.   Includes bibliographical references and index.
ISBN 0-19-507339-8
1. Indians of North America—Health and hygiene—Statistics.
2. Indians of North America—Health and hygiene—Social aspects.
I. Title. [DNLM:
1. Indians, North American—United States.
2. Indians, North American—Canada.
3. Chronic Disease—epidemiology—United States.
4. Chronic Disease—epidemiology—Canada.
5. Communicable Diseases—epidemiology—United States.
6. Communicable Diseases—epidemiology—Canada.
WA 300 Y77ha 1994] RA408.I49Y68   1994
614.4'2'08997—dc20   DNLM/DLC
for Library of Congress   93-20705

9   8   7   6   5   4   3

Printed in the United States of America
on acid-free paper

Preface

This book was written during 1992, a year that marked the 500th anniversary of the arrival of Christopher Columbus in the New World. That this symbolic event has aroused passionate debates highlights the continuing need for, and contentious nature of, "taking stock" of the current state of the indigenous peoples in the Americas.

It is customary to declare one's motives at the outset in writing a book. I write from the perspective of an academic researcher who has felt the need to take a critical and comprehensive look at what is known about the state of health of Native Americans, why certain diseases are common, and how best to prevent and control them. Unlike most academic researchers, I have spent a good part of my professional life practicing, first clinical medicine, and later public health, in Native communities in northern Canada. While I have also visited Alaska and Greenland, the extent of my personal knowledge and experience is still geographically limited. I have relied on the published literature in both the social and biomedical sciences and on assistance from a network of researchers, practitioners, and administrators in Canada and the United States. This is an academic book, for which I make no apologies. There is a time and place for advocacy and activism; there is an equally important time and place for analysis and appraisal. By sifting through the massive amount of data on Native American health, I hope to have something to offer, not just to fellow researchers, but also to those engaged in the delivery of health services in Native communities, from the harassed and burdened front-line workers to the desk-bound bureaucrats.

By invoking the phrase "biocultural epidemiology" in the subtitle, I deliberately hope to forge closer links between the disciplines of epidemiology and anthropology. It is amusing that the "spell-check" program of my word-processing software insists on substituting "bicultural" for "biocultural" whenever the latter appears. In many ways disciplinary boundaries are as formidable as cultural ones. At the University of Manitoba our Department of Community Health Sciences attempts to offer students and faculty both a "biocultural" orientation and a "bicultural" environment. I particularly value the informal collegiality and intellectual stimulation provided to me by my colleagues and students over the years.

That I have been able to pursue an active research agenda in Native American health in the recessionary climate that currently afflicts all academic institutions is due in large part to generous financial support from the National Health Research Development Program of the Department of National Health and Welfare of Canada.

In addition to the anonymous reviewers provided by Oxford University Press, I have benefited immensely from the insightful comments of several colleagues in Winnipeg and elsewhere: Brian Postl, Peter Bjerregaard, Ann Herring, Linda Garro, John O'Neil, and Emöke Szathmary. They cannot be held responsible for any errors in fact or interpretation that I may have committed.

With the advent of the personal computer age, it is no longer necessary for authors to thank their secretaries for long hours of typing and retyping the manuscript. Nonetheless, I am indebted to the secretarial staff of the Northern Health Research Unit, Dawn Stewart and Kathy Bell, for guiding me through the intricacies and awesome capabilities of word processing. Joan Mollins also contributed substantially to most of the computer-generated graphics.

This book would not have come to fruition without the support of Edith Barry, associate editor at Oxford University Press, who saw merit in my proposal and supported it through its evolution from manuscript to book. Susan Hannan, development editor, ably edited the manuscript.

Finally, I owe my emotional sustenance to my wife Valerie and children Steven and Robin, who have wholeheartedly remained my most ardent supporters and in-house critics.

Contents

The Health of Native Americans

1

An Introduction to Native Americans

The health of Native Americans has undergone substantial change from pre-Columbian times to the present. Contact with Europeans had brought along new communicable diseases, often with devastating effects on population size, social organization, and the cultural life of various peoples on the North American continent. Between the seventeenth and nineteenth centuries there was considerable variation between tribes with regard to onset, severity, and duration of disease effects. Since the beginning of the twentieth century there had been a general recovery among native groups in both Canada and the United States. As in the general population, when infectious diseases became better controlled, the disease burden shifted to the chronic diseases. In addition, rapid social changes led to new epidemics of injuries and social pathologies, the control of which has proved far more intractable than for infectious diseases.

Study of the health of Native Americans provides a unique opportunity to apply the methodologic approaches of both anthropology and epidemiology. The genetic origins of Native Americans in the Asian continent and its diversity subsequent to the crossing of the Beringia landbridge, the different intensity and speed of contact, and the acculturation experienced by different tribes inhabiting widely divergent ecological habitats are reflected in the distribution of prevalent diseases among Native peoples. From a global perspective, the health experience of the Native Americans of North America is comparable to that of aboriginal and indigenous populations on other continents (Trowell and Burkitt, 1981; CIBA Symposium, 1977).

This book will develop the theme that the evolution and current pattern of health and disease among Native Americans constitute a case study of "biocultural epidemiology." The traditional tasks of epidemiology, describing the dis-

3

tribution and analyzing the determinants of diseases and health conditions in populations, require an understanding of the interactions of cultural adaptations and genetic susceptibility to disease. Because epidemiology is the basic science of the practice of public health and community medicine, the biocultural approach also has an important application in the planning and evaluation of intervention programs.

The ability to offer solutions, even in situations when "not all the facts are in," is of critical importance to epidemiologists, who should not forget that they are applied scientists. Commenting on the Canadian situation, Postl and colleagues (1987) reminded the public health community that "we now have available a large catalogue of the ill health, socioeconomic disadvantages and cultural stress being experienced by the Native Peoples of this country. A challenge remains as to how to convert this catalogue into improvements in health status."

Organization and Plan

This book is organized into seven chapters. Chapter 1 provides a general overview of Native Americans: their origins and affinities, ecological habitats and adaptations, cultural and historical development, present geographic distribution, and social and economic conditions.

Chapter 2 describes the overall population and health status of Native Americans and how it has evolved historically from before contact with Europeans to the present time.

The remainder of the book is devoted to detailed discussion of three groups of diseases and health conditions:

1. *Infectious diseases,* with special attention to tuberculosis, meningitis, gastroenteritis, pneumonia and respiratory infections, viral hepatitis, sexually transmitted diseases, streptococcal infections, and the parasitoses.
2. *Chronic, noncommunicable diseases,* including cancer, ischemic heart disease, stroke, hypertension, dyslipidemia, obesity, diabetes, and gallbladder disease.
3. *Injuries and the social pathologies,* encompassing unintentional injuries (or accidents), suicide, homicide and violence, and alcohol and substance abuse.

Each group of conditions will be discussed using a consistent format, which addresses a similar set of questions, as follows:

1. *Extent and magnitude of problem.*
   • Do Native Americans suffer more, or less, from these conditions compared to non-Natives in North America?

- Is there variation in disease risk among Native Americans belonging to different geographical, cultural, and linguistic groups?
- Are these diseases/conditions occurring more, or less, frequently in recent times compared to the past?

2. *Etiology and risk factors.*
   - What is known about the etiology and pathogenesis of these diseases, and are there factors unique to Native Americans?
   - What are the relative contributions of environmental and genetic risk factors in accounting for the observed frequency and distribution of these diseases?

3. *Prevention and control strategies.*
   - What prevention and control strategies are available for these diseases and conditions, and has their effectiveness been evaluated?
   - To what extent are these interventions potentially applicable to Native American communities?

The final chapter summarizes the major conclusions of the book and argues for an integration of anthropology and epidemiology, perhaps in a new subdiscipline called "biocultural epidemiology." The needs for future research and the implications for health care are identified.

A Note on Nomenclature

The geographic focus of this book is North America, defined here as including Canada and the United States but excluding Mexico. Some data from Greenland, as the homeland of Eskimos, are also included, even though for much of its recent history Greenland has been linked more with Europe than with North America.

The term *Native American* is used throughout to refer to the indigenous populations of North America that occupied the continent when members of various European nations first arrived, and their descendants. It encompasses North American Indians (Amerindians, Amerinds), Eskimos (Inuit), and Aleuts. In the anthropological literature, the first term is often used in generic sense to include the Eskimos and Aleuts. *Native American* is widely accepted as the "correct" term in the United States, corresponding to such other usage as *African American* and *Asian American*. The expanded term *American Indian and Alaska Native (AIAN)* is often used in U.S. government publications. *Alaska Native* is the collective term for Eskimos, Indians, and Aleuts living in that state. I have also used *Native American* when referring to Native citizens of Canada in general. [I hasten to add that *American* here applies to North America and not to the United States alone.] In some usages, the term *Native Americans* also includes Native Hawaiians, a practice clearly not appropriate for this book.

In Canada, the term *Native* continues to be used by some Native organizations and their leaders, although *Aboriginal* seems to be preferred, as reflected in official communications from the late 1980s. In constitutional negotiations over self-government, three Aboriginal groups are recognized in Canada: Indians, Inuit, and Metis. The term *Indian,* while still used widely by many Indians themselves, is being replaced by *First Nation.* As an adjective, this term is awkward (as in First Nation people), and I have therefore retained the term *Indian* when this group needs to be distinguished from the other Native groups. In Canada, a further distinction is made between "status" ("Treaty," "registered"), and "nonstatus" Indians, which is defined legally by the Indian Act. Such status could be lost in the past through enfranchisement or, in the case of Indian women, through marriage to a non-Indian. All registered Indians are members of a "band," a political and administrative unit created by the federal government.

The term *Eskimo* is almost never used today in Canada, where it is perceived to be a derogatory term. Instead, *Inuit* is preferred by the people. (Inuit is the plural form; the singular is Inuk.) In Alaska, *Eskimo* is still widely used for self-identification. In this book I used *Inuit* when referring to those in Canada, and *Eskimos* when referring to them elsewhere. I have opted for *Eskimo/Inuit* when describing the group "continentally."

Metis is used only in Canada, and refers to a distinct cultural group that originated from mixed Indian-white marriages in the early settlement of the Canadian West. Although officially considered as Native, little of the health and population data available in Canada refers to this group specifically.

I have retained Indian tribal names that have had long usage in the anthropological and popular literature, rather than substitute for them the less familiar names in their individual Native languages (e.g., Papago rather than Tohono-O'odham, Ojibwa rather than Anishinabe, Kwakiutl rather than Kwakwaka'wakw).

Many Native Americans live in legally designated territories called *reservations* in the United States and *reserves* in Canada. One or more reserves may be occupied by members of an Indian band. There are other enclaves inhabited predominantly by Natives that are not officially considered reservations or reserves. Many Native Americans also live in cities, towns, and villages intermingled with members of other ethnic groups.

The issue of "who is Native" is extremely complex, and has legal, historical, cultural, social, and political connotations and ramifications that almost defy resolution. The inability to distinguish individuals or groups based on "genetic" vs "sociocultural" definitions (a problem by no means unique to Native Americans) does not represent a "fatal flaw" in studies of Native American health and population. One of the tasks in compiling data for this book is the sorting of biological and cultural influences on health. It is clear that many studies have had to grapple with the "population denominator" issue, and not always successfully.

Origins and Genetic Diversity

The Asiatic origin of Native Americans is not seriously in dispute—what is in dispute is the date of the migration, how many "waves" of migration, the point(s) of entry in the Americas, and how long it took for humans to populate a land mass that stretches from the North Shore of Alaska to Tierra del Fuego. A detailed discussion of this topic is beyond the scope of this book. It would require an intimate knowledge of, and the ability to synthesize, a diversity of data—archeological, geological, linguistic, genetic, cultural, dental etc. An extensive literature on the subject includes several recent, very informative, reviews, monographs, and symposia [see for example, Laughlin and Harper (1979), Kirk and Szathmary (1985), Dillehay and Meltzer (1991)].

To the extent that the issue of origins affects our understanding of the current cultural and genetic diversity of Native Americans—and thus indirectly the distribution of diseases—epidemiologists with an interest in Native American health need to be familiar with some basic facts and theories. Thus, if there were only one ancestral group common to all Native Americans, their genetic and cultural differentiation would necessarily have occurred within the Americas. The interpretation of genetic susceptibility to certain diseases would then be different from that if there were two or more ancestral groups who were already genetically distinct and who "crossed over" at different times.

Archaeologists seem to compete with one another in uncovering evidence of ever-earlier human habitation in North America. [For a highly readable guide, see Fagan (1987)]. The geological evidence points to the Beringia landbridge, exposed during various times during the last glaciation (the Wisconsin) of the Pleistocene Ice Age, as the most likely route and time over which migration occurred. Dispersal of migrants southwards occurred as the ice sheets receded. Greenberg and associates (1986), in marshalling the archeological, linguistic, and dental evidence, proposed that three migrations of biologically differentiated groups entered North America: the Amerind (also called Paleo-Indian), the Na-Dene (primarily Athapaskan Indians), and the Aleut-Eskimo (or Eskaleut). Various ranges of dates of entry have been proposed: 16,000–40,000 BP (before present) for the Paleo-Indians, 12,000–14,000 BP for the Na-Dene, and 4,000–9,000 BP for the Eskimos. Evidence from studies of Gm and Km allotypes (serum proteins used in measuring genetic distance) has also been found to support the three-migration theory (Williams et al., 1985; Schanfield et al., 1990).

Meltzer (1989) raised the possibility that these migrations were not discrete episodes involving small founding peoples, but instead may have been migratory "dribbles" spread over thousands of years.

With the development of new techniques involving mitochondrial DNA, there is now evidence to indicate that Paleo-Indian and Na-Dene populations were founded by two independent migrations and that the present Native American population may have ultimately derived from four primary maternal lineages (Torroni et al., 1992).

The rapidly developing and exciting line of research involving mitochondrial DNA has opened up an entirely new perspective on the origin and evolution of *Homo sapiens* itself, of which the origin of Native Americans in the Western Hemisphere is but one scene in a larger drama. A lively debate has raged, primarily between geneticists and archeologists, over whether all present-day human beings could be traced along maternal lines to a single woman dubbed "Eve" who lived in Africa some 200,000 years ago (Wilson and Cann, 1992), or derived from multiple stocks as indicated by different fossils at sites around the world (Thorne and Wolpoff, 1992).

With the re-submersion of the Beringia landbridge, the human populations in the Americas became isolated from the Old World. As they penetrated new ecological zones, natural selection in response to environmental stresses operated on existing genetic variability, produced by past mutations and perhaps also as a result of genetic drift and founder effect.

The older physical anthropology literature on Native Americans is replete with detailed descriptions and measurements of racial characteristics—hair color, texture, and distribution; cranial and facial dimensions; anthropometric indices; epicanthic folds; skin pigmentation; dermatoglyphic patterns; and dental morphology. Of more recent vintage is the analysis of inherited biochemical traits, the prevalence of which may demonstrate divergence or affinity between populations (e.g., inactivation of the drug isoniazid, ability to taste phenylthiocarbamide, presence of enzyme variants, and capacity to secrete specific chemicals in the urine and saliva). [For a summary of findings relating to Native Americans, see Sievers and Fisher (1981)].

There is also a large body of data on polymorphisms of blood groups and other genetic markers such as HLA and serum proteins, which form the basis of genetic distance analysis to determine the "relatedness' of different populations, both between Native Americans and the other races, and among Native Americans (Roychoudhury, 1978; Szathmary, 1984).

Native American languages offer some clues to the genetic relationship of the different population groups. While language per se is not inherited (although most of us do learn our mother tongue from genetically related family members), the process of genetic differentiation is akin to that of linguistic differentiation as a people migrate into and populate new lands. Except where military conquest

Table 1.1 Classification of Major Native American languages in North America

PHYLUM American Arctic-Paleosiberian

FAMILY Eskimo-Aleut
e.g., Aleut, Eskimo

PHYLUM Na-Dene

FAMILY Athapaskan
e.g., Dogrib, Chipewyan, Kutchin, Sekani, Beaver, Sarcee, Carrier, Chilcotin, Tahltan, Navajo, Apache

ISOLATE Tlingit

ISOLATE Haida

PHYLUM Macro-Algonkian

FAMILY Algonkian
e.g., Cree, Montagnais, Naskapi, Fox, Sauk, Kickapoo, Shawnee, Ojibwa, Saulteaux, Delaware, Penobscot, Malecite, Micmac, Blackfoot, Piegan, Blood, Cheyenne, Arapaho

FAMILY Muskogean
e.g., Choctaw, Chickasaw, Alabama, Creek, Seminole

PHYLUM Macro-Siouan

FAMILY Siouan
e.g., Crow, Hidatsa, Mandan, Dakota

FAMILY Iroquoian
e.g., Seneca, Cayuga, Onondaga, Mohawk, Oneida, Huron, Tuscarora, Cherokee

FAMILY Caddoan
e.g., Caddo, Pawnee, Arikara

PHYLUM Hokan

FAMILY Yuman
e.g., Walapai, Havasupai, Yavapai, Mohave, Maricopa, Yuma, Cocopa

ISOLATE Washo

PHYLUM Penutian

FAMILY Sahaptin-Nez Perce

ISOLATE Tsimshian

ISOLATE Zuni

PHYLUM Aztec-Tanoan

FAMILY Kiowa-Tanoan

FAMILY Uto-Aztecan
e.g., Northern Paiute, Bannock, Shoshone, Comanche, Southern Paiute, Ute, Chemehuevi, Hopi, Luiseno, Cahuiilla, Pima, Papago, Tarahumara

OTHER ISOLATES/FAMILIES

ISOLATE Kutenai

FAMILY Salish
e.g., Lillooet, Shuswap, Thompson, Okanagan, Colville, Spokane, Quinault, Lummi, Songish, Halkomelem, Squamish, Comox, Bella Coola

FAMILY Wakashan
e.g., Nootka, Nitinat, Makah, Kwakiutl, Bella Bella, Heiltsuk, Kitamat, Haisla

had forcibly imposed a different language on the conquered, or when a people decided to adopt a wholly foreign language as their own, language families tend to reflect genetic differences. This has been demonstrated in many studies of genetic distance around the world (Cavalli-Sforza et al., 1988), including Native Americans north of Mexico (Spuhler, 1979).

There are hundreds of mutually unintelligible Native American languages in North America. The viability of many of these, unfortunately, is in serious doubt. In Canada, only three languages—Inuit, Cree, and Ojibwa—still have large enough numbers of speakers not to be threatened with extinction. There is, not unexpectedly, no agreement among scholars in linguistics on the precise number and classification of distinct Native American languages. Table 1.1 lists some of the more important languages, particularly of those tribes mentioned in this book, based on the system developed by Voegelin and Voegelin, reprinted in Driver (1969). Particularly controversial is the larger groupings of families and language isolates into higher-order "phyla" [analogous to zoological and botanical taxonomy]. At the most radical, Greenberg hypothesized that all Amerindian languages were ultimately derived from three stocks: Amerind, Na-Dene, and Aleut-Eskimo, corresponding to the three migrations (Greenberg et al., 1986). There are also attempts to link Amerindian languages to various Indo-European and Asiatic languages in sweeping, global schemes (Greenberg and Ruhlen, 1992).

The gene-disease relationship of course has long been the subject of much research, from classical medical genetics to the relatively recent genre, genetic epidemiology. Diseases can be viewed as agents of natural selection, resulting in microevolutionary changes, while genes can predispose or protect individuals or populations from certain diseases. Increasingly the interest has shifted from single-gene diseases to the polygenic or complex diseases. The relatively small and isolated Native American populations offer unique opportunities for the delineation of such gene-disease relationships (Chakraborty and Szathmary, 1985).

Ecological Habitats and Adaptations

Several types of physical environments in the New World can be considered "extreme" in terms of climate and physiography, such as the cold regions in the tundra and boreal forest, the hot, dry desert, and high altitude areas with their rarefied atmosphere. Human populations that occupy these habitats have, over thousands of years, developed a complex array of biological and behavioral adaptations to permit not only survival but also the conduct of a rich cultural life. Such adaptive mechanisms, however, can be altered by acculturation or modernization. Although adaptations occur to some extent in all environments, it is in these habitats that they are most evident and hence most studied. It should be recognized that there are an infinite variety of environmental stresses to which humans adapt, and the available mechanisms for adaptation are equally varied and diverse. Each population can be considered to be unique in the adaptive pattern that has evolved (Baker, 1966). The diversity of ecological habitats is reflected in the delineation of "culture areas," of which there are at least ten in North America (see below).

The Eskimos/Inuit in the Arctic and various Algonkian and Athapaskan Indians in the subarctic boreal forest of Alaska and Northern Canada are faced with severe winter climates. A substantial literature in human physiology is available on the body's ability to maintain its core temperature under cold ambient temperatures. A variety of biological and behavioural adaptations have been recognized (So, 1980; Moran, 1981). Biological factors include the distribution of body fat, body shape (long body, short extremities), more actively functioning sweat glands in the face than on the body, and rapid rewarming of fingers after cooling. Such features have been found in the Eskimo/Inuit (Shephard, 1980; Auger et al., 1980; Schaefer et al., 1974). Northern Algonkian Indians have also been shown to maintain high finger temperatures during cooling and to rewarm rapidly. Furthermore, white genetic admixture appears to reduce the level of such protective cold responses (Hurlich and Steegman, 1979).

Perhaps more important in cold adaptation are such behavioral strategies as shelter, clothing, work/activity pattern, diet and eating habits, and risk avoidance/safety precaution practices (Moran, 1981; Steegman et al., 1983). That such adaptations have been remarkably successful is illustrated by the relatively low frequency of cold injuries among Native Americans inhabiting cold climate regions, provided there is no impairment by alcohol.

In contrast to the scientific interest in cold adaptation in the Arctic and Subarctic, relatively few studies have been conducted among Native Americans who inhabit the other climatic extreme, such as the hot and arid Southwest and Great Basin. Here the problem is one of efficient heat dissipation. Hanna (1970) found that Papagos in Arizona had a lower rate of sweating and lower rectal temperatures than migrant whites after induced heat stress (walking two hours per day for one week in the hot desert sun), while Yaqui Indians in Mexico had a physiological response similar to that of *mestizos* who were lifelong residents of the desert but whose parents came from other parts of the country.

Few Native Americans in North America inhabit high altitudes, unlike some Andean Native populations in South America, who have also evolved specific adaptations to the low-oxygen pressures in the atmosphere, particularly in the respiratory and hematologic systems [see, for example, studies among the Quechua in Peru (Baker and Little, 1976)].

Cultural and Historical Development

While the Native Peoples in North America did not develop empires comparable in scale and complexity with those of the Aztecs and Incas in Mesoamerica and South America, highly stratified societies living in large, agricultural villages could be found in some areas. Terms such as "simple" and "primitive" have been applied to societies lacking in complex social and political organization, such as "bands" of hunter-gatherers. However, the ability to survive, and thrive, in their particular environments required a high degree of technological innovation, detailed knowledge, and diverse skills which were anything but simple.

Prior to the arrival of Europeans, a variety of Native societies existed. These can be broadly grouped according to shared sociocultural traits into large contiguous geographical zones called *culture areas*. Culture areas are useful conceptual tools. As they reflect ecological habitat, subsistence patterns, social organization, population size and structure, religious beliefs and practices, they should also, at least indirectly, affect nutritional status and disease patterns. The re-creation of precontact culture areas and their comparison with known historical and present circumstances can provide clues to the extent, magnitude, and direction of cultural change—which also has health implications.

The authoritative handbook series on Native Americans published by the Smithsonian Institution (Sturtevant, 1978–90) is organized according to ten culture areas: Arctic, Subarctic, Northwest Coast, Great Basin, California, Plateau, Plains, Southwest, Southeast, and Northeast (Fig. 1.1). It should be recognized that the boundaries depicted are at best approximate, and they imply more of a physical reality than intended.

The *Arctic* stretches across the top of the continent from Alaska to Greenland. Located above the treeline, the tundra offers one of the most inhospitable environments on earth. It was here that North America's original inhabitants, the Eskimo/Inuit and Aleuts, developed the most ingenious adaptations. The main subsistence activity was the hunting of sea mammals (seals, walruses, whales) along the coast; in specific locations, fishing or caribou hunting were also important.

The *Subarctic,* which also spans North America, from the interior of Alaska to the Atlantic coast, is dominated by the boreal forest. Athapaskan and Algonkian Indians lived as nomadic hunters of large game such as moose and caribou. The large number of lakes and rivers provided a variety of fish, an important part of the diet.

The *Northwest Coast,* extending from the Alaska "panhandle" south to Oregon, offered a mild and moist climate and plentiful resources on its numerous islands, peninsulas and inlets, particularly salmon fishing. Various Indian linguistic groups such as the Haidan, Tsimshian, Tlingit, Salishan and Wakashan

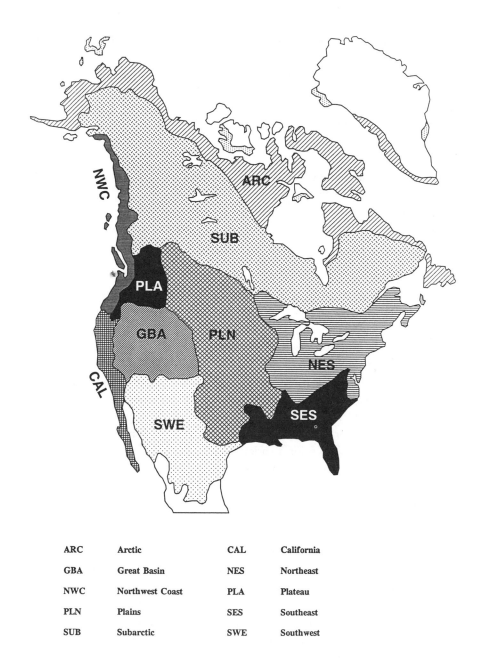

ARC	Arctic	CAL	California
GBA	Great Basin	NES	Northeast
NWC	Northwest Coast	PLA	Plateau
PLN	Plains	SES	Southeast
SUB	Subarctic	SWE	Southwest

Figure 1.1. Map of North America showing culture areas.

developed highly complex, affluent, and sedentary societies (including the development of social classes and slavery).

The *Plateau,* in inland British Columbia, Washington, and Idaho, were inhabited by Salishan and Kutenaian speakers who fished salmon from the fastflowing Columbia and Fraser river systems. Towards the north, the lifestyle resembled that of the Subarctic.

The grassy *Plains* occupy the central part of the continent. Buffalo hunting by Siouan speakers in the north and Caddoan speakers in the south was the dominant lifestyle. The introduction of horses in historic times enhanced the efficiency of the hunt and also transformed the culture.

The *Northeast* encompasses the woodlands around the Great Lakes, the valley of the St. Lawrence River and the Atlantic seaboard. Various Iroquoian and Algonkian tribes lived in villages and developed horticulture, particularly the growing of maize, the main food staple, and other crops such as beans and pumpkin. The Iroquoians also instituted the largest political units north of Mexico.

In the *Southeast,* with its wet and mild climate, agriculture was well developed. Mostly Muskogean speakers lived in a rich, fertile region that once supported the Mississippian culture characterized by huge temple mounds and large cultivated fields. However, by the 16th century, the culture of the mound-builders declined after initial contact with the first Europeans.

The arid and dry *Great Basin* includes all of Nevada and Utah and areas in surrounding states. It was inhabited mainly by tribes belonging to the Uto-Aztecan language family, who led a rather precarious existence from the gathering of nuts and digging for wild vegetables, supplemented by hunting of small game.

The *Southwest* is known for a variety of terrains—plateau, sierras, and canyons. As much of the region is dry desert, villages were founded along streams. They represented a highly developed agricultural society but had declined from an earlier period, when advanced cultures such as the Mogollon and Anasazi flourished. The people were Uto-Aztecans, Yumans, and Athapaskans, the last group (represented by the Navajo and Apache) were the most recent migrants (around the tenth century) from the northern reaches of the continent who had retained their ancestral languages but adopted the culture of surrounding tribes.

The diverse peoples of *California* generally led a settled village life and had the densest population north of Mexico, although they did not practice agriculture. The main food was prepared from pounding acorns into meal.

The history of Native Americans took a new turn after the arrival of Europeans. In their general history, Leacock and Lurie (1971) characterized the following phases:

1. Early contact occurred either directly with explorers, traders, and missionaries, or indirectly with goods traded through neighboring tribes. Much of Native-white contact was on an equal footing and mutually beneficial.

2. Period of large-scale settlement by, and serious conflict with, newcomers, characterized by massive disruptions caused by epidemics and warfare. In some regions, Native Americans were forced into servitude, while in others, the military carried out a policy of genocide. Treaties were signed and repeatedly broken, and whole nations were encroached upon and forcibly displaced.
3. Period of relative stabilization and institution of government controls, such as the establishment of reservations and the withdrawal into geographic and cultural enclaves.
4. Period of cultural revival and emergence of new forms of political organization within the context of modern industrial society.

It should be noted that these periods are gross simplifications. They occurred at different times in different regions, and some peoples bypassed some of these stages altogether. Much of Native American post-contact history is dominated by relationships with non-Native immigrants/settlers and the impact such relationships had on Native American culture. Depending on the geographical location and historical era, the peoples with whom Native Americans interacted included Spanish, French, English, Russians, Scandinavians, Americans, and Canadians.

One concept that has been used to characterize the change in Native culture is "acculturation." A much quoted and still useful definition is that proposed by anthropologists Redfield, Linton, and Herskovitz (1936):

> Acculturation results when groups of individuals having different cultures come into continuous first-hand contact, with subsequent changes in the original pattern of either or both groups.

This concept has been much expanded since then, and different types of contact and processes of change can be distinguished. [For selected Native American case studies, see Spicer (1961).] Some social scientists objected to the whole concept of acculturation for its emphasis on how indigenous peoples had to accommodate, adapt to, and ultimately become assimilated by the dominant external, colonizing power. A concept similar to that of acculturation, one that is ecologically based, is "delocalization," which was defined by Pelto as:

> The tendency for any territorially defined population to become increasingly dependent on resources, information flow, and socioeconomic linkages with the systems of energy and resources outside their particular area. (cited in Waldram, 1985)

Other terms such as "development," "modernization," or "westernization" have been used to describe the complex social, economic, cultural, and political changes experienced by Native Americans, particularly in the second half of the twentieth century.

Present Geographical Distribution

United States

According to the 1980 Census, there were about 1.4 million Native Americans in the United States, only 0.6 percent of the total population of the country. About 37 percent of Native Americans lived in designated areas, including reservations, Alaska Native villages, tribal trust lands, and "historic areas of Oklahoma" [former reservations with legally established boundaries at the beginning of the century].

The ten largest reservations accounted for almost 50 percent of the population of all reservation Indians. They are, in descending order of population size: the Navajo reservation with 105,000 people located in the border regions of Arizona, Utah, and New Mexico; the Pine Ridge, South Dakota, reservation (Oglala Sioux), with 12,000; various reservations in Arizona with populations in the 6,000–7,000 range (Gila River, Papago, Fort Apache, Hopi, and San Carlos); and other reservations also with 6,000–7,000 population each (Zuni, New Mexico, Rosebud, South Dakota, Blackfeet, Montana). A map of U.S. Indian reservations and Alaska Native corporations is shown in Figure 1.2.

The Native American population in the United States has become increasingly urbanized. In 1980 54 percent of the population lived in central cities and their peripheral urbanized areas, compared to 45 percent a decade earlier. The 10 metropolitan areas with the largest Native population in 1980 were, in descending order: Los Angeles-Long Beach, California (48,000), Tulsa (39,000) and Oklahoma City, Oklahoma (25,000), Phoenix, Arizona (23,000), Albuquerque, New Mexico (21,000), San Francisco-Oakland (18,000) and Riverside-San Bernadino, California (17,000), Seattle, Washington (17,000), Minneapolis-St Paul, Minnesota (16,000), and Tucson, Arizona (15,000).

The present distribution of Native Americans reflects the consequences of the historical "opening up" of the country for settlement by European migrants. In 1980 only 6 percent of Native Americans could be found in the northeastern states, whereas just under one-half resided in the West, 27 percent in the South, and 18 percent in the Midwest. The ten states with the largest Native populations were: California (202,000), Oklahoma (170,000), Arizona (153,000), New Mexico (108,000), North Carolina (65,000), Arkansas (64,000), Washington (61,000), South Dakota (45,000), Texas (40,000), Michigan (40,000).*

---

*Data are from the U.S. Bureau of the Census, summarized in the document *Indian Health Care* (U.S. Congress, 1986). A full discussion of the various sources of population data and their limitations is provided in Chapter 2].

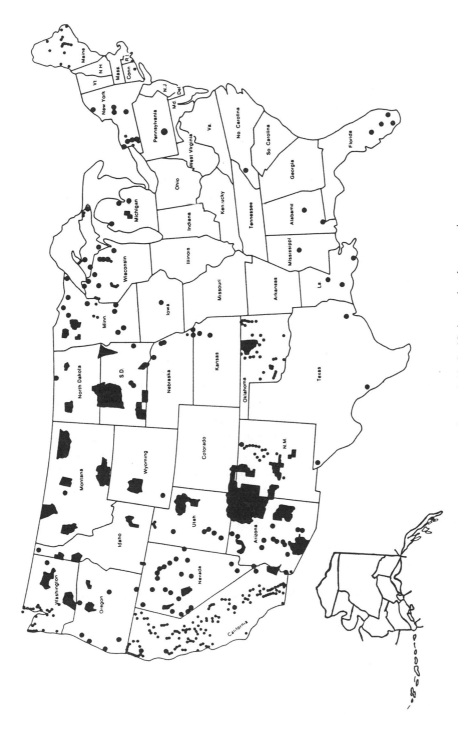

Figure 1.2. Map of United States showing Indian reservations and Alaska Native regional corporations.

Canada

According to the 1986 Census, 760,000 Canadians claimed single Native or multiple (i.e., Native and non-Native) origins, about 3 percent of the country's population. Of those, 570,000 were Indians, 130,000 Metis, 34,000 Inuit, and 24,000 of mixed Native-Native heritage. The approximately 45,000 residents of Indian reserves who were incompletely enumerated in the census were included in the Indian total.

Native Canadians were the majority in only one jurisdiction—the Northwest Territories, where they accounted for 58 percent of the population. The Yukon had the second largest proportion of Natives in its population, with 21 percent. In the provinces, Natives represented approximately 8 percent of the population of Manitoba and Saskatchewan, almost 5 percent in Alberta and British Columbia, but only between 1 and 2 percent in central and eastern Canada.

Within the Native population itself, almost one in four Natives resided in the largest province, Ontario. When broken down into the three major categories, almost two-thirds of Indians could be found in Ontario and British Columbia, while two-thirds of Metis were in the Prairie provinces. More than half (55%) of the Inuit lived in the Northwest Territories, with substantial numbers in northern Quebec (21%) and Labrador (12%).

While more than three-quarters of the total Canadian population were urban, 54 percent of Natives (single and multiple origins) lived in urban areas. Once again, the proportion of urban residents differed among the three major Native groups: 53 percent among Indians, 65 percent among Metis, and 26 percent among Inuit. In general, most rural Natives reported only single Native origins, whereas urban Natives were more likely to be of mixed or multiple origins.

Approximately 60 percent of Canadian Indians lived on Indian reserves and settlements. Canadian reserves were generally much smaller in population than those in the United States. Only three reserves had population exceeding 5,000: Kahnawake (Mohawk), Quebec; Six Nations, Ontario; and Blood, Alberta.*

Greenland

Although Greenland, located entirely north of the sixtieth parallel, is the world's largest island, 84 percent of its land surface is covered by the permanent ice cap and is uninhabitable. Settlements occur in a narrow coastal strip, mostly in the southern and middle part of the west coast. In 1988 the population was 55,000, 82 percent of whom were indigenous Inuit with varying degrees of European

*Data are derived from tables published by the Aboriginal Peoples Output Program of Statistics Canada (1989) and the demographic review by Norris (1990). A full discussion of the various sources of population data and their limitations is provided in Chapter 2].

genetic admixture. Greenland was first a colony of Denmark, and then an integral part of that nation until 1979, when Home Rule was introduced, ushering in the first self-governing Eskimo/Inuit state in the world. Greenland had literally been isolated from the outside world until 1950, but since then rapid socioeconomic and cultural changes have occurred (Bjerregaard, 1991).

Social and Economic Conditions

The disadvantaged socioeconomic conditions of Native Americans in both the United States and Canada are evident when standard census-based social indicators are compared (Table 1.2 and Fig. 1.3). In terms of income, education, housing conditions, and labor force activity, Native Americans fared worse than their national counterparts. For Canadian Indians living on reserves, the proportion of the population who were recipients of social assistance ranged between 15 and 20 percent during the 1980s, compared to 6–8 percent among all Canadians, and this trend increased throughout the decade (Hagey et al., 1989).

The poor socioeconomic conditions affecting Native Americans could be expected to have an important impact on their health status. Socioeconomic differences in mortality have been observed in many populations for a variety of diseases. In some diseases, the association has changed over time. Thus, from a

Table 1.2 Selected Social Indicators for Native Americans, United States 1980 Census

Indicator	Native Americans	U.S. All Races
Median age	22.6 yr	30.0 yr
Mean no. persons/family	4.6	3.8
Median family income	$13,700	$19,900
Mean family income	$16,500	$23,100
Per capita income	$ 3,600	$ 7,300
% below poverty line	28.2	12.4
% high school graduates	55.4	66.5
% college graduates	7.4	16.2
% in labor force		
Male age 16 +	68.6	75.1
Female age 16 +	47.7	49.9
% labor force unemployed		
Male age 16 +	14.5	6.5
Female age 16 +	11.9	6.5

Source: U.S. DHHS, *Indian Health Trends 1990.*

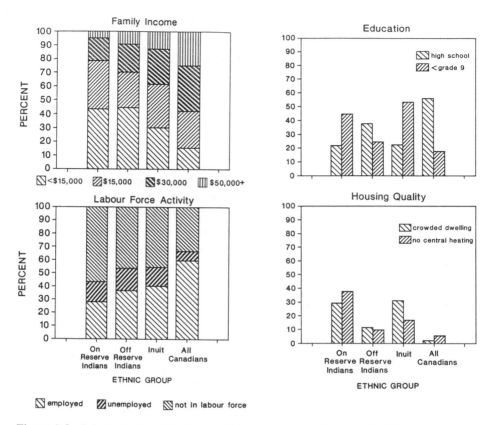

Figure 1.3. Selected social indicators for Native Americans, Canada, 1986 Census.

"disease of affluence," ischemic heart disease has become a disease affecting mainly the "lower" socioeconomic status groups (Marmot et al., 1987).

Although socioeconomic data are routinely collected in epidemiologic studies, there are considerable problems associated with their measurement and conceptualization (Liberatos et al., 1988). Social factors are usually measured to be "controlled for," as confounders, and their role as explanatory variables in their own right is often neglected. The precise mechanisms of how social factors influence health remain to be elucidated, although considerable research has been devoted to such concepts as stressful life events, social networks, social support, and status inconsistency (Marmot et al., 1987; House et al., 1988). Apart from gross social indicators like those provided in Table 1.2 and Figure 1.3, little is known about more refined measures of social relationships among Native Americans.

A particular interpretation of the impact that socioeconomic factors have on health sees ill health as generated by the economic inequities between an oppressed group and the dominant group in society. The "political economy" model has been adopted by "critical" medical anthropologists (e.g., Singer, 1989) and applied to Native Americans, such as Canadian Inuit (O'Neil, 1986). Disparities in such indicators as education, income, and employment are considered mere symptoms of the unequal—in fact, internal colonial—power relationship between Native Americans and the "modern capitalist state."

That socioeconomic status (SES) and ill health are associated is beyond dispute. In the sociological literature, particularly that relating to mental health, two explanations are generally offered. The "social causation" school attributes the relation to adversity and the stress of low SES, whereas the "social selection" school asserts that genetically predisposed persons drift down to or fail to escape from low SES. While there are some empirical data from other populations (Dohrenwend et al., 1992), little work has been done among Native Americans to test the applicability of these models.

Race and Ethnicity

Are Native Americans a race or an ethnic group? While the use of race and ethnicity permeates epidemiologic research, researchers who use such concepts have been criticized for a common failure to specify their meanings or acknowledge their theoretical and methodologic deficiencies (Cooper, 1985; Wilkinson and King, 1987). In his study of ethnic and racial differences in disease, Polednak defined races as natural units or populations that undergo evolutionary change and that differ slightly from one another in gene frequencies while they share distinct biological characteristics. In contrast, ethnic groups are seen as being culturally distinct (Polednak, 1989:3). The two classifications obviously overlap. Race can be used to characterize human evolution below the species level, reflecting time separation, breeding isolation, and environmental contrasts (Baker, 1967). The biological concept of race aggregates information relating to multiple genetic systems and can serve as a general indicator of the genetic makeup of populations and individuals.

The population genetic approach to the concept of race differs substantially from the pre-World War II, since discredited, racist notion of "race" based on superficial typologies and the moral and intellectual superiority of one race over another. But the aversion to the use of *race* is such that the term rarely crosses the lips of a social scientist today! Much of the objection lies in the policy implications of using race as an explanatory variable. While racial differences in disease rates are generally acknowledged, there is some controversy over the relative importance of *race* vs *racism* as the cause of such differences. Some social scientists believed that the notion of race had been abandoned by anthropology and that its persistent use in epidemiology was a case of "scientific anachronism." Rather than being a biological entity, *race* is a social category, its definition the result of economic and historical, not evolutionary development (Cooper, 1985). Others have argued that *race* is but a proxy measure of *class* (at least in the U.S. context), and that there are far more commonalities among races of the same class than between classes in the same race (Navarro, 1989).

Despite the confusion and controversy surrounding its use, or even existence, *race* can be a useful term for teaching and research in both human biology and epidemiology. It has utility in descriptive studies of variation in disease risk, it can assist in the generation of etiologic hypotheses, and it allows the targeting of special programs designed to assist those in greatest need.

In the context of disease variation, the terms *race* and *ethnic group* have often been used interchangeably, particularly when it is difficult to disentangle determinants that are primarily genetic—hence *racial*—and those that are sociocultural—hence *ethnic.*(Often the issue is avoided altogether by substituting less emotionally tinged terms such as *population, group,* or even *gene pool* for the word *race.*) In terms of programs to improve health, it is possible to intervene only at the social and cultural level, not—at least in any practical scale—at the genetic level.

For Native Americans, whether they are called a race or an ethnic group is not as important as it is to recognize their internal diversity. While Natives do share broadly common experiences as a group, particularly vis à vis the dominant North American society, they also live in different geographical areas, speak different languages, lead different lifestyles, and have different values, customs, and traditions.

The term *tribe* also needs clarification. It is used throughout this book to denote cultural/linguistic subgroups of Native Americans such as Cree, Pima, or Mohawk. Yet the term implies a certain degree of political organization that was not present in all Native American groups. Many nomadic, hunting-gathering peoples did not coalesce into tribes, but led their existence in small family groups that from time to time gathered into larger conglomerations for specific purposes. In the modern era, however, *tribe* has taken on a different meaning that is defined in terms of the political relationship between Native Americans and the larger American or Canadian state, particularly in such usages as tribal government or tribal council.

2

An Overview of Population and Health

A major task of epidemiology is the measurement of health in a population. There are, however, many definitions of *health*. Nearest to a universally accepted definition is the much-quoted World Health Organization (WHO) definition, which first appeared in the preamble to its charter in 1948. This definition emphasizes that health is not just the absence of disease, but something much broader: a state of complete physical, mental, and social well-being. While grand in rhetoric, this definition is difficult to "operationalize" in health research or health care delivery. Nevertheless, it serves to emphasize the "positive" aspects of health, away from the traditional preoccupation with death, disease, and disability.

Much effort has been directed at developing health indicators and indices that would provide the most comprehensive picture of the health of a population. Little attempt has been made, however, to construct a health status index specifically for Native American populations. A rare example is that of Connop (1983), who combined traditional mortality and hospitalization data in an index but weighted those data by values of health priorities as expressed by community members in a survey of Indian communities in northern Ontario.

The "health field concept," first propounded in 1974 by the Canadian Department of National Health and Welfare and is usually attributed to the then-Minister, Marc Lalonde, has gained wide international acceptance. As broad determinants of health, the four fields include human biology, the environment, lifestyles, and health care organization. In terms of impact on health status, the first three fields are far more important than the last, but it is to the last field that the largest share of health care resources have been directed.

The focus of this book is on health status overall, and three groups of diseases and conditions in particular—infectious diseases, chronic diseases, and injuries. The respective contributions of human biology, the environment, and lifestyles are emphasized. The organization and administration of health services is not discussed to any extent, either as a determinant of health or as a potential solution. While specific strategies to prevent and control the three groups of health problems are discussed, they do not necessarily involve the existing health care system. Increasing physician supply or building more hospitals are not seen as having a direct role in disease causation or health improvement. Such general issues in health care as accessibility, equity, cost, and community control, while important in their own right, are only peripherally relevant to the objectives of this book.

If *health* is difficult to define, *disease* would seem at first glance to pose no problem at all. This ease of definition is only so if one considers disease within the "Western, biomedical model." In a book on Native American health and disease, a case can be made for viewing disease in its "ethnomedical" context. This I have not chosen to do, perhaps to the chagrin of my cultural anthropological colleagues. If diseases like tuberculosis and diabetes are modern public health problems affecting Native Americans, then incorporation of ethnomedical definitions of such diseases is not relevant to the accurate assessment of disease burden or determining its causal factors. At the same time, however, understanding a people's cultural knowledge of such diseases is extremely important to their control. I have thus taken a stance that in this particular situation, public health makes use of ethnomedicine to serve its purpose without adopting the Native worldview. Indeed, as Alland commented, an ethnomedical perspective tended "to obscure the ecological relationships which [constituted] the *real* epidemiological patterns of a population (Alland, 1970:9).

I would make an analogy. In some cultures, the death of an infant before baptism or naming does not "count"—the infant has not "lived." An ethnomedical infant mortality rate would thus be lower than the Western biomedical version. Yet, this does not mean the death has not occurred, that risk factors contributing to that death have not been operating in that household or community, and that the recent delivery has no impact on the health and future reproductive risk of the mother. It is the Western biomedical concept and definition of infant death, and not the ethnomedical one, that has to be used to determine and investigate the state of maternal and infant health in that community.

By focusing on three groups of diseases and causes of ill health, this book would be considered by some as being "disease-oriented," instead of "health-oriented." Within public health there is a curious dichotomy between the "disease prevention" and "health promotion" schools, as though the two are incompatible and cannot both be accommodated in the global struggle to improve human health. Surely, health cannot but improve if diseases are prevented, whether singly or "holistically." For much of the world, it would be a major achievement if the greatest causes of mortality and morbidity were controlled. The state of well-being of large numbers of people would be improved immeasurably, even if nothing were done to promote positive and holistic health. Singling out three important groups of diseases would, in fact, focus attention on practical, specific solutions.

Historical Perspective

To understand fully the current health status of Native Americans, it is important to trace the historical development in health and population, particularly the changes that have occurred since the arrival of Europeans, or "contact." Yet, to evaluate the demographic and epidemiologic impact of that contact, one needs to know the situation before contact occurred.

The estimation of precontact Native American populations is fraught with difficulties and uncertainties, and the results show wide-ranging variation. Various approaches have been used, all of which require special assumptions and have inherent problems, such as nonrepresentative sampling and large margins of error in dating. One could perhaps compare paleodemographic exercises to solving several unknowns in one equation in algebra. Archaeological specimens in the form of skeletal remains, cultural artifacts, and food remains provide some clues to the size and characteristics of prehistoric populations. Other types of archaeological evidence include habitation space: the number of rooms and houses and the area occupied by such units. Other methods bypass archaeology altogether but instead rely on simulation models and ethnographic analogy. A review of such methods can be found in Schacht (1981).

Leading anthropologists of the 1920s and 1930s, such as James Mooney and Alfred Kroeber, estimated the aboriginal population of North America on the eve of Columbus to be around 1 million (Ubelaker, 1976). In an influential paper, Dobyns (1966) argued that the population was closer to ten times as high, around 10–12 million. He considered epidemic diseases to be the most important agents of depopulation after contact. Using selected case studies where sufficient archival records from the early contact period existed, he suggested that Native American populations were reduced by a ratio of 20–25:1. By applying such a depopulation ratio to the nadir (i.e., lowest) population after contact, it was possible to arrive at an estimate of the population before contact. In a later book, Dobyns revised his estimate upwards to 18 million Native Americans in North America (Dobyns 1983:298). He suggested that contact between tribes through an extensive trade network could have promoted the long-distance transmission of infectious diseases long before the actual arrival of Europeans in a particular locality.

It is not my intention to enter into a detailed (and likely contentious) debate on the relative merits of the various estimates. The size of the precontact population in North America is often interpreted to indicate the degree of technological capability and social complexity of aboriginal peoples. It also becomes entangled with philosophic and political positions on various issues, including the following: did Europeans simply occupy a "near-empty" continent, or did Native Americans suffer a "holocaust" of catastrophic proportions after 1492?

Regardless of the true extent and magnitude of depopulation after contact, introduced diseases are believed to have played an important role. This role was studied and well documented in a variety of Native populations in the postcontact era [see for example, Ashburn (1947), Crosby (1972), Dobyns (1983) and Thornton (1987)]. This process was repeated among groups that were more recently contacted, such as Eskimos and Athapaskan and Algonkian Indians in Alaska and northern Canada (Krech, 1978; Young, 1988a; Fortuine, 1989).

If disease was the major factor in regulating population size, it is important to know the type and frequency of diseases in prehistoric and historic times. Apart from extrapolation from existing hunter-gatherer peoples (Dunn, 1968; Eaton and Konner, 1985) to precontact Native Americans, paleopathology provides the only direct evidence. Unfortunately, skeletal remains are capable of demonstrating only a limited number of pathologies (e.g., trauma, osteomyelitis, syphilis, tuberculosis, metabolic bone disease, tumors, and arthritis), although nonspecific osteologic indicators of stress have been useful in providing a population perspective on nutritional and health status rather than diagnosis in individual specimens. More recent techniques of carbon isotope ratios and trace mineral analyses have provided clues to the sources of plant foods and contribution of animal proteins to the diet (Buikstra and Cook, 1980). Mummified tissue remains, coprolites, and cultural artifacts provide additional evidence of prehistoric diseases (Inhorn and Brown, 1990).

Even if paleopathological specimens were all immaculately preserved, accurately dated and sexed, diagnostically certain, and representative of all dead people at a point in time, they could never be representative of people *at risk* for disease or death at a certain age. Any attempt to reconstruct rates would be misleading, and the only appropriate epidemiologic indicator would be proportionate mortality. Even so, one would be faced with the problem of competing causes of death. For prehistoric populations, any competing causes that left no trace would never be known, and the role they played in the changing proportions of those causes that did leave a trace could not be estimated (Wood et al., 1992).

In the face of unreliable and incomplete data, it is tempting to ascribe an "halcyon age" to aboriginal peoples prior to contact. An example of such a romantic notion of a "paradise lost" can be found in Dobyns (1983:35), who wrote:

> The near-absence of lethal pathogens in the aboriginal New World allowed the native peoples to live in almost a paradise of well-being that contrasted with their historic purgatory of disease.

In a similar, and more graphic, vein, Ashburn (1947:5) wrote:

> Into this Arcadian continent came the white man. . . . Arcady was no more. Death stalked from Canada to Patagonia, pestilence walked in darkness, and destruction wasted at noonday.

Such a view conceived traditional societies to be well adapted by cultural and biological means to those aspects of their environments that were relevant to health and survival, including disease-causing microorganisms and vectors, and the flora and fauna from which all necessities of life (food, clothings, shelter, etc.) were derived. Rather than an absence of disease, a state of benign chronicity and endemicity was maintained at bearable levels. With acculturation, such adaptations were compromised, resulting in environmental alterations and cultural intrusions that culminated in epidemics and malnutrition (Wirsing, 1985).

Some scholars have disputed the impact of introduced diseases in depopulation. Helm (1980) concluded that there were no severe epidemics among northern Athapaskans before the nineteenth century. Instead, intermittent starvation and female infanticide kept the population at low levels. There is also documentary evidence to indicate that depopulation after contact was by no means a universal phenomenon among Native Americans. Meister (1976) reviewed historical demographic data for various southwestern tribes and found that the model of initial continuous decline to a population nadir applied to the Pueblo, Maricopa, Ute, and various California tribes. That model was not applicable to the Navajo or Pima, tribes that had been growing since contact except for short periods in the nineteenth century, and whose population decline was associated with the loss of land and water resources, not any lack of immunity to European diseases.

The demographic history of Native Americans can be broadly divided into several periods (Johansson, 1982), bearing in mind that intertribal differences and deviation from this scheme may be considerable. During precontact, the birth rate was slightly higher than the death rate, and the population remained more or less stable. During the "contact shock" period, birth rate declined, while mortality rate increased, resulting in depopulation. By the end of the nineteenth century, most Native populations began to undergo a recovery period, which saw the birth rate eventually overtaking the death rate. In the latter half of the twentieth century, a period of "modernization" has occurred, with mortality rate leading birth rate in a downward trend, in the classical "demographic transition" fashion (Johansson, 1982).

Kunitz (1976) suggested that ecological adaptation and social organization in the postcontact and early reservation periods was predictive of the relative ranking of mortality and fertility rates among tribes. Because of their differing response to mechanisms of social control, semi-nomadic tribes were more likely to have higher mortality rates than semi-sedentary and sedentary tribes. Among semi-nomadic tribes, periodic dispersion, which had been used to resolve conflicts, was no longer feasible once the reservation system was introduced. They were thus less adapted to the geographic and psychologic "space" constraints imposed by the reservation system.

Thornton (1987) attached numbers to the demographic history of Native Americans in the area covered by the 48 coterminous U.S. states. He estimated that the population was 5 + million at the beginning of the sixteenth century, a figure that was lower than the one arrived at by Dobyns. This population was halved approximately every 100 years, and reached its nadir toward the end of the nineteenth century, when there were about 250,000 Natives, less than 5 percent of the population at contact. In addition to diseases, other negative factors include warfare and genocide, removal and relocation, and the loss of the traditional way of life, as caused, for example, by the extermination of the bison on the Great Plains.

Sources of Data

In this book "national" estimates of rates of occurrence of a variety of health conditions are reported, in both the United States and Canada. It is important to note that no "true" national estimates are possible, and special assumptions and limitations are associated with different sources of data and their statistical manipulation. Studies conducted in a specific regional or tribal group may also employ sources of data different from those reported routinely by official agencies.

United States

The U.S. Census (taken once every ten years on a year ending in "0") categorizes American Indians, Eskimos, and Aleuts based on self-identification. The Census remains the most important source of estimate of the total Native American population, regardless of legal status, residence, or degree of admixture. The Indian Health Service (IHS) uses a different population denominator in its official statistics. The "IHS service population" covers those Native Americans who are eligible for IHS services (but who may or may not actually use the services). This is derived from the Census-based counts of self-identified Native Americans living in counties on or near a reservation or other officially designated Native communities. During inter-census years, the population is adjusted based on data on births and deaths obtained from the National Center for Health Statistics (see below). States containing Indian reservations and in which IHS has responsibility are called "reservation states," and the number of such states increased from 25 in 1955 to 33 in 1988. In this book data on population and vital rates relating to Native Americans in the United States are obtained from the IHS unless otherwise specified. In the 1980 Census, of all Native Americans in the United States, there were 940,000 (or 61%) in the IHS service population, 480,000 (31%) in the nonservice population within reservation states, and 130,000 (8%) in nonreservation states (U.S. Congress, 1986). In 1990, the estimated total IHS service population was 1.1 million (U.S. DHHS, *Trends in Indian Health 1990*).

Additional sources of population data include the Bureau of Indian Affairs and individual tribal governments. Different criteria exist for tribal memberships, such as "blood quantum" and residence, and they not only vary between tribes but also over time within the same tribe as a result of political changes.

Heightened cultural pride and perceived benefits (e.g., entitlement to government services, land claims settlements) may increase the number of self-identified Natives. Passel (1976) identified increases in American Indian age cohorts over the decade between the 1960 and 1970 Censuses, which he attributed to the increased social acceptability of Native heritage.

Births and deaths of all U.S. residents are recorded by each state health department and reported to the National Center for Health Statistics (NCHS). The NCHS extracts Native American data and forwards them to the IHS. In IHS publications, it is the Native American population in the reservation states that serve as the denominator for vital rates. The quality of data depends on the accuracy of the original birth and death certificates. For some regions, significant underreporting of Native American status exists, for example in California, where many Native Americans have Hispanic surnames (U.S. Congress, 1986).

Canada

As in the United States, the sources of data for the Native population in Canada include the national census, the Indian health service agency [Medical Services

Branch (MSB) of the Department of National Health and Welfare], and the Department of Indian Affairs and Northern Development (DIAND).

The national census in Canada has been conducted every 10 years on a year ending in "1." Prior to the 1980s an abbreviated census was also conducted at mid-decade in a year ending in "6." The 1986 Census, however, was a full-fledged one, and one that broke new ground in its scope (for example, by including questions on health and disability). The Census remains the only source of data for non-status Indians, Metis and Inuit, while for status or registered Indians, MSB and DIAND can serve as additional data sources. Although they are acting in violation of the Statistics Act, more and more Indian bands have refused to cooperate with the census. For example, in 1981, six bands refused to be enumerated, and in 1986, 136 bands with an estimated 45,000 residents were incompletely enumerated and thus not counted. In 1991, 59 bands did not participate, estimated to be 17 percent of the total on-reserve status Indian population in the country. In some provinces, such as Ontario, less than half of the Indian population took part in the 1991 Census (unpublished data, Statistics Canada). Even where there was cooperation, under-enumeration, particularly in remote areas with poor access, likely occurred (Hull, 1984).

For the Census determination of ethnic status is based on self-identification and is therefore influenced by social experience and cultural ties of the respondents. Failure to identify with any of the Native categories, particularly by people of mixed heritage or non-reserve residence, will result in an undercount.

DIAND maintains an Indian population register, which is updated by notices of births and deaths. The quality of this system, however, is compromised by such problems as late reporting and underreporting (Piché and George, 1973). The service population of MSB covers about 75 percent of status Indians living on reserves in the country, and residents of all ethnic groups in the two northern territories. After 1987, health services in the Northwest Territories were transferred to the territorial government and excluded from further reporting by MSB.

There is no convenient single source of fertility and mortality data for Canadian Natives. Data reported by MSB on its service population are derived from a variety of sources, depending on the region. Some regions obtain birth and death certificate data from the provincial vital statistics system, while others act as their own vital statistics agency in collecting primary data. Counts of births and deaths (the latter not broken down by cause), are also available from DIAND.

Unlike the practice in the United States, ethnic or racial origins are not available from the national vital statistics system in Canada. It is possible, however, to extract data from the Canadian Mortality Database (CMD) for residents of

Indian reserves, which are assigned special residence codes. One drawback of this source is that the two northern territories are not covered because there are no official reserves, and some provinces are not covered because their Indian reserves are not assigned separate codes (e.g., British Columbia before 1985). In this book previously unpublished special analyses of the CMD for Indian reserves in six provinces over two periods 1979–83 and 1984–88 [British Columbia is included in the second period only] are presented to provide a "national" perspective on mortality.

Data on the Inuit in the Northwest Territories are available from MSB and territorial government publications. At the moment it is not possible to obtain health statistics on nonstatus Indians and Metis (except when they are specially enumerated in a local study).

Comparison Groups

In this book various comparison groups are used. For the United States this is usually the national "all-race" population, but also sometimes the "White" population. For Canada, the total Canadian population is used. For specific regional studies, the local non-Native populations are also sometimes used. Because of the different age structures of different populations and of the same population at different times, age-standardized rates (by the direct method) are reported wherever possible. Unless otherwise specified, U.S. IHS data were standardized to the 1940 U.S. national population, while Canadian data were standardized to the 1970 Canadian national population. While it would make logical sense to restandardize all rates in the United States and Canada to the same "standard," the necessary raw data are not available. It is therefore not appropriate to compare age-standardized mortality rates of Native Americans in the United States and Canada; instead, comparisons should be made between the Native population and its respective national population in each country.

The above discussion highlights the many difficulties involved in exercising even the most basic of demographic and epidemiologic analyses of Native Americans in Canada and the United States. The choice is between making inferences based on flawed and incomplete data or not studying the issue at all. On balance, the limitations of existing data do not invalidate conclusions on broad trends in Native American health and population. Generally, small-scale, disease-specific studies of local populations are more likely to provide a more accurate definition and estimate of the "numerator" and "denominator." In this book large summary tables of local and regional studies of specific diseases and health conditions are provided in each chapter.

Demographic Features

Population Size and Growth

With the onset of the reservation system toward the end of the nineteenth century and the inclusion of Native Americans in the national censuses of both Canada and the United States, more accurate description of the Native American population became possible. Even to this day, however, such demographic accounts are beset with problems. While a reconstruction of the population growth of the Native population in Canada and the United States in the last century is possible, its validity cannot be assured. One is faced with a different set of difficulties from those faced by scholars attempting to reconstruct Native American populations in those misty prehistoric and early contact times. While the national censuses provide for ethnic identification, over the years the methodology has changed. Data collection and processing procedures may not be comparable from census to census, for example, those relating to the number of Native categories, the reporting of multiple origins and mixed heritage, and differences between information obtained by self-enumeration and that solicited by enumerators (Kralt, 1990).

Table 2.1 summarizes the total Native American population in Canada and the United States during the twentieth century as determined by the decennial national census (rounded to the nearest 1,000). In Canada, between 1931 and 1981 the total Native population almost quadrupled. Included in the totals in Table 2.1 are the Eskimo/Inuit. Prior to statehood for Alaska in 1959, census data for Alaska Natives are tabulated separately from the continental United States. The population of Alaska Natives in censuses before 1960 has been added to the American Indian population. In 1980, there were 42,000 Eskimos and 14,000

Table 2.1 Native American Population in Canada and the United States, 1900/01–1980/81

Census Year	Canada	United States
1900/1901	127,941	267,000
1910/1911	106,000	291,000
1920/1921	114,000	271,000
1930/1931	129,000	362,000
1940/1941	161,000	366,000
1950/1951	166,000	379,000
1960/1961	220,000	552,000
1970/1971	313,000	827,000
1980/1981	492,000	1,423,000

Sources: Canadian Census data obtained from tables in Leacy (1983) and Norris (1990); U.S. data from Bureau of the Census, summarized in U.S. Congress (1986)

Aleuts in the United States, of whom 80 percent and 60 percent, respectively, live in the state of Alaska (U.S. Congress, 1986). Canadian Inuit numbered around 6,000 in 1931 but had increased to 25,390 in 1981 (Robitaille and Choinière, 1985).

Coincident with the population recovery of the Native American population was the increase in admixture with other racial groups, who now constitute the majority in the continent. In the 1910 U.S. Census, about 57 percent of American Indians were considered "full-blood." By 1930, the proportion of full-blood American Indians declined to 46 percent (Thornton, 1987). There is of course considerable geographical variation, due to such factors as urbanization, security of the land base, and community cohesion, among others. In the 1986 Canada census, those with mixed Native and non-Native origins accounted for 46 percent of Indians and 18 percent of Inuit (Statistics Canada, 1989).

Fertility Trends

Figure 2.1 shows the trend in crude birth rate (CBR) for Canadian Indians and Inuit from 1921 to the late 1980s, and for Alaska Natives and American Indians since 1955. It can be seen that the birth rate among U.S. and Canadian Natives consistently exceeded that of the national, all-race population, and maintained a relatively constant ratio of about 2:1. In both jurisdictions, the Native rate peaked during the 1960s and then began a precipitous decline. Among Alaska Natives, however, an upward trend since the late 1970s can be observed, whereas among Indians in the "lower-48" the decline has also stopped, and the birth rate appears to have leveled off. Among Canadian Indians there are also indications that the birth rate again began to rise again in the 1980s. The Canadian Inuit rate started off at a substantially higher level and has retained its position relative to Indians and all Canadians. The period of decline was also shorter and began to increase again in the mid 1980s.

The CBR is not an accurate measure of fertility since it includes in its denominator men and women who are not in the reproductive age range. The total fertility rate (TFR) represents the sum of all age-specific fertility rates for women in the child-bearing ages. It can be interpreted as the number of children that would be born to a woman who experienced each of the age-specific fertility rates as she aged. The TFR usually follows the same trend as the CBR. In the late 1960s, the TFR for all Canadians was 2.5 children per woman, compared to 6.1 for Canadian Indians and 9.2 for Inuit. By the early 1980s, the TFR in all three groups had declined, to 1.7 for all Canadian women, and more drastically, to 3.1 and 4.1 among Indians and Inuit, respectively (Norris, 1990).

Romaniuk (1974) reconstructed the historical trend in CBR for the James Bay Cree from 1927 to 1972. It increased from about 40/1000 in the pre-World War

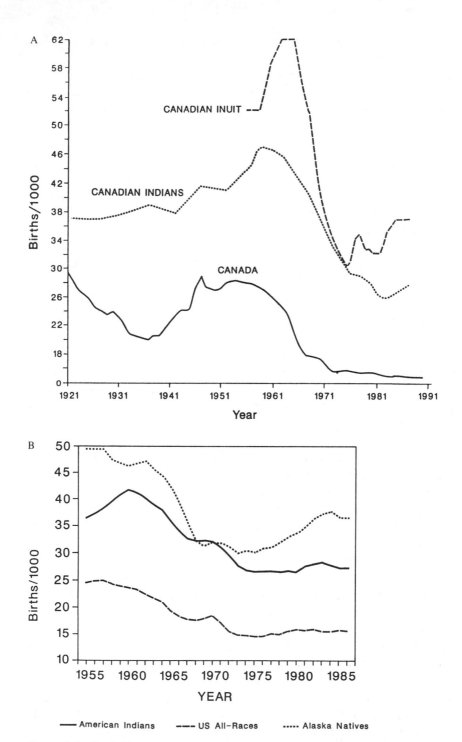

Figure 2.1. Crude birth rate: (*A*) USA, 1955–87, American Indian, Alaska Native, and all-race populations (*B*) Canada, 1921–87, Indian, Inuit, and national populations.

II years to just under 50/1000 in the early 1960s, corresponding to the early modernization period of this population and the accompanying weakening or removal of biocultural inhibitions of childbearing in traditional societies. A shortening of birth intervals was believed to be the main mechanism of fertility increase. Several factors were believed to have operated: the decline in breast-feeding frequency and duration, reduced pregnancy wastage due to improved medical care and living conditions, and reduction in spousal separation due to sedentarization and improved transportation (Romaniuk, 1974). Romaniuk later generalized the observation on the impact of modernization on fertility to the total Canadian Indian population, reconstructing birth rates from the early years of the twentieth century (Romaniuk, 1981).

The rise in fertility reaching a peak in the early 1960s was also observed in the Alaska Native population. The decline after that time was attributed to the beginning of family planning programs (Blackwood, 1981). The resurgence in increased fertility (or at least, the cessation of the decline) observed in various Native populations in the 1980s (Fig. 2.1) can be explained by the large number of women born during the "boom" of the 1960s entering the reproductive age themselves.

Broudy and May (1983) remarked that the continued high rate of growth and fertility among the Navajo reflected the rapid implementation of modern medical care and public health on the reservation, independent of intrinsic Navajo values and the process of modernization. The low fertility associated with modernization has not caught up with the rapid mortality decline.

Age-Sex Distribution

The age-sex distribution of Native Americans reveals a much younger population than the national populations of Canada (Fig. 2.2) and the United States (Table 2.2). The age-sex pyramid of Native Americans resembles that of developing countries today or that of the general North American population of a century ago. In the United States the median age of Native Americans in the 1980 Census was 23 years, compared to an all-race figure of 30 years. In Canada the proportions of Natives with ages under 15 and over 65 were 37 percent and 3 percent, respectively, in 1986. the Inuit tend to be the "youngest" (40% under 15) and the Metis "oldest," with only 33 percent under 15.

Generally, women outnumber men slightly. This pattern was observed in Canadians nationally as well as among Natives as a whole (1986 Census, 964 M to 1000 F). Among the Inuit, however, the reverse sex ratio is observed (1029 M to 1000 F). Schaefer (1982) suggested that the sex differential in disease mortality, such as tuberculosis and post-partum hemorrhage was responsible, particularly among the cohort of women born during the late 1920s. In the

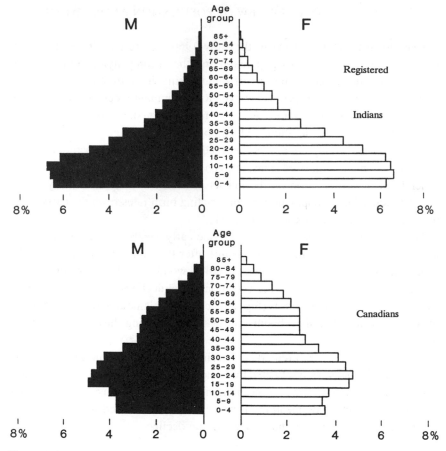

Figure 2.2. Age-sex distribution of population: Canada, 1981 Census, Registered Indians and all Canadians.

Table 2.2 Age-Sex Distribution of Population: United States, 1980 Census, Native American and U.S. All-Race Populations (in percent)*

Age Group	Native American		US All-Races	
	Male	Female	Male	Female
<10	10.8	11.5	7.5	7.1
10–19	11.8	11.5	8.9	8.5
20–29	9.5	9.7	9.0	9.0
30–39	6.5	6.8	6.9	7.1
40–49	4.3	4.6	4.9	5.2
50–59	3.2	3.5	4.9	5.4
60–69	2.0	2.3	2.8	4.6
70+	1.4	1.9	2.8	4.6
Total	49.3	51.7	48.6	51.4

*Percentages may not sum to 100 due to rounding.
Source: U.S. DHHS, Trends in Indian Health 1990.

United States, for every decade until 1970, Native American men outnumbered women, in contrast to the national population. In 1970 the M:F ratio was 962/ 1000 and in 1980 975/1000. Still, The ratio was higher than the 950/1000 ratio in the national population (Thornton, 1987).

Patterns of Mortality

Life Expectancy

Life expectancy has often been used as an overall measure of health status, although it is entirely based on the mortality experience of the population. It can be directly compared between populations as it is independent of the age structure of the population.

In her bibliographic review of Native American demography Johansson (1982) cited a skeletal-based estimate for a life expectancy of about 23 years among precontact Native Americans, comparable to most primitive hunter-gatherers around the world. This is in fact not very different from the Canadian Inuit figure of only 29 years during the decade 1941–50 (Robitaille and Choinière, 1985). The steady increase in life expectancy at birth since the 1940s is shown in Figure 2.3.

In the United States the gap between Native Americans and Whites narrowed from 10.8 years among men and 14.7 years among women in 1940 to 3.6 years and 3.0 years, respectively, in 1980. Over the four decades, Native American men gained almost 16 years and women 23 years (U.S. DHHS, Trends in Indian Health, 1990). A similar improvement can be observed among Canadian Indians over the two periods 1978–81 and 1982–85 (Canada, DNHW, Health Indicators, 1988). The life-expectancy of the Inuit in the Northwest Territories more than doubled between 1941–50 and 1978–82, when it was 66 years (Robitaille and Choinière, 1985). This is a most remarkable achievement, since it took many modern populations centuries to attain such a doubling.

The major contribution to the reduced life expectancy at birth among Native Americans is their higher infant mortality rate. The improvement in life expectancy in recent years can also be attributed to the much reduced risk of death in childhood. Among Canadian Indians during 1982–85, the difference in life expectancy from the national average was 8 years in males and 7 years in females at birth. By age 30, the gap was reduced to 4 years in males and 5 years in females. By age 60, the difference was less than a year in men and slightly over a year in women. Thus, Native Americans who survive into adulthood have a life expectancy similar to that of their national counterparts.

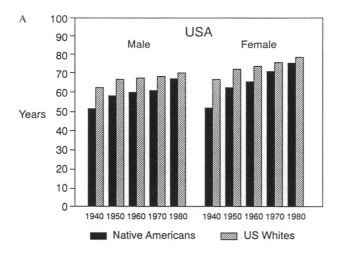

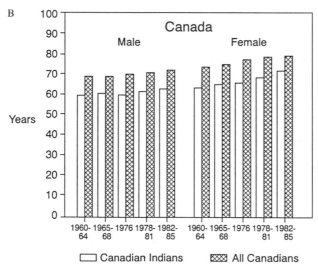

Figure 2.3. Life expectancy at birth by sex: (*A*) USA, 1940–80, Native Americans and Whites; (*B*) Canada, 1960–1985, Canadian Indians and all Canadians.

Infant Mortality Rate

The decline in infant mortality (IMR) among Native Americans in both Canada and the United States has been impressive (Fig. 2.4). The IMR in 1985 was less than one-fifth that in 1955. The American Indian IMR has in fact converged with that of the U.S. all-race rate, while that of Alaska Native was still about 40 percent higher. In Canada, the Indian rate during the 1980s was twice the national IMR. The Inuit in the Northwest Territories have started off with the highest IMR of all Native groups (145/1000 livebirths during 1961–66). While a

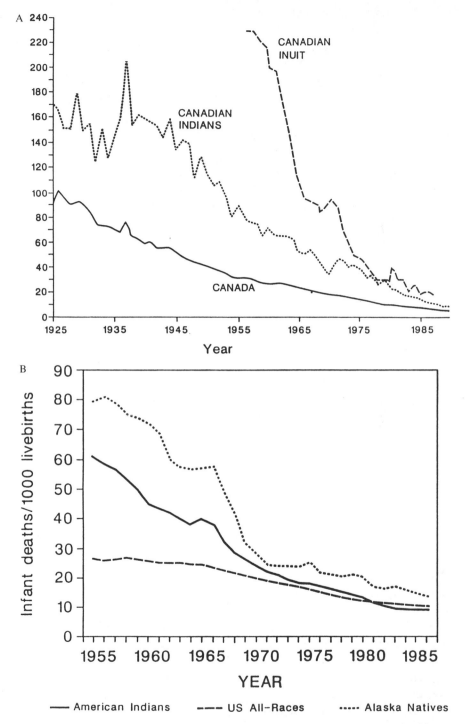

Figure 2.4. Infant mortality rate: (*A*) USA, 1955–86, American Indian, Alaska Native, and all-race populations; (*B*) Canada, 1925–88, Canadian Indian, Inuit, and national populations.

similar dramatic decline has occurred, the Inuit IMR remained higher than that of Canadian Indians (Table 2.3).

IMR can be broken down into neonatal (under 28 days) and post-neonatal (from the twenty-eighth day up to the end of the first year of life) mortality rates. The former is generally considered to be more sensitive to medical care measures while the latter is reflective of socioeconomic conditions. Table 2.3 shows that

Table 2.3 Birth, Infant Mortality, Neonatal Mortality, and Postneonatal Mortality Rate: United States and Canada, 1956–1985, Native Americans and All-Race Populations

Year	Am Ind	Ak Nat	USA	Can Ind	Inuit	Canada
Birth Rate						
1956–60	40	48	24	46	54	28
1961–65	39	45	22	45	62	24
1966–70	33	34	18	40	50	18
1971–75	29	31	15	33	33	16
1976–80	27	32	15	25	34	16
1981–85	28	37	16	27	35	15
Infant Mortality Rate						
1956–60	53	76	26	75	223	30
1961–65	48	60	25	63	144	26
1966–70	30	42	22	46	95	21
1971–75	20	24	18	43	67	16
1976–80	15	21	14	29	36	12
1981–85	10	16	11	19	28	9
Neonatal Mortality Rate*						
1956–60	22		19	NA	NA	19
1961–65	18		18	NA	48	18
1966–70	14		16	NA	33	15
1971–75	10		13	14	26	11
1976–80	8		10	12	16	8
1981–85	5		7	8	13	6
Post-Neonatal Mortality Rate*						
1956–60	33		7	NA	NA	11
1961–65	25		7	NA	97	8
1966–70	16		6	NA	63	6
1971–75	10		5	25	41	5
1976–80	8		4	17	19	4
1981–85	6		4	11	15	3

NA = not available, Am Ind = American Indian, Ak Nat = Alaska Native, Can Ind = Canadian Indian.
*Am Ind and Ak Nat combined.

among Native Americans in the United States the neonatal mortality rate has dropped below the national rate since the late 1970s. In Canada, the Indian rate approached the national rate, while the Inuit rate was still twice as high as the national rate in the most recent period. For post-neonatal mortality rate, the U.S. Native rate was still slightly higher than the all-race rate, while in Canada, the Indian and Inuit rates were, respectively, 4 and 5 times the national rate during 1981–85.

Causes of Mortality

The percent distribution of mortality by cause according to ICD-9 chapters for Canadian Indians is shown in Figure 2.5. Among men, diseases of the circulatory system accounted for about one-third of all deaths during 1979–88, followed closely by injuries, at 28 percent. Neoplasms occupied third place with 12 percent. For women, the proportion of deaths from circulatory diseases was similar (34%), but the order of neoplasms and injuries was reversed. A similar pattern is observed among Native Americans in the United States. Compared to non-Natives; circulatory diseases and neoplasms were less important among Natives in proportionate terms, whereas injuries were much more important causes of mortality among Natives than non-Natives.

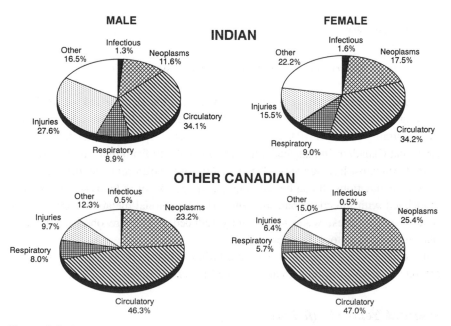

Figure 2.5. Percent distribution of causes of mortality: Canada, 1979–88, Canadian Indians and other Canadians.

Table 2.4 Standardized Mortality Ratio by Major Cause: Canada, 1979–1988, Canadian Indians Compared to Other Canadians

ICD-9 Chapter	Disease	Male	Female
1	Infectious/parasitic	2.6**	2.7**
2	Neoplasms	0.4**	0.7**
3	Endocrine/nutritional/metabolic	1.4*	1.5**
4	Blood	0.4	0.3
5	Mental	2.2**	2.9**
6	Nervous system/sense organs	0.9	0.4**
7	Circulatory	0.7**	0.7**
8	Respiratory	1.1	1.7**
9	Digestive	1.0	1.9**
10	Genitourinary	1.2	1.9**
11	Pregnancy/childbirth	NA	1.0
12	Skin/subcutaneous	0.8	3.0
13	Musculoskeletal	1.6	0.6
14	Congenital	1.0	0.6*
15	Perinatal	1.3	1.1*
16	Symptoms/ill-defined	2.3**	2.6**
17	Injuries/poisoning	2.6**	2.5**
All causes		1.0	1.1

NA = not applicable.
*p < 0.05.
**p < 0.01.
Canadian Indian data refer to residents of Indian reserves in six provinces.

In addition to comparing proportions of death, the relative risk of death according to various causes can also be determined. Table 2.4 shows the standardized mortality ratios (SMR) for all ICD-9 chapters. A SMR greater than 1 indicates that Canadian Indians had a higher risk of death from that cause compared to all Canadians, having adjusted statistically for the different age distribution of the two populations. It can be seen that elevated risks of at least two times were associated with infectious/parastic, endocrine/nutritional/metabolic, mental disorders, and injuries, while significantly reduced risks were observed in neoplasms and circulatory diseases.

In Chapters 3–6 mortality and morbidity relating to infectious diseases, chronic diseases, and injuries are analyzed in further detail.

Potential Years of Life Lost

In health planning, a useful index of *premature* mortality that gives more weight to deaths among younger people (and hence is more "useful" to society on the

Table 2.5 Potential Years of Life Lost by Major Cause: United States, 1981–1983, and Canada 1982–1985, Native American and All-Race Populations

Cause	Native Americans		US All Races		Canadian Indians		All Canadians	
	Rate	%	Rate	%	Rate	%	Rate	%
Injuries	52.8	47	18.5	32	70.6	45	16.9	30
Circulatory	8.0	7	10.0	16	16.3	10	10.1	18
Cancer	4.9	4	9.3	15	8.5	5	11.9	21
All causes	113.9	100	60.6	100	157.2	100	56.5	100

Rates are per 1000 population per year. PYLL in the United States calculated based on an upper age limit of 65 for the 1981–83 period, whereas in Canada it was 70 years for the 1982–85 period
Source: U.S. DHHS, Indian Health Conditions 1990; Canada, DNHW, Health Indicators 1988.

whole) is the "potential years of life lost" (PYLL). It measures the years of life "lost" by individuals who die prematurely (i.e., between the ages of 1 and 65, or 70). For the United States as a whole, Table 2.5 shows the greater importance of injuries in premature mortality among Native Americans, and the lesser role played by cancer and circulatory diseases. Overall, the rate of PYLL for all causes was 114/1000, compared to the U.S. all-race rate of 61 (U.S. DHHS, Indian Health Conditions 1990).

Similar patterns of PYLLs are also observed in regional studies, for example among the Senecas in New York. In this population, injuries accounted for 50 percent of all PYLLs during the period 1955–1984, with circulatory diseases a distant second at 15 percent (Mahoney et al., 1989a).

A different approach investigates the gain in life expectancy that would result if specific causes were eliminated. Carr and Lee (1978) constructed life tables for the Navajos and found that eliminating motor vehicle accidents would add 5.2 and 2.7 years to the life expectancy of a male and female Navajo, respectively, at birth. By comparison, circulatory diseases would add 3.3 years in the male and 3.7 years in the female. For adults in the working ages of 15–65, the elimination of motor vehicle accidents would add 3.1 years in men and 1.1 years in women.

Morbidity and Disability

Hospital Morbidity

Unlike mortality, there is no overall measure of morbidity. The pattern of hospitalization can provide data on the frequency and causes of morbidity, although not all illnesses result in hospitalization, and many factors other than disease incidence contribute to a population's utilization of hospital services. In several

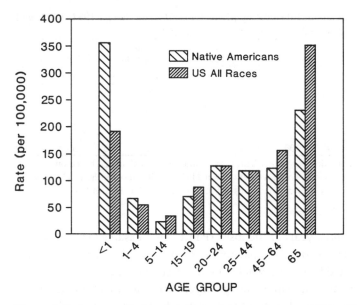

Figure 2.6. Age-specific hospital discharge rate, all causes: USA, 1987–88, Native American and U.S. all-race populations.

Canadian provinces it is possible to extract Native and non-Native hospitalization data from the universal health insurance plan databases. For example, in Manitoba, the age-standardized hospitalization rate for infectious diseases, circulatory diseases, respiratory diseases, and injuries were 4.3, 1.8, 3.0, and 3.3 times higher among Natives than non-Natives (Young, 1988b:53).

In the United States data from all IHS-operated and contract hospitals can be compared to all U.S. general hospitals. The age-specific hospital discharge rates for all causes combined in fiscal year 1987/88 are shown in Figure 2.6. It can be seen that it was among those under five years of age that an excess of hospitalization by Native Americans occurred. In the other age groups, Native Americans were less likely to be hospitalized than Americans in general. While one explanation of the lower hospitalization rate is a lower level of morbidity, this could also result from reduced access to health services among Native Americans.

Activity Restriction

Morbidity can also be assessed in a population health survey setting, both in terms of the prevalence of specific health conditions and the number of restricted activity days. In the United States, the Survey of American Indians and Alaska Natives (SAIAN), conducted in 1987 on a nationally representative sample of the IHS service population as part of the National Medical Expenditure Survey, provided useful data on the self-reported prevalence of various diseases. Such data are cited throughout this book under the various disease categories.

Native Americans are also sampled in the regular National Health Interview Surveys (NHIS) conducted by the U.S. National Center for Health Statistics. Data from those identified in the household survey as American Indian and Alaska Native can be compared with the U.S. national average. It should be noted that Native Americans were not oversampled in such national surveys, and subgroup comparisons (e.g., by regions or specific diseases) would be affected by small cell size. Figure 2.7 compares the number of restricted activity days—

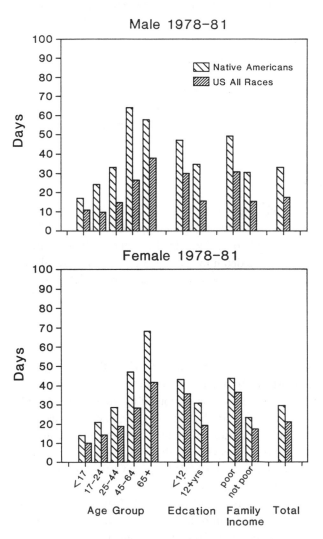

Figure 2.7. Mean number of restricted activity-days per year: USA, 1978–81, Native American and U.S. all-race populations.

an aggregate measure of morbidity and disability—between Native Americans who were sampled in NHIS from 1978 to 1981 and the U.S. national rate for 1981. It is evident that at all age-sex groups, the Native American rate was higher than the U.S. national rate. As expected, the number of restricted activity days per year increased with age and was higher among the less educated and those with lower income (U.S. DHHS, Indian Health Conditions 1990:185).

Disability

In Canada, the Health and Activity Limitation Survey (HALS) conducted in 1987 specially sampled residents of Indian reserves in the provinces and Natives in the two northern territories. It found 12 percent of Native Canadians to be disabled, defined as those having "any restriction or lack of ability to perform an activity in the manner or within the range considered normal for a human being," which must have lasted six months or more and is not eliminated by the use of technical devices. Disabilities can further be divided into those affecting mobility, agility, sight, hearing, and speaking, among others (Hamilton, 1990).

Behavioral Health Risks

Many personal behaviors or "lifestyles" have been shown to be determinants of a variety of diseases. As smoking and diet are often implicated in diverse health problems, they are discussed in this overview chapter. Other individual health risk behaviors are discussed in more detail in subsequent chapters, e.g., alcohol and drug abuse, safety knowledge and practices (Chapter 6), sexual behavior (Chapter 3), and physical activity (Chapter 5).

Smoking

Of all the human behaviors that have an adverse impact on health, tobacco smoking can be considered the most important. It has been estimated that each year one in six deaths in the United States can be attributed to smoking-related diseases, including a variety of cancers (lung, larynx, oral cavity, esophagus, bladder, cervix, etc.), cardiovascular diseases (ischemic, cerebrovascular, and peripheral vascular diseases), chronic respiratory diseases, intrauterine growth retardation, and fetal loss. In addition, many deaths from fires and burns can also be attributed to smoking (CDC, *MMWR*, S-2, 1989).

It is perhaps ironic that tobacco was part of the "Columbian exchange," one of the many species of New World flora introduced into the Old World (Crosby, 1972). Across the continent, different species of the plant were cultivated or

gathered wild, and its product traded far and wide. The ceremonial use of tobacco was integral to the culture of many Native American tribes, with the exception of those in the Arctic, Subarctic, and parts of the Northwest Coast, where
its use was introduced much later by European explorers, traders, and settlers.
By the end of the nineteenth century, the use of tobacco was universal among
all Native Americans (Driver, 1969). The increase in tobacco use is no where
more dramatic than in the Greenlandic population, which had been "opened up"
only since the 1950s. In 1950 it was estimated that the per capita consumption
was two cigarettes per day among adults. By 1987, it had increased to about
thirteen cigarettes per day, one of the highest tobacco consumption rates in the
world (Prener et al., 1991).

In the United States, SAIAN found that the prevalence of smoking among
adults over the age of 18 was 33 percent, only slightly higher than the 27 percent
for the U.S. all-race rate. The prevalence was higher among the young, the less
educated, and men (Lefkowitz and Underwood, 1991). In 1990, a national survey of smoking among Canadian adults in urban centers found that 59 percent
of Natives were regular smokers—the highest observed prevalence of all ethnic
groups—which compared with 23 percent for all Canadians (Millar, 1992).

The modern tobacco "epidemic," however, affects Native Americans differ-
entially. Some tribes in the southwestern United States are known for their low
smoking prevalence (Sievers, 1968a). Elsewhere, regional and community surveys have shown the prevalence to be much higher, for example, in southern
Manitoba (Longclaws et al., 1980) and northwestern Ontario (McIntyre and
Shah, 1986). The 1985 Health Promotion Survey found that 64 percent of the
Indians and 78 percent of the Inuit in the Northwest Territories were current
cigarette smokers, compared to only 39 percent among non-Natives in the Territories and 34 percent among Canadians nationally (Imrie and Warren, 1988).
Among urban Indians in Minneapolis, some 70 percent smoked cigarettes, al-
though the amount smoked was generally lower than that reported from whites
(Gillum et al., 1984).

The situation, however, was much more serious among adolescents. Surveys
of national samples of Native American students in grades 7–12 showed that 78
percent had smoked cigarettes and 58 percent used smokeless tobacco (Beauvais
et al., 1989). Among high school seniors, the prevalence of any smoking during
the past month, daily smoking during the past month, and smoking half a pack
or more per day was higher among Native American than whites. The prevalence
was in fact higher among girls than boys. Comparing 1980–84 with 1976–79,
overall cigarette use among Native American youths had declined, although they
continued to maintain their leading position among all ethnic groups (Bachman
et al., 1991). In Canada, a 1987 survey of smoking among students in the Northwest Territories found exceedingly high rates among Inuit and Indian youths. By

age 19, 71 percent of Inuit and 63 percent of Indians, compared to only 43 percent of non-Natives, were current smokers (Millar, 1990).

As an addiction, the determinants of smoking are multiple and complex, and involve both genetic and environmental factors. Twin studies have suggested the presence of some genetic influences on the initiation and maintenance of smoking, on the level of dependence, and on the ability to quit smoking, perhaps mediated through differential pharmacologic responses to nicotine. Social factors encompass exposure to smoking by family members and peers, cost and availability, advertising, and social acceptance, among other factors.

It has been established that smoking cessation confers major and immediate health benefits in all age-sex groups, and that former smokers tend to have reduced disease risk compared to continuing smokers (CDC, *MMWR*, RR-12, 1990). Native Americans would benefit from any smoking-control strategies directed at the larger Canadian and American societies to which they belong. Such global measures as increasing taxation (and thus prices), restrictions on smoking in public places, elimination of cigarette sales to minors, advertisements in mass media, and public and school health education campaigns would have an impact on Native Americans, because more and more aspects of North American society permeate Native American communities, even in the remote Arctic and Subarctic. The smoke-free policy of all U.S. IHS facilities (Welty et al., 1987), by setting an example among health professionals and government employees, should have a positive impact on Native community members who use such facilities.

Nutrition and Diet

Diet and nutrition are part of the pattern of human adaptation to a particular habitat. Native American foodways have been amply described in the ethnographic literature. In aboriginal times, the diet of Native Americans consisted of fish, game, wild plants, or cultivated plants. Fish was the staple food on the Northwest Coast and various other coastal, riverine, and lacustrine zones. Game predominated in a huge area, including most of the Arctic, Subarctic, and Plains. Wild plants were the principal source of food in California and the Great Basin. Native Americans invented agriculture independently of the Old World, and cultivated plants predominated in the Northeast, Southeast, and Southwest (Driver, 1969:54). Of course, more than one food constituted the diet, and local and regional ecological conditions accounted for the considerable variations.

Diet and nutrition are also sensitive to the effects of acculturation, which are reflected in the changing proportions of "traditional" ("from the land") and "modern" (i.e., imported or store-bought) foods. In the Arctic and Subarctic, traditional foods such as game and fish still constitute an important proportion of the people's diet (e.g., Draper, 1977; Berkes and Farkas, 1978; Winterhalder, 1983; Szathmary et al., 1987). This pattern, however, can be rapidly altered as a result of large-scale natural resources development projects. Waldram (1985) found that in one northern Manitoba community, a hydroelectric project resulted in a substantial reduction in the proportion of food from the land, from some 80–90 percent to 18 percent. The high cost of imported foods and inadequate income from employment and social assistance meant that the nutritional value of the land foods could not be substituted and compensated in full.

It is becoming recognized that dietary change is a major factor in the changing pattern of disease experienced by Native Americans. Dietary and nutritional correlates of specific diseases are discussed in Chapters 3–5.

Many studies have been conducted to assess the composition and nutrient value of Native American diets as well as the nutritional status of the population. These are summarized in Table 2.6. The only national study was the Nutrition Canada Survey of 1972, which included a sample of 1,800 Indians from 29 reserves across the country, both rural and urban, as well as 366 Inuit from four communities in the Northwest Territories (Canada, DNHW, 1975a, b, c). A comparison of the median intake of calories and proteins among Indians, Inuit, and all Canadians from this survey is shown in Figure 2.8.

Epidemiologic Transition

The long-term temporal changes in the pattern of health and sickness in a population has been described as its "epidemiologic transition" (Omran, 1971). Most populations supposedly undergo three "ages"—the age of pestilence and famines, the age of receding pandemics, and the age of degenerative and man-made diseases. The pace of transition differs between populations, and Omran distinguished between the classical or Western model, exemplified by western Europe and North America; the accelerated model, characterized by Japan and eastern Europe; and the delayed model where most developing countries in the world would belong. The concept has found general acceptance, at least its broad outlines, if not its detailed propositions.

No mention was made in Omran's original papers regarding the Native American population. Presumably it would fall under the contemporary delayed model, among other countries of the Third World, where massive modern medical technology heralded the relatively recent mortality declines. Several authors have specifically investigated the applicability of the epidemiologic transition theory to some Native American populations, specifically, among the Navajo (Broudy and May, 1983; Kunitz, 1983), and Canadian Indians (Young, 1988a).

Table 2.6 Regional Studies of Dietary Intake and Nutritional Status among Native Americans

Author	Date	Population[a]	Methods	Results[b]
USA Indians				
Darby et al. (1956)	1955	Navajo: 2 communities within Navajo Res., AZ	n = 1,246 M/F; Qualitative diet; Biochemical	Diet derived from traditional economy based on sheep grazing and cereal growing; no quantitative dietary intake data. Adequate Prot, Fe, and VitA; low VitC
Mayberry and Lindeman (1963)	1960s	Seminole; OK (pop: 2,400)	n = 54, M/F adults; 24-hr recall	Compared to whites in county: higher Kcal; Prot 12%–14%, CHO 41%–44%, Fats 44%–45% of energy; P/S: 0.23
Reid et al. (1971)	1960s	Pima, Papago; Gila River, AZ	n = 277 F, 25–44 yr; Dietary history	Prot 12%, CHO 44%, fats 44% of energy; P/S 0.35; High kcal (3,200/day); adequate minerals, no data on vitamins
Bass/Wakefield (1974)	1970	Dakota; Standing Rock, ND/SD (pop: 4,700)	n = 94 F; 24-hr recall	Prot, VitA, Thia, Niac adequate; Kcal, Ca, Fe, Ribo < RDA; Prot 14%, CHO 50%, fats 36% of energy; wild fruits/vegetables not extensively used; 74% of families received government foods
Kuhnlein/Calloway (1977)	1974	Hopi, AZ (pop: 7,500)	n = 420 F + children; 24-hr recall	<25% included 1 traditional food item, much less variety; Kcal lower (2/3) of RDA: Ca, VitA, B-6, Fola < RDA
Canadian Indians				
Lee et al.; Desai/Lee (1971)	1968	2 BC communities: coastal Nootka (pop: 644) interior Chilcotin (594)	n = 514; 24-hr recall; Biochemical	Low Kcal, VitA, Ca, Fe (< 2/3 of CDS); Low hematological indices
Desai/Lee (1974)	late 1960s	2 Athapaskan villages, Yukon	n = 310; Biochemical	Low Fe status; adequate vitamins except VitC
Canada DNHW (1975b,c)	1972	29 bands across Canada urban/rural/remote, 6 culture areas	n = 1,800, M/F; Biochemical; 24-hr recall	Marginal/inadequate intake of VitA, VitD, Ca, Fola Kcal, Prot, and other minerals/vitamins adequate Fe: low Hgb esp. F, poor iron reserves, deficient intake
Johnston et al. (1977)	1973–76	Micmac, NS	n = 120 F, 15–50 yr	Kcal, Ca, Fe, VitA, Ribo, Thia < CDS; Prot 14%, CHO 45%, fats 41% of energy

Reference	Year	Location (population)	Sample	Findings
Hoffer et al. (1981)	1978	Cree, N. Quebec (pop: 2,300)	n = 592, M/F, 30 + yr; Biochemical	Low VitA (10% moderate risk) and VitC (41% high, 33% moderate risk); other nutrients not different from Nutrition Canada
Kuhnlein (1984)	1981–82	Bella Coola, BC (pop: 675)	Qualitative; 24-hr recall; n = 40 F, 19–49 yr	Traditional foods used more often by reserve residents than urban residents; low intakes of Fola, Ca, VitD/C, Fe (<2/3 RNI)
Wein et al. (1991a,b)	1986–87	Chipewyan, Cree, Metis, Northern AB and NWT (pop: 3,500)	n = 178 M/F, 13 + yr; 24-hr recall	Land food important in diet: 4 ×/week, ⅓ total meat/fish; Ca, VitA, Fola <RDA; Fe low in F; Prot 13%–18%, CHO 46%–54%, Fats 35–38% of energy; land foods better quality, higher nutrient density/kcal, lower fat, but deficient in Ca

Eskimos/Inuit

Reference	Year	Location (population)	Sample	Findings
Mann et al. (1962)	1958	Alaska: members of National Guard + villagers	n = 97 M, 16–75 yr; 3–7 day diary + weighing/analysis	High Prot, bu: low Kcal, Thia, and Vit C. Fat 35% of energy
Sauberlich et al. (1972)	1969	Wainwright, AK (pop: 308)	n = 129 M/F, 2 + yr; Biochemical	18% at risk for anemia (36%–52% in children <5); Vitamins, Prot, and minerals adequate (B-6 marginal)
Canada DNHW, (1975,a)	1972	NWT: 4 communities	n = 346, M/F; Biochemical; 24-hr recall	Low Kcal, high Prot; marginal/inadequate VitA/C/D, Fola, Ca; Adequate Thia, Ribo, Niac, Fe
Bang et al. (1980)	1976	W. Greenland	n = 50, M/F; Weighing/analysis	Prot 23%, CHO 38%, fats 39% of energy; rich in PUFA; P/S: 0.84 (cf. 0.24 in Denmark)
Verdier et al. (1987)	1976–80	Arctic Bay, NWT	n>300, M/F; Biochemical	1976, 1978, 1980 compared to 1972 Nutrition Canada data: fewer deficiencies except for VitA; improved VitC, Fola

aStates/Provinces: AZ Arizona; AB Alberta; AK Alaska; BC British Columbia; ND North Dakota; NS Nova Scotia; NWT Northwest Territories; OK Oklahoma; SD South Dakota.

bStudies on serum lipids and prevalence of obesity not included.

Abbreviations: B-6 = vitamin B-6; Ca = calcium; CHO = carbohydrates; Fe = iron; Fola = folate; Kcal = kilocalories (energy); Niac = niacin; Prot = proteins; PUFA = polyunsaturated fatty acids; Ribo = riboflavin; Thia = thiamine; VitA = vitamin A; VitC = vitamin C; VitD = vitamin D; P/S Polyunsaturated/saturated fatty acid ratio; CDS Canadian Dietary Standards; RDA Recommended Dietary Allowance; RNI Recommended Nutrient Intake.

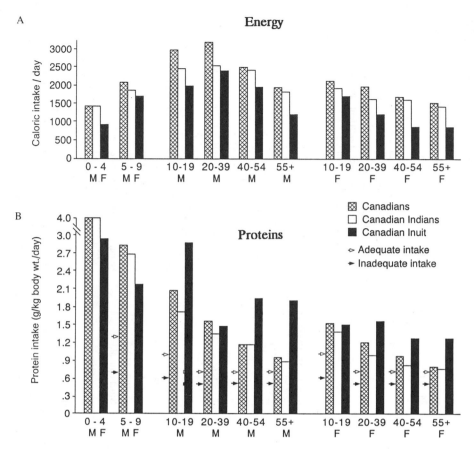

Figure 2.8. Dietary intake: Canada, 1972, Canadian Indians, Inuit, and all Canadians (*A*) Energy, (*B*) Proteins.

Except for the second half of the twentieth century, it is difficult to reconstruct the pattern of health and disease among Native Americans, even within historic times. Official statistics were incomplete and unreliable. The Southwest perhaps has the longest history of medical investigations, beginning with the noted physician-anthropologist Hrdlička's seminal report to the Smithsonian Institution (1908). Clements (1931) analyzed mortality data of the Chemehuevi and Mojave of western Arizona from 1910 to 1930 and noted the preeminence of infectious diseases. In the 1940s an American Medical Association team investigated health conditions among the Navajo and the Hopi and reported the high incidence of such infectious diseases as tuberculosis, syphilis, diarrhea, and trachoma (Moorman, 1949).

The recent epidemiologic history of Native American populations appears to be characterized by several key features: decline but persistence of infectious diseases, stabilizing at a level still higher than non-Native population; rise in chronic diseases but not quite rampant; and the overwhelming importance of social pathologies. Figure 2.9 provides an illustration of these mortality trends among Canadian Indians since the 1940s.

The decline in infectious diseases in the developed countries since the late nineteenth century has generally been attributed to an improved standard of living, particularly nutritional status, rather than to specific medical and public health interventions, or to a change in disease virulence. Such a view has been propounded since the 1960s by such scholars as McKeown (1988). While ini-

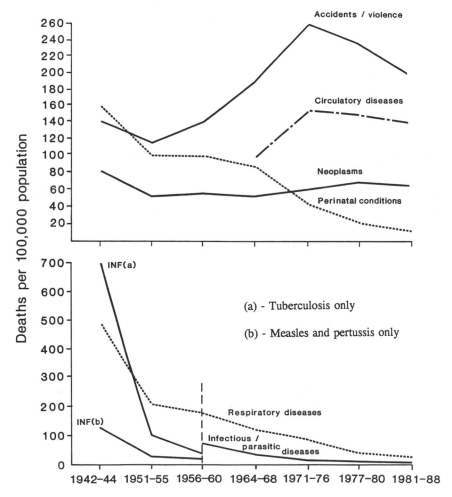

Figure 2.9. Change in crude mortality rate for selected causes among Canadian Indians, 1944–88.

tially this thesis represented a radical departure from the conventional wisdom of the time, these views have since become the mainstream in public health thought. More recently, Wilson, analyzing trends in tuberculosis mortality, challenged the accepted explanation and instead attributed the substantial decline to the practice of isolating active cases, beginning in the late nineteenth century. Even in the absence of effective antibiotic treatment, such public health measures reduced the spread of the disease (Wilson, 1990).

The mortality experience of Native Americans can be viewed in terms of the "mortality convergence" and "minority status" hypotheses. Trovato (1988) found evidence in support for both. Under the former theory, modern society is seen as creating a general homogenization of values, norms, and lifestyles relating to health behavior, thus minimizing mortality differentials among social groups in the population. Under the latter concept, it is predicted that continuing socioeconomic disparities along ethnic lines will prevent disadvantaged minority groups from completely assimilating the survival probabilities of the majority group.

*   *   *

Beginning with Chapter 3, the discussion moves from the general to the specific. Three groups of diseases or health conditions have been selected on the basis of their historical significance and current contribution to the burden of ill health among Native Americans. The existing literature and statistical data available on Native Americans in terms of the extent of the problem, etiology and risk factors, and strategies for prevention and control are reviewed.

3

Decline and Persistence of Infectious Diseases

Infectious diseases have played a major role in the epidemiologic history of Native Americans, as the previous chapter has shown. While pre-contact Native Americans were not free from infections, those infections that were present were likely persistent zoonotic parasitic diseases associated with low virulence (Black, 1975). With the arrival of Europeans, Native Americans underwent a transition from "small band" epidemiology to "large herd" epidemiology, often with devastating results (Neel, 1968).

Throughout human history, infectious diseases have served as agents of natural selection and cultural transformation (Inhorn and Brown, 1990). Pathogens can be considered as coevolving with their human hosts. Every change in the environment or culture is reflected in the patterns of the infectious diseases of the population (Cockburn, 1971). The development of agriculture, increase in population size, sedentarization in villages, domestication of animals, inter-tribal trade and warfare, all played a role in determining the rise and fall of specific diseases. Epidemics may facilitate military conquests and hasten acculturation. "Virgin-soil" epidemics characteristically kill off or debilitate a high proportion of adults in their prime years, people responsible for food procurement, defense, and procreation (Crosby, 1976). In post-contact North America the social disruption that followed such epidemics involved changes in kinship pattern, band membership, and clan organization (Krech, 1978). The impotence of indigenous religious and healing systems to counter the new catastrophes prepared the way for European missionaries.

The success of immunizations had reduced the epidemiological significance of such diseases as measles, rubella, mumps, poliomyelitis, tetanus, and diphtheria in Native American communities. It should be remembered that, as late

55

as the 1950s, virgin-soil epidemics of these diseases still occurred in some areas in the Arctic. The building of the Alaska Highway during World War II by the U.S. Military resulted in a series of epidemics among Natives in the Yukon Territory (Marchand, 1943). In Chesterfield Inlet, Northwest Territories, eight percent of the Inuit population contracted polio from white workers stationed in Churchill, Manitoba, to the south, and 2 percent of the population died (Adamson et al., 1949). In 1952, a measles epidemic swept through Baffin Island, Northwest Territories, and the Ungava peninsula in northern Quebec, with an attack rate of 99 percent and mortality rate between 2 percent and 7 percent. This epidemic was traced to Inuit visitors to the Armed Forces base at Goose Bay, Labrador (Peart et al., 1954).

Despite the great reduction in mortality and morbidity attributed to infectious diseases over the past several decades, Native Americans generally are still at higher risks than non-Natives. The distribution and frequency of specific infections reflect local ecological, socioeconomic, and cultural factors. While in the past certain diseases were considered "racial" characteristics of Native Americans—a view that has largely been abandoned—genetic factors remain important determinants of many diseases, and new research sheds light on the existence of "host" susceptibility factors in infectious diseases.

Most official statistics on mortality and morbidity use the International Classification of Diseases (ICD) system. The ninth edition, ICD-9, has been in use since the late 1970s. It should be noted that the ICD-9 is a mixed system of classification based on a combination of disease etiology, anatomical site, and specific age-sex group. The majority of infectious diseases are classified in Chapter I "Infectious and Parasitic Diseases." Included in this category are diseases caused by specific microbial agents such as tuberculosis, poliomyelitis, and pertussis. Certain important conditions are classified elsewhere in ICD-9, however. Thus meningitis and otitis media are in Chapter VI "Nervous System and Sense Organs;" influenza and pneumonia, under Chapter VIII "Respiratory System;" pyelonephritis and cystitis, under Chapter X "Genitourinary System;" and cellulitis and impetigo, under Chapter XII "Skin and Subcutaneous Tissues." While intestinal infections or diarrheal diseases should be coded as 001-009 under Chapter I, sometimes they are included incorrectly in Chapter IX "Digestive System." Awareness of the coding scheme is important, if underestimation of the true burden of infectious diseases is to be avoided.

The excessive burden of infectious diseases as a group among Native Americans is reflected in national data for both the United States and Canada. In Canada, analysis of the National Mortality Database for the periods 1979–83 and 1984–88 indicates that Indian reserves experienced a higher risk of infectious diseases (ICD-9 Chapter I, inclusive of codes 001-139) during both periods. However, the rates were lower during the more recent period (Table 3.1).

Table 3.1 Age-Standardized Mortality Rate for Selected Infectious Diseases among
Residents of Indian Reserves in Six Canadian Provinces, 1979–1983 and 1984–1988

	1979–1983[b]				1984–1988			
	Male		Female		Male		Female	
ICD-9 code[a]	IR	PR	IR	PR	IR	PR	IR	PR
001-139	13.2	4.5	9.6	2.8	10.3	6.3	11.2	3.4
001-009	0.7	0.2	0.7	0.2	0.2	0.2	0.4	0.2
480-486	42.1	26.9	33.0	15.0	29.8	29.8	25.2	16.0
320-326	2.2	0.7	0.9	0.5	1.6	0.6	1.7	0.4
Total[c]	60.5	34.8	46.0	20.7	42.9	37.2	41.5	21.6

[a]001-139, infectious and parasitic diseases; 001-009, intestinal infections; 480-486, pneumonia;
320-326, infections of central nervous system.
[b]IR = residents of Indian reserves in six provinces; PR = other Canadians in same provinces
[c]Total refers to sum of 001-139, 480-486, and 320-326

Regional variation in the Native American age-standardized mortality rate for infectious diseases can be demonstrated in both Canada (between provinces) and the United States (between IHS Service Areas; Fig. 3.1A, USA, and Fig. 3.1B, Canada). Within regions, interethnic differences in mortality risk are usually also present. In New Mexico, for example, a study of vital statistics during 1958–87 indicated that, compared to Hispanic and non-Hispanic whites in that state, Native Americans showed the highest mortality rates from infectious diseases, including tuberculosis, pneumonia, and meningitis. All three ethnic groups, however, experienced substantial declines during this period (Becker et al., 1990).

In this chapter, several infectious diseases are presented for detailed review: tuberculosis, meningitis, gastroenteritis, pneumonia and acute respiratory infections, hepatitis, sexually transmitted diseases, streptococcal infections, and the parasitoses.

Tuberculosis

Extent and Magnitude of the Problem

The "pre-Columbian" origin of tuberculosis (TB) in North America has been the subject of debate among archeologists and paleopathologists. Artifacts depicting human deformities and skeletal remains suggestive of tuberculosis of the spine, as well as isolation of acid-fast bacilli in a Peruvian mummy have been cited as evidence of the endemicity of TB among Native Americans in prehistoric times. [For a review of this literature, see El-Najjar (1979), Paulsen (1987), and Clark et al. (1987)]. Pfeiffer (1984) analysed lytic lesions in the skeletal remains in a large ossuary dating to the mid-fifteenth century in Huron territory in south-

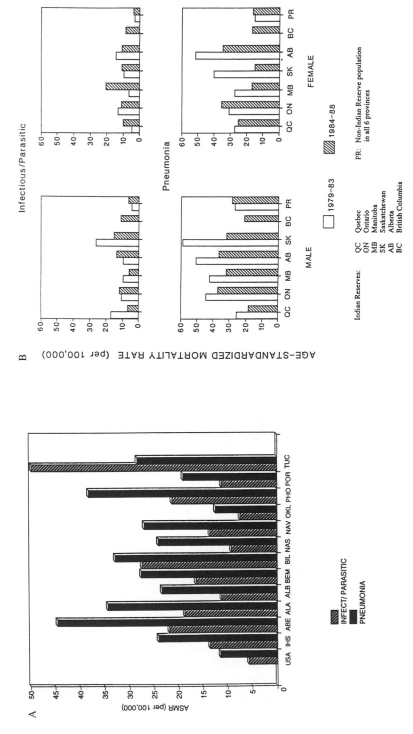

Figure 3.1. Regional variation in age-standardized mortality rate for infectious diseases among Native Americans: (A) USA, 1980–83; (B) Canada, 1979–88.

ern Ontario. On the assumption that skeletal TB represented a small proportion of all TB cases, she estimated that the entire settlement of over 1,000 people could have been infected, perhaps in an epidemic wave abetted by warfare, crowding, and nutritional deficiency. Regardless of the extent of pre-contact infection rates, there is little doubt that after the influx of European settlers into the continent the impact of the disease became devastating (Rieder, 1989; Wherrett, 1977; Ferguson, 1955). In fact, at the beginning of the twentieth century many physicians believed that TB was a "racial" characteristic of Native Americans.

It has been speculated that the high incidence of TB was the result of enforced changes in ecological factors rather than exposure to a new, introduced infectious disease. Clark and others (1987) hypothesized that pre-Columbian TB had only a relatively mild impact among Native American populations because of cross-immunizations by atypical mycobacteria. The severity of the disease in post-contact times could be due to the evolution of a new, and more virulent strain, although it is more likely a result of changes in social conditions such as crowding and poor nutrition, or the loss of "natural vaccination" due to drastic changes in the natural habitat (Clark et al., 1987).

During the twentieth century, the mortality from TB has declined substantially (Fig. 3.2). The decline, in fact, preceded the availability of effective antituberculosis therapy, although it steepened with the large-scale control efforts of the 1950s.

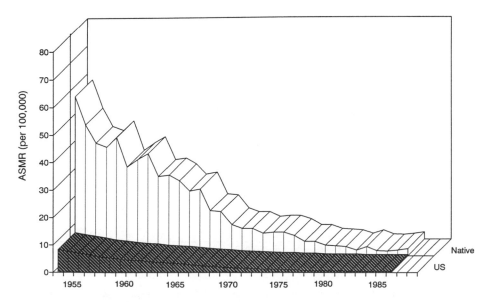

Figure 3.2. Age-standardized mortality rate for tuberculosis: USA, 1955–87, Native American and U.S. all-race populations.

Despite such improvements, the disparity between Natives and non-Natives remains great, with Natives having an incidence as much as ten times higher than non-Natives in Canada. The rates were lowest in eastern Canada and highest in the Prairie provinces and the northern territories (Enarson and Grzybowski, 1986). Figure 3.3 compares the decline in incidence among Canadian Indians, Inuit, and the national population. It can be seen that by the late 1970s the Inuit rate had declined to a level below that of Indians, among whom the rate had remained stable at a relatively high level.

In the United States the mean incidence among Native Americans during 1984–1988 was about 25/100,000. While this was almost three times higher than the U.S. all-race rate, the improvement had been dramatic when comparisons are made with rates of 90/100,000 during 1973–76, 138 during 1969–72, and over 250 in the early 1960s (data from CDC and IHS).

Regional studies, for example those among the Cree-Ojibwa in northwestern Ontario (Young and Casson, 1988), supported the national trend toward levelling off in the decline. Sporadic outbreaks of TB still occurred in Native communities throughout the 1980s, highlighting the need for continuing surveillance and control measures. Natives are also at higher risk for reactivations of TB that has been treated and that remained inactive for some time (Johnson et al., 1985).

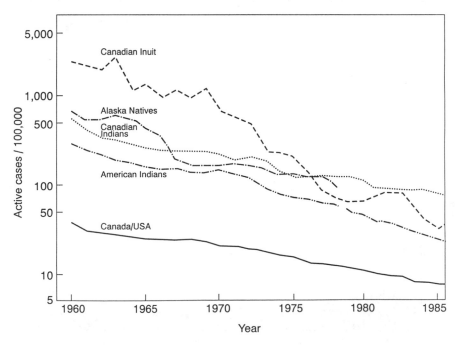

Figure 3.3. Incidence rate of active tuberculosis: USA and Canada, 1960–85, Native Americans and all-race populations.

The incidence and mortality rate of TB do not present a complete picture of the extent and magnitude of the infection in populations. TB epidemiologists have emphasized the need to measure both the risk of infection and the incidence of active disease (Sutherland, 1976). The risk factors associated with these two stages of TB are significantly different (Comstock, 1975). Apparently new TB cases may in fact be reactivations of disease in people who were infected many years ago. It is also possible to have a high case rate and a low rate of new infection. The case rate cannot measure current transmission of the tubercle bacilli, and it is dependent on the case-finding efforts of the health care system.

Whereas statistics on TB incidence and mortality are routinely collected by official health agencies, estimates of risk of infection can only be made through special testing surveys with tuberculin (PPD—purified protein derivative). The risk of infection could be determined directly by following a cohort of uninfected individuals or indirectly through single surveys or a series of cross-sectional surveys the results of which are fitted against mathematical models under various assumptions (Sutherland, 1976).

Among the Inuit in Frobisher Bay, Northwest Territories, the annual risk of infection was estimated to be 3–4 percent in 1971, and 1.5–2 percent in 1974 (Grzybowski et al., 1976). Among Alaska Natives, five surveys over a span of 20 years in the Yukon-Kuskokwim delta showed a marked decline in the prevalence of tuberculin sensitivity (Kaplan et al., 1972b). A survey of the total population of Manitoulin Island, Ontario, in 1957 included 1,475 unvaccinated Indians. The prevalence of tuberculin positivity was much higher than in whites in all age groups. Among the Indians (predominantly Algonkian-speaking Ojibwa and Odawa), 18 percent of the under-15, 63 percent of the 15–39, and 82 percent of the over-40 age group were tuberculin-positive (Grzybowski and Dunaj, 1959). Historical time series of tuberculin surveys among Native Americans, other than those from Alaska, are not readily available from the published literature.

Etiology and Risk Factors

Comstock (1975) distinguished different sets of risk factors for the two stages of tuberculosis, the acquisition of infection and the development of the disease. The risk factors for tuberculous infection are *extrinsic,* and related to the probability of having prolonged close contact (i.e., crowding) with an infectious source case and the degree of infectiousness of that case. Once infected with the bacillus, the risk of developing the disease varies according to such *intrinsic* factors as age, sex, race, and body build. Other rare risk factors include HIV infection, silicosis, immunosuppressive therapy, and diabetes (Rieder et al., 1989). It should be noted that most people who are infected never develop the disease. The bacilli are harboured in the body and kept in check by the immune defenses. When host defenses are compromised, however, the bacilli begin to multiply and clinical disease develops.

The older literature often assumed racial differences in susceptibility to tuberculosis, with Native Americans the most susceptible population because of their extreme high case rate in the past. The evidence for genetic susceptibility derived from animal models, twin studies, and human lymphocyte antigen (HLA) markers is not conclusive, and the observed "racial" differences may well be explainable by other determinants (Kushigemachi et al., 1984). The association of genetic markers such as HLA with TB have been demonstrated in some Asian populations (Rieder et al., 1989), but data on Native Americans are lacking. Overfield and Klauber (1980) found that the prevalence of TB was higher among Eskimos with blood groups AB/B than among those with groups O/A.

There seems to be a resurgence of interest in genetic and racial susceptibility, particularly to the acquisition of infection. Black and white residents of nursing homes, who were initially tuberculin-negative, differed in tuberculin conversion rates, unaffected by those factors associated with progression to clinical disease (Stead et al., 1990). Data from laboratory studies in mice suggest that variability in infectivity can be attributed to differences in the genetically determined ability of unstimulated macrophages in ingesting and destroying the tubercle bacilli. The regulation of macrophage activation was found to be controlled by a single, dominant, autosomal gene, *Bcg,* located on mouse chromosome 1, which is homologous with a region of the human chromosome 2 (Skamene, 1989).

Prevention and Control Strategies

Several strategies are available in the prevention and control of TB: vaccination with Bacille-Calmette-Guérin (BCG), prophylaxis or preventive treatment with isoniazid (INH), mass screening with tuberculin skin tests and/or chest x-rays, and definitive treatment of active cases. All or some of these methods are used by different jurisdictions around the world, the selection to some extent dictated by the financial and human health care resources available. Among Native Americans, under the jurisdiction of the U.S. Indian Health Service, BCG vaccination has never been an important component of TB control policy, whereas in Canada, mass neonatal BCG vaccination has been established practice since the 1960s.

Tuberculosis is a treatable disease, and a variety of efficacious drugs are available. Guidelines have been established for their use (American Thoracic Society, 1986). The former practice of prolonged hospital treatment, often at centers far removed from the home community which imposed severe personal and family disruption among Native Americans, has since the 1970s been generally superseded by shorter courses of intermittent and supervised therapy. An early trial in an Apache reservation indicated that the then new approach was well tolerated, effective, and economical (Mikkelson et al., 1973).

Poor compliance has often been cited as responsible for treatment failures among Native Americans and other minority populations. In a key informant survey in 31 Indian reserves in British Columbia, there was a widespread belief among the respondents that TB was a disease of the past and little knowledge of recent improvements in treatment. There was also substantial resentment toward and mistrust of non-Native health professionals (Jenkins, 1977). Better cultural understanding of the Native response to illness, beliefs regarding causation, and treatment choices is essential in any TB control program among Native Americans.

Much controversy still surrounds the effectiveness of BCG vaccination. Eight major randomized controlled trials of BCG in various parts of the world have produced variable and conflicting results, with protective efficacy ranging from negative to over 80 percent (Clemens et al., 1983). Two of these trials were conducted among Native Americans—among infants in Saskatchewan (Ferguson and Sime, 1949) and among Indians in five states belonging to seven tribes who were aged 20 and under (Aronson et al., 1958). Both trials were initiated during the 1930s and both showed high protective efficacy in the 80 percent range. However, both were also done at a time when the risk of infection, the case rate, and the mortality rate were all extremely high.

Case-control studies have been recommended to evaluate vaccine effectiveness, particularly where an expensive, large, and prolonged trial is not feasible. Several case-control studies on BCG have been conducted, and most reported a protective effect (Fine, 1988). Two case-control studies conducted among Canadian Indians in Manitoba (Young and Hershfield, 1986) and Alberta (Houston et al., 1990) showed a protective effect of at least 60 percent.

The Alberta case-control study showed that the protective effect was higher among those vaccinated after age 6 months (63%) than among those immunized at 6 months or less (42%). However, a clinical study conducted in a group of Cree infants, also in Alberta, found that increasing the age at vaccination from birth to 9 months or more actually enhanced the sensitization to PPD as measured by lymphocyte response (Pabst et al., 1989). This study further showed that breast-feeding enhanced the cell-mediated immune response to BCG given at birth but had no significant effect if the vaccine was given after one month (Pabst et al., 1989b). It should be noted that immunogenicity is not always equated with efficacy.

Whether BCG is effective or not is only one of the issues to be considered in the decision regarding the use of the vaccine on a mass scale, other issues being the significance of the problem, safety of the vaccine, interference with tuberculin testing, and availability of alternative methods of control (Young, 1985).

Preventive therapy or prophylaxis using the drug INH is surrounded by less controversy than BCG vaccination. Contacts of patients with active disease and people found to have recently "converted" (i.e., increased in the size of reaction to tuberculin) are generally put on INH for one year. [This is different from definitive therapy in confirmed cases, where at least two, sometimes as many as four, antituberculous drugs are used]. The effectiveness of chemoprophylaxis is well established. Ferebee (1970) reviewed 13 controlled trials in seven countries, two of which were conducted among Eskimos in Alaska (Comstock et al., 1979) and Greenland (Horwitz et al., 1966). One trial in Frobisher Bay, Northwest Territories, used a supervised regimen of INH and ethambutol three times weekly for 18 months. After ten years of follow-up the chemoprophylaxis was 87 percent effective (Dorken et al., 1984).

Although public health professionals are ideologically committed to "prevention," TB may be one disease where "cure" (the use of drugs to kill bacilli) is better than "prevention" (the use of vaccine). The key to the control of TB lies in the reduction of the risk of infection rather than the incidence of actual disease. Chemotherapy of diagnosed disease has an effect on the risk of infection that is complete and rapid. Vaccination allows infection to occur but prevents the progression to disease and infectiousness to others, which may not occur until some years later (Sutherland, 1981).

WHO recommends the use of mass BCG vaccination in developing countries (1982), and BCG is included as one of the six vaccines in the WHO Expanded Program of Immunizations (EPI). Among Native Americans, where the amount of resources devoted to health services is many times that available for most third world countries, and where a well-organized system already exists for diagnosis, treatment, and follow-up of TB cases, the more expensive but highly effective method of supervised chemotherapy of diagnosed patients, thorough contact tracing, and selective use of chemoprophylaxis may suffice. The use of mass neonatal BCG vaccination may offer additional benefits, particularly in providing protection among those who may at some time fall outside the surveillance of the organized health system. Mass screening procedures such as tuberculin testing and/or radiography may not be justified because of the low yield of cases and the diversion of scarce resources from other more productive public health programs.

The goal of eliminating indigenous (i.e., non-imported) tuberculosis in North America is achievable with existing technology. The U.S. Department of Health and Human Services has established a strategic plan to eliminate tuberculosis in the United States by the year 2010 (CDC, MMWR 1989;38:S-3). The control of this disease among such high-risk groups as Native Americans will be essential if that goal is to be accomplished.

Infections of the Nervous System

Extent and Magnitude of the Problem

The high incidence of meningitis has been demonstrated in many Native communities in Canada and the United States. The most prevalent causative organism is *Hemophilus influenzae* type b (Hib), followed by meningococci, pneumoccocci, mycobateria, and other bacterial and viral agents. The case-fatality rate for meningitis varies according to the organism, from about 34 percent in cases caused by Gram-negative organisms, to 26 percent in pneumococcal, to 10 percent in meningococcal, to 6 percent in Hib cases (Schlech et al., 1985). Patients who survive may develop residual disabilities.

H. influenzae exists in both an unencapsulated and an encapsulated form. The former is associated with mild infections such as otitis media, bronchitis, and sinusitis. Several serotypes (a to f) can be distinguished among the encapsulated form. The b serotype is responsible for over 90 percent of serious, invasive diseases caused by *H. influenza* (including meningitis, epiglottitis, septicemia, cellulitis, pneumonia, and septic arthritis; Shapiro and Ward, 1991).

Compared to bacteria, viruses are much less important etiologic agents of central nervous system infection, although outbreaks of echovirus meningitis were reported in two Yupik Eskimo villages in Alaska in 1970 (Kaplan et al., 1972a).

A study of infant mortality on Indian reserves in five Canadian provinces during 1976–83 showed that the standardized mortality ratio (SMR) for meningitis (from all causes) was 4.3 during the post-neonatal period (Morrison et al., 1986). Table 3.1 shows the age-standardized mortality rate (ASMR) for infections of the central nervous system among Canadian Indians during the periods 1979–83 and 1984–88. Estimates of incidence in various Native populations are provided in Table 3.2. The high Native rates for Hib meningitis can be compared with the Canadian national notification rate of 0.9 to 1.7/100,000 for all ages during 1979–84, and an under-5 rate of 20/100,000 (Hammond et al., 1988). In the review by Shapiro and Ward (1991), the incidence rate reported from various non-Native populations in the United States ranged from 65 to 190/100,000 among the under-1 age group and from 20 to 80/100,000 among the under-5 age group.

In Manitoba, the Indian rate was 1.4 times the non-Indian rate among the

Table 3.2 Regional Studies of Meningitis among Native Americans

Population	Years/No. Cases	Reference	Organism[a]	Incidence Rate (per 100,000) All Ages	< 5 yr	< 1 yr
Alaska	1971–74	Gilsdorf	Total	94	—	3242
Natives	39 cases	(1977)	H.flu	63	474	2323
(Bethel area)			Pneumo	19	—	602
			Meningo	2	—	—
Alaska	1971–77	Ward et al.	Total	84	570	—
Natives	73 cases	(1981)	H.flu	58	409	—
(Bethel area)			Pneumo	8	—	—
			Meningo	9	—	—
Alaska	1980–82	Ward et al.	H.flu	33	282	871
Natives	64 cases	(1986)				
Alaska	1980–86	Davidson et	Pneumo	13	99	—
Natives		al. (1989)				
(Bethel area)						
Inuit,	1972–77	Wotton et al.	Total	202	—	—
Keewatin	30 cases	(1981)	H.flu	46	—	—
zone, NWT[b]			Pneumo	7	—	—
			Meningo	43	—	—
Inuit, northern	1980–85	Proulx	Total	—	800	—
Quebec	29 cases	(1988)	H.flu	—	568	—
			Pneumo	—	88	—
Inuit,	1981–84	Hammond et	H.flu			
Keewatin	9 Inuit	al. (1988)	Inuit	80	530	2333
NWT,	22 Indian		Indians	16	35	126
Indians, MB[b]	cases					
Navajo Res	1968–73	Coulehan et	H.flu	18	173	—
AZ[b]	219 cases	al. (1976)	Pneumo	8	57	—
			Meningo	2	14	—
Navajo Res	1974–80	Coulehan et	Total	—	216	—
AZ	341 cases	al. (1984)	H.flu	—	153	—
			Pneumo	—	46	—
			Meningo	—	1	—
Arizona	1978–83	Yost et al.	Total	—	180	—
Indians	102 cases	(1986)	H.flu	—	136	—
Apaches AZ	1973–82	Losonsky et al. (1984)	H.flu	—	254	1170

[a]H.flu = *Hemophilus influenzae*; Pneumo = pneumococcal; Meningo = meningococcal.
[b]NWT = Northwest Territories; MB = Manitoba; AZ = Arizona.

under-5 age group and 1.8 times among infants. For Inuit in the Keewatin region of the Northwest Territories, the excess was 20 times among the under-5 age group and 33 times among infants (Hammond et al., 1988). In Alaska, Eskimos and Indians had similar age-adjusted relative risks (about 4) of Hib meningitis compared to non-Natives in the same state (Ward et al., 1986).

In a follow-up study of the Northwest Territories Perinatal and Infant Mortality Study (PIMMS) which involved a birth cohort of all infants born in that region during 1973–74, it was found that of 444 Inuit livebirths, 7 percent had experienced meningitis by the age of 8 (Postl et al., 1985).

Studies from Alaska indicate that Native Indians and Eskimos not only suffer from a high incidence of invasive *Hemophilus influenzae* disease, but also a high rate of recurrence (3.5%). The younger the age of an infant at initial infection, the greater the risk of recurrence. Increased host susceptibility—due to the inability of young infants to mount an adequate immune response to the capsular polysaccharide—was believed to be the reason (Brenneman et al., 1987).

The high case rate of meningitis may be associated with a high carriage rate of the organisms in the general population in Inuit communities. In a 1980 survey of nasopharyngeal carriage of meningococci and *H. influenzae* in Baker Lake in the central Arctic, 32 percent of Inuit were found to carry the former and 16 percent the latter. While the attack rate of meningococcal meningitis was highest among children, the highest carriage rate was found in adolescents and in the elderly (Nicolle et al., 1982a and b). Among Yupik Eskimos in four villages in southwestern Alaska, only 7 percent had pharyngeal cultures positive for Hib during a 12-month period, a finding that was not associated with age, sex, season, or prior incidence of disease in the village (Hall et al., 1987). The mechanism for a high incidence of disease even while carriage rate in a community is low remains obscure.

Etiology and Risk Factors

Susceptibility to Hib infections varies according to age. The peak incidence of Hib meningitis occurs during infancy, between the ages of 6 and 12 months. A study among the Navajos indicated that 79 percent of neonates had transplacentally acquired significant maternal capsular type b antibody titers. Yet, by 4 months of age, only 14 percent still maintained this level (Coulehan et al., 1984). A similar pattern was observed among Yupik Eskimos (Ward et al., 1981). Thus it would appear that disease occurs when the infants are at their most vulnerable, with little protection from maternal antibodies.

Ethnic differences in susceptibility are also well documented, whether between countries or within countries. However, the effect of medical care, socioeconomic status, and crowding may have been responsible for the observed differences. Other risk factors that have been implicated in susceptibility include passive cigarette smoking and mode of feeding, breast-feeding being protective (Shapiro and Ward, 1991).

In Alaskan Eskimos, genetic markers such as uridine monophosphate kinase 3 (Petersen et al., 1985) and combinations of Gm immunoglobulin allotypes and HLA-DR markers (Petersen et al., 1987) have been associated with susceptibility to Hib infection. However, the presence of these markers was not associated with capsular type b antibody levels, suggesting that disease susceptibility is not mediated through humoral immunity. Host factors are of great interest since, given identical exposure, not all children develop the disease. The association of Hib disease with some genetic markers suggests that genetic factors may confer increased susceptibility (or conversely increased resistance) to disease. Whether such factors mediate susceptibility directly or are chromosomally linked to other genetic elements that have a more direct influence on the development of disease remains uncertain.

Prevention and Control Strategies

Active Immunization.   Primary prevention against Hib disease is available through active immunization with a vaccine against the polysaccharide capsule of Hib (polyribosyl-ribitol phosphate—PRP) developed in the 1970s. A second-generation "conjugate vaccine" is now available, which supersedes the earlier, purely polysaccharide vaccine, the efficacy of which has been demonstrated only among children 18 months of age or older, thus offering little protection to those at highest risk. Studies among Apache children in Arizona at 18 and 24 months showed that they had a lower antibody response than white children, particularly at 24 months, (Siber et al., 1990). On the other hand, a study among Navajo infants aged 1–2 months, using PRP given simultaneously with diphtheria-pertussis-tetanus (DPT), showed that, despite the presence of maternal antibodies, 50 percent developed a definite antibody responses to the PRP (Coulehan et al., 1983a).

The conjugate vaccine improves immunogenicity by linking PRP covalently to an immunogenic protein carrier, such as diphtheria toxoid (PRP-D), the outer-membrane protein complex of the meningococcus (PRP-OMP), and the nontoxic mutant of the diphtheria toxin, CRM_{197} [that vaccine is called HbOC, for oligosaccharide conjugate]. PRP-D is licensed for children 15 months and older, whereas PRP-OMP and HbOC are recommended for those 2 months and older (CDC, MMWR 1991;40:RR-1).

The immune response of Alaska Native infants to PRP-D was compared with that of infants in Albany, New York. Antibody levels prior to immunization at 2 months of age, presumably maternally acquired, were significantly higher among Alaskan infants. There were no significant differences in antibody levels after any of the three vaccine doses (Ward et al., 1988). A randomized controlled trial of PRP-D conducted among Alaska Natives in six health service areas involving over 2,000 infants showed a protective efficacy of only 35 percent. The lack of efficacy was not related to age of disease onset, age at immunization, type of disease, degree of Native heritage, time after immunization, or year of the study. Even after the third dose, less than half of the infants had adequate antibody levels (Ward et al., 1990).

A field trial of PRP-OMP among infants 2 and 4 months old on the Navajo reservation was more encouraging, demonstrating safety, immunogenicity, and a protective efficacy of over 90 percent (Santosham et al., 1991 a and b).

Passive Immunization.   Passive immunization with hyperimmune globulin containing high concentrations of antibodies against PRP prepared from plasma of adult vaccinees has has been tested among Apache infants. The protective efficacy was 100 percent during the first 3 months and 86 percent after 4 months (Santosham et al., 1987). Combined active/passive immunization (immune globulin + HbOC) was also tested among the Navajo. Compared with vaccine alone, the combined preparation was more immunogenic at 2 months. After the third dose of vaccine, however, the two groups were not significantly different (Letson et al., 1988). The use of combined active/passive immunization is recommended for high-risk situations to provide immediate protection until the full effect of multiple doses of vaccine over a period of months can be established.

Chemoprophylaxis.   Another preventive strategy is chemoprophylaxis, which is treatment of potential contacts with antibiotics to eradicate recently acquired infections. A community chemoprophylaxis trial using minocycline and/or rifampin was conducted in Baker Lake, Northwest Territories (Nicolle et al., 1982a). Although this study did not examine reduction in disease incidence, it did demonstrate a substantial reduction in nasopharyngeal carriage of meningococci, which persisted for nine weeks. No antibiotic-resistant strains emerged. This study simultaneously examined the effect on nasopharyngeal carriage of *H. influenzae,* which was less successful. While carriage rate fell from 14 percent to 5 percent after one week, it returned to 12 percent by nine weeks. Furthermore, 10 percent of the strains at one week and 7.5 percent at nine weeks were rifampin-resistant (Nicolle et al., 1982b).

Infections of the Intestinal Tract

Extent and Magnitude of the Problem

Diarrheal disease, or gastroenteritis, is a worldwide problem in children, particularly in developing countries. Even in developed countries large numbers of children become sick, are hospitalized, and some even die. Many bacterial and viral agents are responsible for the diarrheal diseases. With the increasing sophistication of diagnostic techniques, the proportion of previously labeled "nonspecific" causes has been steadily reduced as more and more organisms, particularly viruses, are identified. Rotaviruses are by far the commonest etiologic agent, but the list of viruses now includes Norwalk virus, enteric adenovirus, calicivirus, astrovirus, and a host of other viruses of uncertain public health significance (Blacklow and Greenberg, 1991). In the Navajo reservation, about a quarter of children under the age of 2 with gastroenteritis of "unknown" etiology has been found to be positive for the *pestivirus,* a pathogen usually associated with animals (Yolken et al., 1989). Among bacterial pathogens are *Shigella, Salmonella, Escheridria coli, Yersinia,* and *Campylobacter.* (Protozoa such as *Entameba histolytica* and *Giardia lamblia* also produce diarrhea; these are discussed under the section on parasites later in this chapter.)

The declining trend in age-standardized mortality from gastroenteritis among Native Americans in the United States from 1955 to 1987 is shown in Figure 3.4. The ASMR for intestinal infections in Canada during 1979–83 and 1984–88 are shown in Table 3.1.

Outbreaks have occurred in a variety of settings, such as Alaska (Fournelle et al., 1966; Bender et al., 1972), the James Bay coast of northern Quebec (Robinson and Moffatt, 1985), an Apache reservation in Arizona (Woodward et al., 1974; Santosham et al., 1985), and in Buffalo, New York (Elsea et al., 1967). Far more epidemics have occurred than are reported in the literature.

Even in nonepidemic situations, Native Americans suffer a much higher burden of diarrheal morbidity than non-Natives. In southwestern Ontario, Evers and Rand (1982) reported 573 episodes of gastroenteritis and 73 hospitalizations per 1,000 person-years in a cohort of infants during their first-year of life, a relative risk of 3 and 24, respectively when compared with non-Natives in the same area. During the second year of life, the relative risk for office visits for treatment of diarrhea was reduced to 1.7 (Evers and Rand, 1983).

In the United States the annual incidence of shigellosis was 4.7/100,000 during the 1970s, while the rate for Native Americans was 17.4/100,000. There had been a steady decline in shigellosis since the 1940s. This period also experienced the virtual disappearance of *S. dysenteriae,* which causes severe epidemic dysentery, and its replacement first by *S. flexneri,* which was in turn overtaken by *S. sonnei,* such that the disease has become progressively milder. This transition is generally observed as a region develops economically. In the United States nationally, *S. sonnei* comprised 70 percent of isolations, *S. flexneri* 30 percent, and *S. dysenteriae* less than 1 percent. Among Native Americans, *S. flexneri* accounted for a much higher proportion of isolations (58%). The flexneri/sonnei ratio increases with age, being 0.28 under age 20 and 0.45 over age 20. Among Native Americans, the corresponding ratios were 2.1 and 2.9 (Blaser et al., 1983).

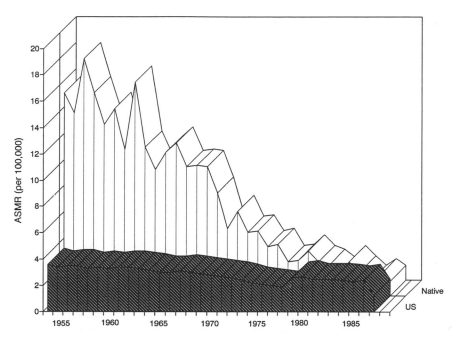

Figure 3.4. Age-standardized mortality rate for gastroenteritis: USA, 1955–87, Native American and U.S. all-race populations.

Among the Cree in the James Bay area of northern Quebec, where during the 1980s several severe epidemics of *E. coli* and rotavirus gastroenteritis were reported, a population-based stool survey found 21 different serotypes of enteropathic *E. coli* in 7 percent of those sampled (as high as 13% in one community), whereas none of the other bacterial pathogens such as *Salmonella, Shigella, Yersinia,* and *Campylobacter* were isolated. This finding raised doubt as to whether strains designated as enteropathogenic were truly pathogenic, or whether such carriers could play a role in episodic outbreaks (Brassard et al., 1985).

Mention must be made of *botulism*, a disease caused by the bacteria *Clostridium botulinum*. While not strictly speaking an infection, but poisoning by the toxin produced by the bacteria, it is caused by ingestion of contaminated food. Its manifestations are more neurological (paralysis) than gastrointestinal. Botulism has special significance in certain Native American populations and can even be considered a "culture-bound" disease. In Canada, between 1971 and 1984, 61 outbreaks involving 122 cases and 21 deaths were reported. Ninety-three percent of the cases were Inuit from northern Quebec and the Northwest Territories and Indians from British Columbia. Prior to 1951 the disease in Canada occurred mostly among people of European origin who engaged in home canning. Since then the disease has been found almost exclusively in the Native population. All Native cases belong to type E (Hauschild and Gauvreau, 1985). Botulism outbreaks, primarily type E but also some type A and B, have also occurred among Alaska Natives, Between 1947 and 1986, there were 59 outbreaks among Alaska Natives, predominantly Eskimos in the western part of the state (Shaffer et al., 1990).

Etiology and Risk Factors

Regardless of the causative organism, gastroenteritis is generally transmitted from person to person through the oral-fecal route. Outbreaks often can be traced to a common source such as food, water, or fomites. Environmental factors that favor the transmission of diarrheal diseases include overcrowding, inadequate sanitation, and a contaminated water supply. In the Fort Apache reservation in Arizona, the diarrheal attack rate rose in tandem with increasing temperature, rainfall, and the bacterial contamination of water sources (Woodward et al., 1974). The respiratory route has been suggested for the transmission of rotaviruses in a later outbreak on the same reservation, due to the rapid appearance of widely scattered cases, the absence of a common source of exposure, and the coexistence of respiratory symptoms, although viruses were not isolated from respiratory secretions (Santosham et al., 1985). Certain foodborne outbreaks can be attributed to "culture-specific" practices, as, for example, salmonellosis from consuming whale meat in an Eskimo village on the Bering Sea coast (Bender et al., 1972).

Several analytical studies have been conducted in Native communities to determine specific risk factors for gastroenteritis. In a Hopi pueblo during the 1960s the community was divided politically and culturally into a "progressive" and a "traditional" faction, providing the setting for a natural experiment. In 1964 the U.S. government installed indoor plumbing in the community, but the traditionalists refused to accept it and continued to use outdoor taps and privies. A study by Rubenstein and others (1969) demonstrated that traditionalists had higher rate of outpatient visits for diarrhea and hospital admission for all causes, and for diarrhea, than the progressives. Among the latter, there was also a decline in all-cause and diarrhea outpatient visits after the plumbing installation, while no significant change could be observed among the traditionalists.

A small case-control study on rotavirus gastroenteritis in an Apache Reservation in Arizona in 1980 showed that the presence of siblings under 2 years of age and the presence of dogs were significant risk factors for the disease. The sample size was not large enough, however, to demonstrate a significant risk associated with the absence of indoor toilets and indoor water supply (Englebert et al., 1982). A larger case-control study in another Apache reservation showed that exposure to other children with diarrhea was the most important risk factor of rotavirus diarrhea, although a high score for poor environmental sanitation was also significant. These factors were independent of mother's education, age, and employment status (Menon et al., 1990).

The relationship between diarrhea and nutritional status is generally accepted. Considerable evidence exists in the world literature (predominantly from the developing countries) to indicate that diarrhea causes poor nutritional status. The evidence for the reverse, that poor nutritional status predisposes to an increased incidence of diarrheal disease, however, is not strong, although there is some support for the association between nutritional status and the severity and duration of diarrhea (Feachem, 1983).

Feachem and Koblinsky (1984) reviewed 35 studies in 14 countries on breast-feeding as a protective factor for diarrheal diseases. Breast-feeding, whether exclusive or partial, offers protection up to 1 year of age but not beyond. Protection is greatest during the first three months of life (with a median relative risk of 2.4) and declines afterwards. During the first 6 months, exclusive breast-feeding is more protective than partial, and partial is more protective than no breast-feeding at all. Among Native American infants, the benefits of breast-feeding in terms of protection against diarrheal disease have been demonstrated in northern Manitoba (Ellestad-Sayed et al., 1979), the Navajo reservation (French, 1967), and among the Pima (Forman et al., 1984a).

The sources of botulism in the Native population are contaminated, traditionally prepared foods. Among the Inuit/Eskimos the most common source is raw, parboiled, or fermented sea mammal meat. Two traditional delicacies *urraq*— uncooked seal flippers soaked in seal oil—and *muktuk*—fermented whale meat with blubber and skin—are particularly susceptible to contamination with *C. botulinum*. Among Indians in the Northwest Coast, fermented salmon eggs or fish are the most common sources (Hauschild and Gauvreau, 1985). In Alaska modifications of traditional fermentation techniques (e.g., using plastic bags and putting containers above ground) have been associated with outbreaks of botulism in a previously unaffected area (Shaffer et al., 1990).

Prevention and Control Strategies

In a series of papers evaluating interventions in the control of diarrheal diseases in developing countries, Feachem and colleagues (1983) grouped them as follows. Many are potentially applicable to Native American communities.

1. Case management: the use of oral rehydration therapy and promotion of appropriate feeding during the illness and its convalescence.

2. Increasing host resistance: improvement of maternal nutrition, infant nutrition (breast-feeding, weaning practices), immunization against rotaviruses, and chemoprophylaxis against bacterial pathogens.
3. Reducing transmission of the agent: improving water supply and excreta disposal, personal and domestic hygiene, food hygiene, control of animal reservoirs and fly population.
4. Epidemic surveillance, investigations and control of outbreaks.

Studies that purport to demonstrate the benefits of improved water and sanitation were beset by methodological flaws (Esrey and Habicht, 1986). Overall, however, the evidence is in favor of a beneficial role for excreta disposal in improving children's health. Increasing water quantity for domestic hygiene use is more important than the bacteriological quality of the water supply.

As infection with rotavirus offers life-long immunity, vaccination offers a potential means of prevention. Several vaccines have been field tested in a variety of populations with inconsistent results. A randomized controlled trial of two vaccines—the rhesus rotavirus vaccine (RRV) and the bovine vaccine RIT 4237—among infants aged 2–5 months was conducted in the Navajo reservation. Compared to placebo, there was little difference in terms of episodes of diarrhea or clinical severity. The serologic response was also weak. No association between serologic response and breast-feeding was found (Santosham et al., 1991b). These prototype vaccines are directed at single serotypes. The next generation of vaccines, which will incorporate all four major serotypes of rotavirus, may offer better protection.

Despite the epidemiological importance of shigellosis in Native communities, chemoprophylaxis is not generally recommended (De Zoysa and Feachem, 1985). The widespread emergence and dissemination of *Shigella* resistant to trimethoprim-sulfamethoxazole has been demonstrated on the Navajo reservation (Griffin et al., 1989).

Health education provided to families by community health workers on preventive practices has been shown to be effective in an evaluation study among the Papagos. Measures of the frequency and severity of diarrheal diseases improved among high-risk infants (based on a variety of clinical and family social variables), while the program had little effect on low-risk individuals (Nutting et al., 1975).

The use of oral rehydration is safe, effective, and inexpensive (Avery and Snyder, 1990). In developing countries its use is supported by UNICEF and WHO and is a centerpiece of international efforts to improve child survival. Its acceptance by health professionals, both in North America and elsewhere, has been slow, probably the result of ingrained bias in favor of complicated and expensive technology. Oral rehydration of course does not prevent the occurrence of diarrhea, but it is a means of treatment of established disease and prevention of complications and fatality.

Oral rehydration, together with immunizations of key diseases and breast-feeding, constitutes "selective primary care," which is believed to provide the greatest reduction in childhood mortality for the least cost (Walsh and Warren, 1979). Its detractors (e.g., Rifkin and Walt, 1986) objected to its "medical" orientation and failure to address issues of equity and community participation that "comprehensive" primary health care and improvement in water and sanitation entailed. The latter was not necessarily cost-ineffective if different assumptions were used in the analysis (Briscoe, 1984). In terms of prevention strategy for Native Americans, there is no dilemma in choosing between "selective" and "comprehensive" primary health care because the existing systems in both Canada and the United States provide all necessary health services. It is imperative, however, that all known effective methods be applied where they are compatible with local conditions.

Pneumonia and Acute Respiratory Infections

Extent and Magnitude of the Problem

Respiratory infections are a serious, and often underestimated, public health problem worldwide, particularly in less developed countries where young children are the chief victims. Respiratory infections are caused by a variety of bacterial and viral infectious agents. Among the bacteria, *Hemophilus influenzae* type b (Hib) and *Streptococcus pneumoniae* or pneumococcus are the more important causes of severe, invasive disease. Among the viruses are rhinoviruses, coronaviruses, influenza, parainfluenza, respiratory syncytial virus, adenoviruses, and enteroviruses (Graham, 1990).

The influenza virus has an illustrious career in world history, having been responsible for pandemics. Morbidity from influenza by itself is not of public health concern—it is the pneumonia mortality among the elderly, chronically ill, and immunocompromised that is of concern. Of the three major types of influenza (A, B, and C), A is the most important epidemiologically. Influenza A has many subtypes based on surface antigens. Major genetic changes in subtype—antigenic *shifts*—have been responsible for new pandemics. Less dramatic variations within a subtype—*drifts*—are more frequent. Immunity acquired through natural infection or immunization with one strain may not protect against another strain of the same subtype (Thacker, 1986).

The traditional clinical classification of respiratory infections is based on anatomic site:

Upper: the common cold, acute otitis media, pharyngitis, tonsillitis, and sinusitis

Middle: croup, epiglottitis, laryngitis, and tracheitis

Lower: bronchiolitis, bronchitis, and pneumonia

Among Native Americans, the age-standardized mortality rate of pneumonia and influenza has been declining steadily. During 1970–75, the Native rate was 41/100,000, compared to a U.S. all-race rate of 19 (U.S. DHEW, 1978). The Native rate declined to 27/100,000 during 1980–82 (U.S. Congress, 1986) and further to 19/100,000 during 1985–87 (U.S. DHHS, 1990b), compared to a national rate of 13/100,000. The rates for Canadian Indians during 1979–83 and 1984–88 are given in Table 3.1. Among Canadian Indian infants in the postneonatal period, the SMR for acute bronchitis was 21.2 and pneumonia 12.1 (Morrison et al., 1986).

The age-specific mortality rate for pneumonia among Native Americans is shown in Figure 3.5.

In Alaska, the risk of Hib pneumonia, as for Hib meningitis, was very high among Eskimos and Indians compared to non-Natives in the same state (relative risk 11.6 for Eskimos and 5.6 for Indians). Epiglottitis due to Hib is extremely rare (Ward et al., 1986). This rarity has also been noted among the Navajo (Coulehan et al., 1984) and also Indians in Manitoba (Moffatt et al., 1991).

A study from the Yukon-Kuskokwim Delta in Alaska showed that the Native (predominantly Eskimo) incidence of pneumococcal pneumonia during 1980–86 was 65/100,000, with 42 percent of the cases occurring in children under the age of 2 (Davidson et al., 1989).

While bacteria such as *H. influenzae* and pneumococcus are common etiologic agents of pneumonia and other respiratory infections, epidemics of respiratory infections from viral causes have also been reported in Native communities, e.g., in Alaska (Maynard et al., 1967). A comparative seroepidemiologic study of several isolated populations in Alaska, Micronesia, and South Africa indicated that all showed high proportions of sera with antibodies against influenza A2 and B; parainfluenza 1, 2, and 3; reovirus 1, 2, and 3; and two M rhinoviruses, comparable to results observed in non-isolated populations (Brown and Taylor-Robinson, 1966).

A high proportion of Native infants can be expected to suffer from lower respiratory infections during the first two years of life. In Alaska more than one-third of infants were diagnosed with pneumonia or bronchitis during their first

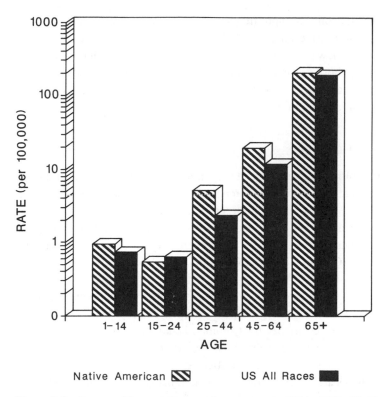

Figure 3.5. Age-specific mortality rate for pneumonia: USA, 1983–87, Native American and U.S. all-race populations.

year of life (Brody, 1965). Among the Navajo, the incidence of pneumonia was estimated to be about 20 bouts per 1000 person-years, with a case-fatality rate of 2 percent. The age distribution was U-shaped, with the highest incidence recorded among the under-fives (Oseasohn et al., 1978).

In rural southwestern Ontario, 46 percent of Indians and 18 percent of non-Indians experienced lower respiratory disease during their first year of life. Indian infants were also more likely to have multiple episodes of illness (Evers et al., 1985). The relative risk was 17.6 for office visits and 5.8 for hospital admissions during the first year (Evers and Rand, 1982). The high risk of hospital admission for lower respiratory infection continued during the second year of life (Evers and Rand, 1983). A study of hospitalization data of children under 5 years of age living in 17 Indian communities in British Columbia estimated rates at 81 and 136/1000 for upper and lower respiratory infections, respectively, 5 and 8 times the corresponding rates for non-Native children (Thomson and Philion, 1991).

Respiratory infections are more frequent among Native Americans, and clinical studies in Alaska (Fleshman et al., 1968), Alberta (Herbert et al., 1967, 1977), and Saskatchewan (Houston et al., 1979) have shown that such infections, particularly those associated with adenovirus, were more likely to be severe, recurrent, and associated with serious sequelae such as bronchiectasis in the Native population than in the general population.

Etiology and Risk Factors

A large number of risk factors for acute respiratory infections have been identified, including outdoor air pollution, smoking (both active and passive), crowding, poor nutrition, indoor air pollution (especially nitrogen dioxide from cooking and heating gas stoves), psychosocial stress, weather conditions, and low socioeconomic status. Few data exist for genetic factors, except for a family history of asthma (Graham, 1990), a factor that is not believed to be important among Native Americans.

Most respiratory viruses are associated with the winter season in the temperate zone. While there may be biological reasons such as virus survival and host defenses in the upper respiratory tract, human behavior associated with winter indoor living may also be responsible (Thacker, 1986).

Wood-burning stoves have been identified as a source of indoor pollutants. Because such stoves are the chief source of heat in many Native homes in remote and rural communities, their use may be a risk factor for the high prevalence of respiratory disease in children. One case-control study of Navajo and Hopi children with pneumonia or bronchiolitis showed that, on multivariate analysis, wood-burning stove use and recent exposure to respiratory illness in the home were independent risk factors (odds ratio of 4.9 and 4.2, respectively; Morris et al., 1990).

Among Greenland Eskimos, Bjerregaard (1983) used primary care contacts for respiratory infections as indicators and found elevated rates among those in poor housing and lowest social class.

According to the Pima Infant Feeding Study, breast-feeding is protective of respiratory infections. The odds ratio for upper respiratory infection and otitis media, comparing infants who were exclusively breast-fed for four months with those exclusively bottle-fed, was 0.64, adjusted for season, birthweight, and socioeconomic status. Little benefit could be demonstrated beyond nine months. For more serious conditions such as pneumonia, only a marginal reduction was associated with breast-feeding (Forman et al., 1984b).

Multiple food allergies (particularly to milk and dairy products) were found to be associated with recurrent pneumonia in a case series of Indian children in Saskatchewan (Upadhyay and Gerrard, 1969). However, population-based data are lacking on the extent to which allergies are responsible for the high risk of recurrent respiratory infections among Indians.

Prevention and Control Strategies

As described earlier, under the discussion of meningitis, the Hib vaccine has a role in the prevention of pneumonia caused by Hib. A polysaccharide vaccine for pneumococcal infections has been available since the late 1970s. The CDC's Immunization Practices Advisory Committee strongly recommended the widespread use of the vaccine among the elderly (CDC, MMWR, 1989;38:64–76). That committee included Native Americans as a high-risk group. Unfortunately, an effective vaccine against infections in children under 2 years of age is still needed. Formulations that are being developed include only the few serotypes that most frequently cause invasive disease in children. The wide geographical, temporal, and age-related variations in the distribution of pneumococcal serotypes emphasizes the importance of identifying species-wide antigens that are protective in all high-risk individuals (Broome and Breiman, 1991).

Vaccination against influenza A may offer protection against pneumonia secondary to the viral infection. An inactivated vaccine is available, although each season's vaccine is different depending on the prevalent strains. Alternatively, prophylaxis with anti-viral drugs (e.g., amantadine) can be offered to those at risk (CDC, MMWR, 1990;39:RR-7).

Viral Hepatitis

Extent and Magnitude of the Problem

The epidemiology of the viral hepatitides is a rapidly changing and expanding field. Whereas at one time only two types were recognized—*serum hepatitis* and *infectious hepatitis*—five distinct hepatitis viruses, named from A to E, have since been identified.

Hepatitis A outbreaks are common in Native American communities. The incidence rate in South Dakota reservations during 1980–85 was 212/100,000, 40 times that of whites in the same state and 23 times the U.S. national rate. Over 90 percent of affected patients were under 20 years of age, compared to 40 percent of whites (U.S. DHHS Indian Health Conditions, 1990). Various seroprevalence surveys of antibodies to hepatitis A virus (HAV) have been conducted in several Native communities across the continent: in Arctic Canada (Minuk et al., 1982a; Minuk et al., 1982b), Greenland (Skinhøj et al., 1977), Sioux reservations in South Dakota (Shaw et al., 1990), and a Navajo boarding school

(Williams, 1986). These surveys consistently showed extremely high prevalence (in the order of 70% and above), comparable to the situation in many developing countries. Seroconversion occurs at an early age, and by middle age, most if not all members of the community would be HAV-positive.

Hepatitis B has a causal association with hepatocellular cancer. Its prevalence has been extensively studied in various Inuit communities in the circumpolar region. Table 3.3 summarizes the prevalence of HBsAg (the surface antigen), anti-HBs (antibody against the surface antigen), and other serological markers of infection.

Although the prevalence of HBV infection among Inuit is generally high, there are important regional differences. The Greenland rate was the highest, suggestive of hyperendemicity (Skinhøj, 1977). The Canadian Inuit rates were lowest (Minuk et al., 1982b; Minuk et al., 1985; Larke et al., 1987; Baikie et al., 1989). HBV infection was uncommon before age 20 and increased in prevalence with age, reaching 80–90 percent in those over age 50. Within the Canadian Arctic,

Table 3.3 Regional Studies of Hepatitis B among Native Americans: Prevalence of Serological Markers

Region/ Population	Years	Reference	Sample Size	Prevalence (%)		
				HbsAg	anti-HBs	Any Markers
Greenland: 3 districts	1965–66	Skinhøj (1977)	1450	16.6	45.8	62.5
Alaska: 2 Eskimo villages	1973	Barrett et al. (1977)	418	13.9	—	54.8
Alaska: 12 Eskimo villages	1973–75	Schreeder et al. (1983)	3053	6.4	17.8	24.2
NWT Inuit village	1980	Minuk et al. (1982a)	720	4.0	23.0	27.0
NWT Inuit village	1982	Minuk et al. (1985)	172	2.3	20.0	22.0
NWT: all communities	1983–85	Larke et al. (1987)	Inuit: 8283	3.9	24.5	—
			Indians: 3140	2.9	21.5	—
			Others: 2776	0.3	8.5	—
Labrador	1986	Baikie et al. (1989)	Inuit: 766	6.9	—	26.4
			Indians: 516	0.4	—	7.6
			Others: 723	1.9	—	10.0

NWT = Northwest Territories.

the Baffin region reported the highest prevalence. In Alaska the prevalence was 18 percent even among children under the age of five, slowly increased with age, but did not exceed 45 percent among people over the age of 60 (Schreeder et al., 1983). The "e" antigen, which indicates recent infection, was present in 69 percent of those positive for HBsAg in Alaska (Schreeder et al., 1983), whereas in the Northwest Territories it was only 9 percent, clustered in a few communities with the highest HBV marker rates (Larke et al., 1987). The persistence rate (measured by the number of individuals positive for HBsAg divided by those positive for either HBsAg or anti-HBs) in the Northwest Territories was less than 15 percent (Minuk et al., 1982b; Larke et al., 1987), but in Alaska it was 30 percent (Schreeder et al., 1983).

Compared to Eskimos/Inuit, Indians have been much less studied. A low prevalence of HBV markers was reported from the Montagnais-Naskapi in Labrador (Baikie et al., 1989) and the Sioux in South Dakota (Shaw et al., 1990).

The possible adverse effects of an acute HBV infection are the chronic carrier state, chronic active hepatitis, cirrhosis, and hepatocellular cancer. A longitudinal study of over 1000 seronegative Alaskan Eskimos showed that the risk of becoming a carrier was inversely related to the age of the person at the time of infection (McMahon et al., 1985). The actual risk of developing primary liver cancer was about 2 percent among 150 HBsAg carriers followed for 8–10 years, a risk some 300 times that which could be expected from the U.S. population adjusted for age and sex (Alward et al., 1985). The Alaskan investigators have further reported on the outcome of 1,400 HBsAg carriers followed from 1983 to 1987: the incidence rate of hepatocellular cancer was 387/100,000/yr in males and 63/100,000/yr in females; the rate for chronic active hepatitis was 193 (M) and 107 (F); and for cirrhosis 158 (M) and 95 (F) (McMahon et al., 1990a).

Few data are available for the more recently identified viruses. The seroprevalence of *hepatitis C* (formerly "non-A, non-B, post-transfusion hepatitis") was found to be very low (0.3%) in one Inuit community in Canada (Minuk et al., 1991).

Etiology and Risk Factors

Hepatitis A virus may be spread through contaminated water supplies and foods, which are responsible for many common-source epidemics. Most infections, however, are acquired through sporadic or endemic transmission, primarily through person-to-person contact via the oral-fecal route. Poor hygiene, poor sanitation, and the opportunity for close contact (overcrowding or sexual) all contribute to its transmission (Lemon, 1985).

The risk factors for HBV are known for about 60–70 percent of cases in the United States. The most important ones include male homosexuality, parenteral drug abuse, and heterosexual contact. Less important are blood transfusions, health care employment, household contact, hemodialysis, and residence in mental institutions. Most occurrences in minority populations are without known risk factors (Alter et al., 1990).

A study in Alaska suggested that the size of the household was correlated with the prevalence of HBsAg (Barrett et al., 1977). The prevalence of HBV markers was also higher among Alaskan Native chronic alcoholics than among age-matched nonalcoholics (McMahon et al., 1990b).

Worldwide there are two basic patterns with regard to HBV marker prevalence: (1) In most developing countries, the pattern is one of high prevalence of markers (>50%) and high persistence of greater than 10 percent. The infection occurs mainly during childhood, primarily from maternal-infant transmission and secondary spread among children. The high chronic carrier rate has been shown to be responsible for the high rate of primary liver cancer. (2) In much of the developed world, the prevalence of HBV markers is low (<20%), as is its persistence rate (<10%). It is mainly an infection of adulthood, transmitted parenterally and sexually.

The Inuit pattern in Canada is interesting and suggests a shift from pattern (1) to pattern (2) and a dramatic decline in transmission over the past 2–3 decades. The usual risk factors for adult infection—drug addiction, homosexuality, use of scarification—are not known to be widespread.

The high seropositivity to HBsAg and HBeAg in Alaskan Eskimo children suggests that they have been recently infected with HBV and are probably mainly responsible for the transmission of the infection in the community. Unlike other hyperendemic populations in the developing countries, perinatal transmission does not appear to be the major route. A probable mechanism is suggested by a study that detected HBsAg in gingival swabs, saliva, and impetiginous lesions of Eskimo children, as well as surfaces frequently touched or objects placed in the mouth (Peterson et al., 1976).

Prevention and Control Strategies

As is the case with many other infectious diseases, viral hepatitis can be prevented through alteration of environmental and behavioral risk factors (e.g., water and sanitation, personal hygiene, crowding, sexual behavior, and drug use). Individuals can also be offered protection through active or passive immunization.

For *hepatitis A* the mainstay of prevention and control has been the use of immunoglobulins (IG). [IG was formerly called immune serum globulin (ISG) or gamma globulin.] Guidelines are available for prophylaxis both before exposure (directed mainly to travelers to endemic areas) and after exposure (used in epidemic control). Vaccines, both live attenuated and inactivated ones, have been developed. A single dose of an inactivated, purified vaccine derived from cell culture has been found to protect children 2–16 years of age. The goal of preventing the disease, however, will not be reached until affordable vaccines are licensed and childhood immunization programs launched (Bancroft, 1992).

For *hepatitis B* passive immunizations using immunoglobulins (HBIG), and since its licensure in 1981, active immunization with the inactivated vaccine, are both available. While IG contains both anti-HAV and anti-HBs, HBIG is the superior preparation for HBV infection since it contains a much higher titer of anti-HBs. HBV vaccine can be considered not only as a vaccine to prevent hepatitis B, but also as a vaccine to prevent liver cancer and the chronic liver diseases that are sequelae of the viral infection.

A statewide program of HBV vaccination was launched by IHS in Alaska in 1983 (McMahon et al., 1987), following a successful demonstration of safety, immunogenicity, and efficacy under field conditions in the Bethel area in 1981 (Heyward et al., 1985). The program has the following components:

1. Serological screening of the entire Native population
2. Vaccination of susceptible persons (i.e., those negative for anti-HBc) and all newborns
3. Screening of all pregnant Native women and administration of HBIG to babies born of HBsAg-positive mothers
4. Twice-yearly testing of all HBsAg carriers for alpha-fetoprotein as a marker of malignant change to hepatocellular carcinoma

A five-year follow-up of the Yupik vaccinees from the original field trial in Bethel showed that 81 percent maintained adequate anti-HBs levels. The incidence of new infections declined from a preprogram level of 50/1000/yr to 0.5/1000/yr (Wainwright et al., 1989). A progress report of the Alaska experience after seven years of follow-up showed that while the level of anti-HBs showed further decline, protection remained adequate (Wainwright et al., 1991).

In other Native populations of North America, vaccination has been directed only at specific groups, for example among the predominantly Inuit populations of the eastern Canadian Arctic and Greenland. In the general population of United States and Canada, there has been growing recognition of the inadequacy of the selective, high-risk approach and the need for universal childhood vaccination against HBV (Alter et al., 1990; CDC, MMWR 1991;40:RR-13).

Because *hepatitis C* is transmitted through blood transfusions, the systemic screening of blood products for antibodies (anti-HCV) is one way to eliminate its occurrence. *Hepatitis D* can be prevented through the use of HBV vaccine. No specific immunologic agent is available for *hepatitis E*. As these diseases are of little or unclear epidemiological significance in the Native American population, public health programs should be directed specifically at hepatitis A and B, for which effective strategies are now available.

Sexually Transmitted Diseases

The sexually transmitted diseases (STDs) are a group of etiologically and clinically diverse diseases that share in common transmission through sexual contact. Traditionally the STDs (or venereal diseases) consisted of syphilis, caused by the spirochete *Treponema pallidum,* and gonorrhea, caused by the gonococcus *Nesseria gonorrhea.* In more recent years, the spectrum of STDs has expanded to include *Chlamydia trachomatis, Trichomonas vaginalis,* herpes simplex, and human papillomavirus, among others. In the periodically updated treatment guidelines for STDs published by the CDC, at least twenty distinct organisms were listed (CDC, MMWR 1989;38:S-8). The latest to join the list was the acquired immunodeficiency syndrome (AIDS), caused by the human immunodeficiency virus (HIV). Despite their diversity, the STDs are closely related. The ulcerative diseases (syphilis, chancroid, and herpes) are associated with increased risk of acquiring the transmitting HIV. The diseases associated with discharges (gonorrhea, nonspecific urethritis, and trichomoniasis) have also been implicated in the transmission of HIV. The immunosuppression of HIV infection, on the other hand, alters the clinical manifestations and therapeutic responsiveness of the other STDs (Cates and Hinman, 1991).

Extent and Magnitude of the Problem

Syphilis is perhaps the oldest of the STDs among Native Americans. Medical historians and archaeologists have long debated whether syphilis was part of the "Columbian exchange," which introduced the disease from the Americas to Europe (Crosby, 1972). With the availability of effective antibiotic treatment, syphilis greatly declined in public health importance in North America. Nevertheless, since the mid-1980s there has been a resurgence of the disease, particularly in certain ethnic and socioeconomic subgroups in the United States, reflecting the same changes in social mores and sexual behaviors that have promoted the spread of HIV/AIDS. The U.S. all-race incidence of syphilis in 1989, at 18/100,000 was the highest since 1949 (Rolf and Nakashima, 1990). Of particular concern is the fact that syphilis, together with other STDs characterized by genital ulcers, appears to be a cofactor in the transmission of HIV. Among Native Americans, despite an occasional outbreak (Berber et al., 1989), the incidence of syphilis in the 1980s was about 2–3 times higher than the rate for whites and yet was considerably lower than the U.S. all-race rate. There also was decline from a peak of 21/100,000 to 5/100,000 by the end of the decade (Rolf and Nakashima, 1990). Compared to the period 1969–1976, when the mean annual incidence was 170/100,000 (U.S. DHEW, 1978a), the improvement has been remarkable.

Although nationally the Native American rate for syphilis was lower than the U.S. all-race rate, the situation was different in specific regions of the country. In a study of STDs in thirteen states with large Native American population, the syphilis incidence rates during 1984–88 were higher among Natives than non-Natives in all but two states (Oklahoma and North Carolina). In Arizona the rate was seven times that of non-Natives, and in New Mexico it was four times higher (Toomey et al., 1989). In Canada, data from Manitoba in the early 1980s indicated that Natives were affected three times more often than non-Natives (Lee et al., 1987).

In the United States, notification rates of *gonorrhea* continued to decline throughout the 1970s, and 1980s. Nationally the rate among Native Americans during 1984–88 was 316/100,000, lower than the all-races rate of 349/100,000. In thirteen states with a large Native population, however, the average rate was 500/100,000, compared to a non-Native rate of 248. Alaska Natives had the highest rate of 1470/100,000 (Toomey et al., 1989). In King County, Washington, gonorrhea surveillance indicated that, in terms of incidence, Native Americans occupied a position between that of blacks and Hispanics, but had higher rates than Asians and whites. This relative ranking remained even when categories of socioeconomic status were considered individually (Rice et al., 1991).

Other infectious agents that can be sexually transmitted account for an unknown proportion of all STDs, since reporting of these diseases in many jurisdictions has only been instituted recently or not at all. Many of these agents are ubiquitous in their distribution. Seroprevalence surveys of antibodies to chlamydia, cytomegalovirus, and herpes, for example, in the Canadian Inuit population, have shown higher levels than among non-Native residents in the same settlements (Nicolle et al., 1986). *Chlamydia* antibodies have been identified in 80 percent of Canadian Inuit in one community (Kordova et al., 1983). Serological testing of placental fluids suggested that the human placenta could be a reservoir of the infection (Wilt et al., 1976).

The incidence of chlamydia infection in the United States has now surpassed gonorrhea, and it is increasingly recognized that it is associated with serious consequences such as endometritis, pelvic inflammatory disease, infertility, and ectopic pregnancy (Cates and Wasserheit, 1991). Among prenatal Navajo women, one in four who were screened were infected with chlamydia (Harrison et al., 1983). Maternal infection resulted in pneumonia and conjunctivitis of the newborns, as well as increased risk of respiratory and gastrointestinal infections during infancy (Schaefer et al., 1985). In Kotzebue, Alaska, chlamydia organisms were identified in just under one-fourth of women who underwent gynecologic examinations for any reason. The presence of infection was poorly correlated with genital signs and symptoms or concurrent gonorrhea (Toomey et al., 1987).

Since its recognition as a clinical syndrome in 1981 and the subsequent delineation of its mode of transmission, the identification of the etiologic agent and the development of serologic tests, the global incidence of AIDS has shown no sign of abatement (Chin and Mann, 1990). While only a very small number of Native Americans have been afflicted, the virus has entered this population across the continent, from the deserts in the Southwest to the Canadian tundra. The potential of devastating epidemics exists, if the experience with other STDs is any guide. In Canada, of the 5,000 cases of AIDS reported up until 1991, fewer than thirty were in people of Native ethnic origin. In the United States of America, over 200 AIDS cases among Native Americans had been reported to the CDC by the end of 1990. The incidence rate for 1990 was 4/100,000, compared to 43/100,000 among blacks, 32/100,000 among Hispanics, and 12/100,000 among whites. While such data would suggest that the problem is least among Native Americans, they had nevertheless experienced the greatest increase between 1989 and 1990 (Metler et al., 1991).

The epidemiological patterns of AIDS cases also differ between ethnic groups in the United States. While among whites, the M:F ratio was 19:1, the Native ratio was only 5:1, comparable to the figure for blacks and Hispanics. In terms of risk categories, the Native pattern generally occupied an intermediate position between the patterns for blacks and whites. Thus over 50 percent of Native AIDS cases were homosexuals/bisexuals—lower than the proportion in whites but higher than in blacks or Hispanics. At the same time, heterosexual intravenous drug users comprised only 16 percent of Native cases, higher than the proportion in whites but considerably lower than in blacks or Hispanics (Metler et al., 1991).

Few populations in North America have undergone systematic screening for HIV infections. One such population was composed of civilian applicants to the U.S. military. Between 1985 and 1990 there were over 3 million applicants, of whom 20,000 were Native Americans. The seroprevalence among Natives was 0.8/1000, compared to 3.3/1000 for blacks, 1.8/1000 for Hispanics, and 0.5/1000 for whites (Metler et al., 1991).

Etiology and Risk Factors

Despite the many causative microorganisms and clinical syndromes, the STDs share common risk factors in terms of individual sexual behavior: early age of

onset of sexual activity, multiple partners, nonuse of protective barriers, trau-
matic sexual practices (particularly involving the anal mucosa), and concurrent
high-risk behaviors such as intravenous drug use and alcohol abuse. Sample
surveys that investigated knowledge, attitudes, and behaviors relating to sexual
practices and risk of STDs have been conducted in few Native American communities.

The Indian Adolescent Health Survey, which surveyed over 13,000 grade 7–
12 students in eight IHS Service Areas in 1987, found that 65 percent of boys
and 57 percent of girls had experienced sexual intercourse by grade 12. Among
the sexually active, the mean age of first sexual contact was 14.2 years in girls
and 13.6 years in boys. Among sexually active adolescents, 49 percent of boys
and 24 percent of girls used condoms (Blum et al., 1992).

A survey of 710 Native Americans from twelve centers in Oregon, Idaho, and
Washington revealed that 7 percent admitted to male homosexual activity or
intravenous drug use, while 30 percent had had two or more sexual partners in
the past year or had relations with a stranger. Between 80 percent and 95 percent
knew of AIDS as a viral disease and its transmission via sexual intercourse or
perinatally, while between 40 percent and 65 percent scored correctly in terms
of the low transmissibility of HIV through casual contact or food handling (Hall
et al., 1990). The pattern of response to the AIDS knowledge questions in this
Native American sample did not differ substantially from the 1988 National
Health Interview Survey.

Surveys among Greenland Eskimos have found a higher number of lifetime
sexual partners and earlier age of first intercourse compared to Danes (Kjaer et
al., 1989).

Prevention and Control Strategies

The traditional approach to STD control rests on the identification and treatment
of cases, contact tracing, and treatment of sexual partners. In terms of prevention, the strategies for all STDs are more or less the same—either abstinence or
careful selection of sexual partners, use of condoms, and periodic examination
for those at high risk. The ability of health professionals to modify behavior is
limited, and evidence demonstrating the effectiveness of patient education is
lacking (Horsburgh et al., 1987). Particularly recalcitrant are "repeaters" or
"core transmitters," who are usually of low education and socioeconomic status,
many of whom also engage in illicit drug use and prostitution.

The advent of AIDS has led to increased emphasis on community-based education aimed at changing sexual behavior and attitudes. Much controversy surrounds the need for and extent of serological screening; the "at risk" vs "population" approach to such screening; individual rights to privacy vs protecting

the public health; isolation, quarantine, and legal sanctions; needle-exchange programs for drug users; and "universal" precautions in handling body fluids. There are few diseases in the field of preventive medicine where so many complex ethical, legal, moral, political, and scientific issues are intertwined.

For Native Americans the control of STDs requires culturally sensitive and appropriate strategies that take into account social relationships, community dynamics, and unique features of the health care and social service systems. In their description of the syphilis epidemic, Gerber et al. (1989) noted that traditional contact-tracing methods had to be modified. Community health workers were used to determine social circles of the infected. Individuals who were identified as being at risk were given presumptive treatment prior to laboratory confirmation of seroconversion.

Native American health professionals have also developed special treatment and prevention manuals for use in their communities, an example of which is one on HIV prevention produced by the National Native American AIDS Prevention Center in California (Rush, 1992).

In Canada, despite the relatively small number of Native AIDS victims, the potentially explosive situation was recognized by both Native political and health care organizations and the federal government. A Joint National Committee on Aboriginal AIDS Education and Prevention was established in 1989. The committee includes all key "stakeholders," and it has embarked on a public education program across the country.

Streptococcal Infections and Their Sequelae

Extent and Magnitude of the Problem

Although diseases caused by Group A streptococci such as pharyngitis and impetigo are not important causes of mortality, they are responsible for potentially serious sequelae such as acute rheumatic fever (ARF) and acute glomerulonephritis (AGN). The virulence of Group A streptococci is determined by the M proteins on the cell wall and the hyaluronate capsule. Strains rich in M proteins and heavily encapsulated are readily transmitted from person to person and tend to cause severe infection. Eighty serotypes have been recognized, based on antigenic differences in the M protein molecule. ARF and AGN are caused by different serotypes, although the M1 serotype can cause both (Bisno, 1991).

The incidence of *acute rheumatic fever* has been declining in the developed countries since the 1920s, even before the advent of antibiotics. This decline was accelerated during the 1960s and 1970s. The disease, however, persists in low-income inner city neighborhoods and among certain minority populations such as Native Americans. A study among Indian and Inuit children in Manitoba and the Keewatin region of the Northwest Territories during the 1970s indicated that the Native incidence rate was 126/100,000, compared to 29/100,000 among non-Natives (Longstaffe et al., 1982).

While ARF has declined, there was no evidence that the prevalence of streptococcal infections themselves has changed, although strains known to be particularly virulent and rheumatogenic in the past might have declined. Interestingly the disease had an unexpected resurgence in the mid 1980s when several outbreaks of ARF occurred across the United States, usually in white, middle-class families (Bisno, 1991). Native Americans were not known to be involved in this new pattern.

The high risk of *acute glomerulonephritis* among Native children has also been documented in various Native American communities. In Minnesota, repeated outbreaks have occurred in the Red Lake Reservation, the name of which has become associated with a particular nephritogenic strain of streptococci (Perlman et al., 1965; Anthony et al., 1969). In this population, impetigo was a more common source of the original infection than pharyngitis was. In southwest Alaska an epidemic occurred among the Eskimos during 1975–77. Almost 70 percent of those affected had impetigo (Margolis et al., 1980).

A cohort of children on the Red Lake Reservation was followed for two years, and repeated throat and nose swabs were obtained for culture and blood samples for serotyping. Almost 90 percent of the cohort developed streptococcal impetigo during the study period, particularly during the summer and fall. Streptococci were recovered from the respiratory tract most frequently in the winter months. It was also possible to distinguish serotypes that are primarily respiratory and others that usually affect the skin (Anthony et al., 1976).

In Canada, a survey of schoolchildren in two communities—one Inuit and one Indian—determined the prevalence of pharyngeal carriage of group A streptococci on three separate occasions, which ranged from 5 percent to 34 percent among the Inuit and 5 percent to 10 percent among the Indians. Impetigo was clinically present in 1–4 percent of the children examined. Increased pharyngeal carriage correlated with larger size of the household and lower school grades. Seasonal variations in the incidence of pharyngitis and impetigo were apparent, with January the peak month for impetigo in both communities; for pharyngitis it was late winter in the Inuit and midsummer in the Indian community. Stereotyping showed consecutive outbreaks of different serotypes in the Inuit community but a persistent low level of endemic infection in the Indian community (Nicolle et al., 1990a).

Etiology and Risk Factors

It is generally believed that overcrowding, poor housing, poor personal hygiene, and low socioeconomic status contribute to the risk of ARF (Bisno, 1991). Studies on genetic markers have linked ARF to HLA class II antigens: DR4 among whites and DR2 among blacks (Ayoub et al., 1986). No data, however, are available for Native Americans.

The role of impetigo in the pathogenesis of AGN also underscores the importance of environmental conditions. Inadequate water supply for washing and laundry, poor personal hygiene, and inadequate sanitation promote secondary infection of bites and scabies.

In Alaska, streptococcal colonization was found to be associated with increasing age, past infection, and health care factors (Brant et al., 1982).

Prevention and Control Strategies

Streptococci remain very sensitive to penicillin, and prompt treatment of streptococcal infection is the main strategy for the prevention of ARF and its recurrence. Antibiotic treatment is not known to abort progression of streptococcal infection to acute glomerulonephritis. For people with a previous attack of ARF, prolonged, periodic penicillin prophylaxis is required.

Streptococcal control programs in various Native American communities, such as in Alaska (Brant et al., 1982) and the Navajo reservation (Coulehan et al., 1982) have consisted of screening with throat swabs in schools and penicillin treatment of people with positive cultures. A randomized controlled trial in one Inuit community and one northern Indian community in Canada showed that both oral penicillin and intramuscular benzathine penicillin were highly effective in eradicating streptococcal carriage (Nicolle et al., 1990b). An evaluation of the program in the Navajo reservation, however, showed that, in terms of cases of ARF prevented, costs far exceeded benefits (Coulehan et al., 1982).

Protozoan and Helminthic Parasites

Extent and Magnitude of the Problem

Among Native Americans, parasitic infections are very sensitive to both ecological factors and cultural practices. Various helminths and protozoa and their animal hosts and reservoirs are limited by such factors as climate, terrain, and the flora and fauna prevalent in an area. Exposure to such parasites, however, is determined by cultural traditions in food gathering and preparation methods, and the relationship to domesticated animals. While the physical environment does not change radically (except, for example, when large tracts of land are flooded by hydroelectric projects), cultural changes as a result of modernization can reduce or eliminate the risk of parasitic diseases.

Trichinosis is caused by ingesting meat infected with the larval cysts of the nematode (roundworm) *Trichinella spiralis.* The larvae hatch in the stomach and eventually reach the muscles and internal organs via the bloodstream. The incidence in the United States has declined substantially since the 1940s. Alaska has the highest incidence, but even there, the incidence decreased threefold between 1975–81 and 1982–86 (Bailey and Schantz, 1990). In Alaska, outbreaks traceable to walrus meat occurred among Eskimos in Barrow during the mid 1970s (Margolis et al., 1979). In Canada, sporadic cases have also been reported from Natives in northern Quebec and Labrador. Foxes and bears are also known reservoirs. A seroprevalence survey in northern Quebec found diagnostic titers in 9 percent of Inuit and 2 percent of Indians (Tanner et al., 1987).

Diphyllobothriasis, or infestation by the fish tapeworm (a cestode), was formerly very prevalent in the temperate regions around the world, but the problem has largely been controlled. It persists, however, in the Native populations in the Arctic and sub-Arctic. *Diphyllobothrium lata,* the predominant species in temperate and sub-Arctic zones, infects pike and perch primarily and is not found in the far north. *D. dendriticum* is found in the salmonids, fish such as salmon, Arctic char, trout, and whitefish (Curtis and Byland, 1991). In the 1950s diphyllobothriasis was widely distributed across northern Canada (Wolfgang, 1954). Older stool surveys in various parts of the Arctic during the 1950s and 1960s showed relatively high prevalence, as high as 80 percent in some localities (Arch, 1960; Rausch et al., 1967), but more recent surveys showed a much reduced prevalence (Freeman and Jamison, 1976; Watson et al., 1979; Sole and Croll, 1980; Brassard et al., 1985). Stool surveys among dogs in northern Quebec have also found *D. dendriticum.* While transmission from dog to man is not possible, the presence of the worm in dogs is indicative of the high level of availability of this parasite in the environment (Desrochers and Curtis, 1987).

Hydatid disease is caused by various species of the cestode *Echinococcus.* In North America, cystic disease of the lungs and liver is caused by *E. granulosus,* of which there are two biologically distinct forms: a northern form occurring in the Arctic and sub-Arctic which is propagated via a sylvatic (i.e., forest) cycle with the wolf as the final host and the deer and moose as intermediate hosts (Rausch, 1992). Domestic dogs become involved when viscera of infected animals killed by hunters are fed to them. In communities where dogs live in close proximity to human beings, poor domestic hygiene increases the likelihood of human infection. A large number of cases have been reported from northwestern Canada and Alaska, characterized by mild clinical illness (Meltzer et al., 1956;

Wilson et al., 1968). With the decline of the dogsled in transportation, this disease has declined substantially. A recent seroprevalence survey in northern Quebec found only 1 percent of Inuit and 3 percent of Indians to have diagnostic titers (Tanner et al., 1987). No evidence of *E. granulosus* was found in a stool survey of dogs, also in northern Quebec, although it still occurred in wolves and caribou in the region (Desrochers and Curtis, 1987).

A "European" form of *E. granulosus* is widely distributed around the world, including the western United States, where the sheep is the chief intermediate host. Navajo and Zuni Indians in New Mexico and Arizona accounted for over 10 percent of the cases reported in the United States between 1900 and 1974. This was a relatively new phenomenon as no cases were reported prior to 1965 (Pappaioanou et al., 1977).

Infection with the protozoans *Entameba histolytica* and *Giardia lamblia* can result in diarrheal diseases, which in the case of *amebiasis* can be severe and fatal. It is manifested clinically as amebic dysentery. During the 1960s, frequent outbreaks of amebiasis occurred in Native communities in northern Saskatchewan (Eaton, 1968). A stool survey in 1964 found that 70 percent of the people sampled had some intestinal protozoa, 31 percent had *E. histolytica,* and 12 percent had *G. lamblia* (Meerovitch and Eaton, 1965). Elsewhere in Canada, more recent surveys have indicated that the prevalence was much lower. In Labrador, *E. histolytica* and *G. lamblia* was found in less than 5 percent of Inuit and Indians. Non-pathogenic ameba such as *Entameba coli* and *E. hartmanni* were found in higher proportions (>10%) (Sole and Croll, 1980). In northern Ontario and northern Quebec, *E. histolytica* and *G. lamblia* were found in less than 10 percent of stool samples. The overall parasite loads were 44 percent and 29 percent, respectively, in the two regions (Watson et al., 1979; Brassard et al., 1985).

Etiology and Risk Factors

While the parasitoses are caused by different pathogenic organisms belonging to different, taxonomically divergent species, with different life cycles, animal hosts, and reservoirs, they share certain common risk factors related to the cultural practices of Native Americans.

The shared living quarters between man and dogs, whether in the Southwestern desert or the Arctic and Subarctic, promote the transmission of *Echinococcus.* In the Southwest home-butchering of sheep provided a link between dog and sheep (Schantz et al., 1977), while in northern Canada and Alaska the traditional Native pursuit of hunting provided dogs access to the viscera of infected ungulates.

In northern Quebec, the prevalence of parasites was highest in the 1–9-year age group, and the infected children serve as a reservoir for infecting others in the community. On multivariate analysis, age, crowding, and community of residence were independent predictors of parasite infection, while piped water and indoor flush toilets were not (Brassard et al., 1985).

Prevention and Control Strategies

Treatment of humans and animals, where treatment is effective and available, should interrupt the transmission and reduce the reservoir of the parasites. This is possible in the case of diphyllobothriasis in man and echinococcosis in dogs.

Health education on the importance of thorough cooking of fish and meat, particularly those obtained from the land, will help control diphyllobothriasis and trichinosis, respectively. Food hygiene practices, such as proper control and inspection of slaughtering of sheep, should also prevent the transmission of echinococcus from sheep to domestic dog.

Proper sewage disposal will disrupt the life cycle of *D. latum,* preventing feces with tapeworm eggs from reaching water courses where they hatch and infect the fish. For *D. dendriticum,* this may be difficult because it is spread by gulls, which will continue to contaminate the waterways regardless of what humans do. Improved sanitation and protection of water supply are also important in the prevention of amebiasis and giardiasis.

The diminution of risk of parasitic diseases among Native Americans is indicative of a general improvement in socioeconomic status, but also of the decline of traditional activities such as hunting and the use of the dog-team in the lifestyle of these people.

4

Emergence of Chronic Diseases (I)

Over the past several decades Native Americans have undergone the "epidemiologic transition," characterized by the decline, though not disappearance, of infectious diseases and the increasing importance of the chronic, noncommunicable diseases, accidents, and acts of violence as causes of mortality and morbidity. In Chapters 4 and 5, several chronic diseases of particular significance among Native Americans are discussed in terms of their frequency of occurrence, risk factors, and methods of control. Included are cancer, cardiovascular diseases (including ischemic heart disease, hypertension, dyslipidemia), obesity, diabetes, and gallbladder disease.

There is no generally agreed definition of "chronic" diseases, apart from the fact that they are of insidious onset, long duration, and not caused by microorganisms. It should be noted that some infectious diseases are also of insidious onset and long duration (e.g., tuberculosis). Some chronic diseases are of slow progression, but their clinical manifestations may be acute in onset, such as acute myocardial infarction. Furthermore, some cancers are now believed to be caused by viruses. Thus the division of diseases into "infectious" and "chronic" is arbitrary and is used for the sake of convenience.

The diseases chosen for review in this chapter and in Chapter 5 have in fact been called "diseases of modernization" or "Western diseases" [see, for example Trowell and Burkitt (1981)]. Their alleged ability to serve as "indicator" diseases makes them interesting subjects for study from a biocultural perspective. There is growing evidence that they share similar risk factors and that they are interrelated in their pathogenesis, which makes them particularly amenable to analysis. Therefore a host of other important chronic diseases have been excluded from discussion, including musculoskeletal (e.g., arthritis), neurological (e.g., dementia), respiratory (e.g., chronic obstructive lung disease), and psychiatric (e.g., schizophrenia) conditions.

Cancer

Extent and Magnitude of the Problem

Cancer is not a single disease but a group of diseases with different etiologies, clinical and pathological features, and affecting different body organs and tissues. Epidemiologists have traditionally found it convenient to study malignant neoplasms according to anatomic site (e.g., lung, cervix, breast, etc.), recognizing that within each site there may well be different histological types (e.g., squamous cell carcinoma, adenocarcinoma, etc.).

Because of the generally high lethality of cancers, mortality rates have often been used as a proxy measure of incidence. Figure 4.1 shows the trend in age-standardized mortality rate for all cancers among Native Americans compared to

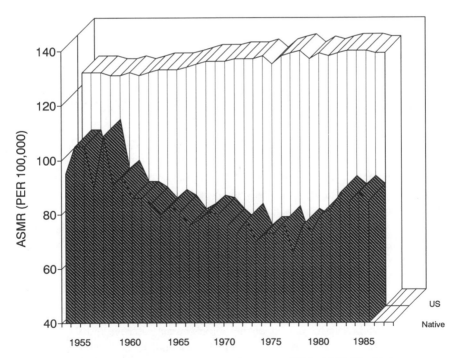

Figure 4.1. Age-standardized mortality rate for cancer: USA, 1955–87, Native American and U.S. all-race populations.

the U.S. all-race rate. It is evident that the Native American rate has been consistently below that of the U.S. national rate.

Incidence for a specific population is far more difficult to ascertain, and its estimation depends on the existence of cancer registries, which employ a variety of data sources, including physician notifications, hospital discharge abstracts, pathologists' reports, and health insurance claims. While all Canadian provinces and selected regions in the United States have had population-based cancer registries for some time, none exist for Native Americans specifically, although in some registries data on ethnic status are available. The U.S. Surveillance, Epidemiology and End Result (SEER) program, which covers five states and four metropolitan areas, is an important source of data on Native American cancer. The majority of Native American cases in SEER were from New Mexico and Arizona at 78%, with 12 percent from Seattle, and 10 percent from the other registries (Young et al., 1984). A word of caution, however, is warranted. A linkage study between the Portland Area Indian Health Service and the Puget Sound SEER indicated that racial misclassification of Native Americans may have contributed to the relative lower incidence of cancer among Native Americans (Frost et al., 1992).

A "national" picture of Native American cancer is difficult to obtain. An early attempt in Canada surveyed all Indian Health Service facilities during 1948–52 and found an overall lower risk of cancer, with the exception of cancer of the cervix, compared to Canadians (Warwick and Phillips, 1954). In the United States, Smith (1957) and Creagan and Fraumeni (1973) reviewed race-specific mortality data from national vital statistics during 1949–52 and 1950–67, respectively, and also reported lower overall risk of cancer among Native Americans. More recent national surveys have not been conducted.

There are, however, studies on the incidence of various cancer sites from several Native American populations. These are summarized in Table 4.1. Viewed together, these regional studies provide an overall view of the distribution of cancer in a variety of geographical and cultural settings. Mahoney and Michalek (1991) conducted a meta-analysis of seven published epidemiologic studies covering Native populations in four U.S. states and two Canadian provinces during various time periods from the mid-1950s to the early 1980s. An overall lower incidence was observed when all sites were combined. For men there was an increased risk for kidney cancer and reduced risks for cancer of the colon, lungs, and prostate, as well as the lymphomas and leukemias. Among women, an increased risk was observed for cancer of the gallbladder, cervix, and kidneys, whereas for cancer of the colon, breast, uterus, and the lymphomas, the risk was reduced. While such a technique has the advantage of increasing sample size and improving the power to detect significant trends, it tends to obscure regional and biocultural differences between various Native populations, which may themselves offer clues to etiology.

Geographical variation in overall cancer mortality is also evident from Canadian and U.S. IHS data (Fig. 4.2 A and B). The Eskimo/Inuit pattern has generally been different from that of Indians. Of particular interest is the extremely high risk of several cancers that are relatively rare in other populations: nasopharyngeal, salivary gland, and esophageal cancer. [The term "Eskimoma" has been coined for the type of salivary gland tumor commonly observed among the Eskimo/Inuit (Hildes and Schaefer 1984)]. For other cancers, there appear to be regional differences among the various circumpolar Eskimo/Inuit groups. The risk for primary hepatocellular cancer (PHC) is elevated in Alaska (Lanier et al., 1987) but not elsewhere in the Arctic, such as Greenland (Melbye et al., 1984b) and the Northwest Territories in Canada (Gaudette et al., 1991). In Alaska, PHC is primarily a disease of young men, and it affects the Yupik more than other Eskimos, and Eskimos more than Indians. In Alaska, gallbladder cancer rates are elevated in all Native groups—Athapaskan Indians, Indians belonging to the Northwest Coast culture area, Inupiat and Yupik Eskimos (Boss et al., 1982). However, gallbladder cancer is not a high risk cancer among Eskimos in Greenland or the Northwest Territories.

Cancer is generally not a significant health problem in childhood. In a study of childhood cancers in New Mexico during 1970–82, Native American children had lower risk of cancer overall, particularly the leukemias and lymphomas, the central nervous system, and the kidneys. The risks, however, were higher for retinoblastoma, cancer of the bones, and genital tumors (Duncan et al., 1986).

Mortality is a function of incidence and survival. Limited available data, especially from the SEER program in New Mexico, indicate that Native Americans generally have poorer survival than white Americans in most cancer sites (Young et al., 1984). The 5-year relative survival rates for several cancer sites are presented in Figure 4.3. This is an actuarially generated ratio of the observed proportion of cancer patients who survive past 5 years to the expected survival rate of persons in the general (i.e., non-cancer) population of the same race, sex, and year of age. In Saskatchewan, an overall lower survival among Indians compared to the province as a whole was also observed. Survival was better among women than men, but decreased with age (Gillis et al., 1991).

In a study of Native American cases from New Mexico and Arizona during 1969–1982, Samet and others (1987) found that compared to whites, Native American cancer patients were more likely to have advanced disease (e.g., with remote metastases) and less likely to have received treatment, although this observation was not consistent across all sites. The hazard ratios (i.e., risk of not surviving), adjusted for stage of disease, treatment, age, and sex,

Table **4.1** Regional Studies of Cancer Mortality (MO) and Incidence (IN) among Native Americans

Region/ Population[a]	Years	Authors		Relative Risk[b]															
				All	SAL	NAS	ESO	STO	COL	REC	LIV	GBD	PAN	LUN	PRO	KID	BLA	LYM	LEU
MEN																			
A. Indians in U.S.																			
All U.S.	1949–52	Smith (1957)	MO	0.5*			0.1*	1.0	0.4*	0.3*		0.8+	0.7*	0.3*	0.5*		0.4‡*	0.2*	0.5*
All U.S.	1950–67	Creagan/ Fraumeni (1973)	MO	0.6*			0.5*	1.0	0.4*	0.4*	0.9	3.0*	0.7*	0.3*	0.6*	1.0	0.3*	0.5*	0.5*
NM	1969–72	Thomas (1979)	IN	0.4	—	3.2	0.7	1.4	0.1	0.6	—	1.9	0.3	0.3	0.3	1.6	0.4	0.8	0.8
NM	1973–77	Key (1981)c	MO	0.6	—	—	1.1	0.9	0.4	0.3	1.1	3.8	0.3	0.2	0.8	1.2	—	0.7	0.5
			IN	0.6	—	—	0.7	1.9	0.3	0.4	1.0	3.3	0.6	0.2	0.7	0.8	0.2	0.3	0.4
NM: Zuni	1969–82	Sorem (1985)	IN	0.5*				4.6*	—		3.7	14		0.1*	0.9	1.1			
NY: Seneca	1955–84	Mahoney et al. (1989b,c)	MO	0.8*				0.7	1.0	2.1	1.0		1.1	0.6	0.9	0.5	0.6	0.8	0.3
			IN	0.6*				0.4	0.6	1.1	2.7	1.1	1.3	0.5*	0.6	1.6	0.1*	0.3	0.5
AK	1969–73	Lanier et al. (1980b)	IN	0.9	—	—	1.0	0.4	1.6	1.7	—	—	0.8	0.5	1.0	2.5	0.2	0.5	0.9
	1974–78	Lanier et al. (1982)	IN	1.0	—	9.1*	0.9	0.6	1.6	1.3	2.7	1.6	0.4	1.2	0.8	1.2	—	0.3	0.3
	1969–83	Lanier et al. (1989)	IN	0.9	1.1	9.8*	1.4	1.1	1.1	1.3	2.0	2.2	0.7	0.8	0.9	1.3	0.2*	0.5	0.8
WA	1974–83	Norsted/White (1989)	IN	0.4*				0.5	0.5*				0.4	0.4*	0.2*	0.9	0.3*	0.5	0.9

B. Indians in Canada

BC	Gallagher/ Elwood (1979)	1964–73	MO	0.5*	—	—	—	0.5*	0.5*	0.8	—	0.9	0.5	0.3*	0.5*		0.6	0.7	0.3
ON: Cree, Ojibwa	Young/Frank (1983)	1972–81	MO	0.7*					0.3			5.9	0.5	0.3*	0.9	6.9*			
			IN	0.5*					0.6			5.4		0.3*	0.7	7.1*	—		
MB	Young/Choi (1985)	1970–79	IN	0.4*				0.4*	0.2*	0.5		0.7	0.1*	0.3*	0.7*	1.2	0.3*	0.3*	0.3*
SK	Gillis et al. (1991)	1967–86	MO																
			IN																

C. Eskimos/Inuit

AK	Lanier et al. (1980b)	1969–73	IN	0.8*	2.9	18*	2.5	1.7	0.8	1.1	6.2*	5.0	1.0	0.8	0.3	0.7	0.5	0.4	0.3*
	Lanier et al. (1982)	1974–78	IN	0.8	—	29*	1.7	2.1*	0.9		5.2*	1.5	1.0	0.8	0.1*	1.5	0.3*	0.3*	0.3*
	Lanier et al. (1989)	1969–83	IN	0.9*	2.2	20*	2.0*	2.6*	0.9	0.9	8.5*	1.5	1.2	0.8	0.3*	1.5	0.3*	0.6*	0.3*
NT, QC, Labrador	Gaudette et al. (1991)	1970–84	IN	1.2	9.2*	22*	3.1*	1.5		0.9	0.7	2.0	0.8	2.4*	0.1*	1.4	0.1*	0.7	1.2
Greenland	Nielsen (1986)	1950–74	IN	0.8*	9.0*	25*	5.4*	1.0	0.8		1.7	1.9	0.6	0.8	0.1*	0.9	0.3*	0.4*	0.7
	Prener et al. (1991)	1973–85	IN	0.7*	8.0*	27*	5.8*	0.5	0.7	0.4*	1.1	2.0	0.9	1.2*	0.1*	0.6	0.2	0.4*	0.2*
	Prener et al. (1991)	1958–85	IN	0.8*	8.3*	24*	6.0*	0.9	0.8	0.6*	1.5	2.1	0.7	1.1	0.1*	0.7	0.3*	0.4*	0.3*

continued

Table 4.1 Regional Studies of Cancer Mortality (MO) and Incidence (IN) among Native Americans (continued)

Region/Population[a]	Years	Authors		Relative Risk[b]																		
				All	SAL	NAS	ESO	STO	COL	REC	LIV	GBD	PAN	LUN	BRE	CEX	UTE	OVA	KID	BLA	LYM	LEU
WOMEN																						
A. Indians in U.S.																						
All U.S.	1949–52	Smith (1957)	MO	0.8*	—	—	1.2	0.7*	0.4*	0.4*	—	1.6*†	1.3	0.9	0.3*	1.9*	—	0.5*	—	0.8‡	0.3	0.6*
All U.S.	1950–67	Creagan/Fraumeni (1973)	MO	0.9*	—	—	0.6	1.3*	0.5*	0.5*	1.8*	3.8*	1.2*	0.7*	0.5*	2.5*	0.9	0.6*	1.0	0.6*	0.5*	0.6*
NM	1969–72	Thomas (1979)	IN	0.6	—	—	—	1.8	0.5	0.7	—	4.1	0.4	0.1	0.3	2.3	0.2	0.2	1.0	0.7	—	1.8
NM	1973–77	Key (1981)[c]	MO	0.8	—	—	—	0.6	0.2	1.2	1.1	3.3	1.4	0.1	0.5	1.3	—	0.5	2.6	—	0.6	0.9
			IN	0.7	—	—	—	1.7	0.4	0.8	1.5	4.7	1.3	0.2	0.3	1.2	0.2	0.9	1.3	—	0.4	0.9
NM: Zuni	1969–82	Sorem (1985)	IN	0.5*					—			19*			0.2*	0.8	0.4*	0.9				
NY: Seneca	1955–84	Mahoney et al. (1989b,c)	MO	0.7*	—	—		1.5	0.5	0.7	0.9		—	1.6	0.4*	2.7*	0.5	0.4	—	—	0.3	1.0
			IN	0.5*	—	—		0.8	0.4	0.6		0.6	—	1.2	0.3*	1.4	0.7	0.3	1.0	—		0.8
AK	1969–73	Lanier et al. (1980)	IN	0.9	0.5	20*	—	4.2*	1.1	1.9	3.3	7.5*	0.8	1.0	0.5*	0.5	0.2	—	4.4*	0.8	0.4	0.5
	1974–78	Lanier et al. (1982)	IN	0.9	7.1	14		0.8	0.7			5.2*	0.7	0.9	1.0	1.5	0.2*	0.3	—		0.4	0.5
	1969–83	Lanier et al. (1989)	IN	0.9	5.1*	14*	0.8	1.9	1.0	1.4	1.0	4.3*	0.5	0.8	0.7*	2.5*	0.2*	0.9	1.7	0.2	0.6	0.4
WA	1974–83	Norsted/White (1989)	IN	0.6*				1.5	0.8				0.7	0.3*	0.5*	1.6*	0.2*	0.3*	0.7	0.2	0.1*	1.1
B. Indians in Canada																						
BC	1964–73	Gallagher/Elwood (1979)	MO	1.0	—	—	—	1.6	0.5	0.8	1.6	5.3*	0.6	0.7	0.7	4.5*	0.6	0.5*	—	—	—	0.5

Region	Period	Reference	Group	Relative risk by cancer site
ON: Cree, Ojibwa	1972–81	Young/Frank (1983)	MO	1.4 · 1.7 · 6.8* · 1.6 · 0.9 · 0.8 · — · 1.3 · 13* · 0.9
			IN	0.8 · 0.9 · 9.0* · 3.0 · 0.8 · 0.3* · 0.7 · 0.8 · 7.7* · 0.1* · 0.3
MB	1970–79	Young/Choi (1985)	IN	0.5* · 0.4* · 0.6 · 3.1* · 1.1 · 0.7 · 0.4* · 0.5 · 0.1* · 2.9* · 0.3 · 0.1* · 0.9
SK	1967–86	Gillis et al. (1991)		0.6 · —

C. Eskimos/Inuit

Region	Period	Reference	Group	Relative risk by cancer site
AK	1969–73	Lanier et al. (1980b)	IN	0.8* · 8.0* · 10 · 2.0 · 0.4 · 1.4 · 1.4 · — · 10* · 1.4 · 0.6 · 0.4* · 0.7 · — · 1.0 · 2.0 · 0.4 · — · 0.2
	1974–78	Lanier et al. (1982)	IN	1.1 · 1.7 · 38* · 5.1* · 1.1 · 1.7* · 4.4 · 4.8* · 2.0 · 1.4 · 0.4* · 1.6 · 0.8 · 3.4* · 0.4 · 0.2 · 0.6
	1969–83	Lanier et al. (1989)	IN	0.9 · 4.4* · 23* · 3.5* · 1.2 · 1.7* · 1.0 · 2.9 · 4.8* · 1.1 · 1.4 · 0.4* · 1.6 · 0.1* · 0.4 · 3.4* · 0.3* · 0.2* · 0.4
NT, QC, Labrador	1970–84	Gaudette et al. (1991)	IN	1.3 · 21 · 27* · 5.6* · 0.8 · 0.9 · 1.8 · 2.7 · 4.8* · 2.0 · 6.4* · 0.2* · 3.0* · 0.1* · 0.4 · 1.8 · 0.3 · 1.8 · 0.3
Greenland	1950–74	Nielsen (1986)	IN	0.9* · 11* · 23* · 8.2* · 0.9 · 0.7 · 0.6 · 2.3* · 1.2 · 0.9 · 1.2 · 0.5* · 1.3* · 0.2* · 0.2* · 1.1 · 0.4 · 0.4 · 0.6
	1973–85	Prener et al. (1991)	IN	0.9 · 11* · 48* · 9.5* · 1.1 · 0.8 · 0.5 · 0.8 · 1.0 · 1.1 · 1.7* · 0.5* · 3.2* · 0.2 · 0.8 · 1.2 · 0.5 · 0.5 · 0.5
	1958–85	Prener et al. (1991)	IN	1.0 · 13* · 35* · 9.4* · 1.1 · 0.8 · 0.6 · 1.6 · 1.1 · 1.1 · 1.6* · 0.5* · 2.2* · 0.3* · 0.8 · 1.1 · 0.6 · 0.3* · 0.7

a States/Provinces/Territories: *Canada*—BC, British Columbia; MB, Manitoba; NT, Northwest Territories; ON, Ontario; QC, Quebec; SK, Saskatchewan. *USA:* AK, Alaska; NM, New Mexico; NY, New York; WA, Washington.

b Relative risk based on SMR, SIR, or ratio of ASMR, ASIR comparison groups may be white/all-race in same region or nationally. *Abbreviations of cancer sites:* BLA, bladder; BRE, breast; CEX, cervix uteri; COL, colon; ESO, esophagus; GBD, gallbladder; KID, kidney; LEU, leukemias; LIV, liver; LUN, lung; LYM, lymphomas; NAS, nasopharynx; OVA, ovary; PAN, pancreas; PRO, prostate; REC, rectum; SAL, salivary glands; STO, stomach; UTE, corpus uteri.

"All" refers to all cancer sites excluding non-melanoma skin cancers.

Blank space indicates data not reported; dash indicates zero cases.

*p <0.05, significantly different from unity; †combined LIV/GBD; ‡combined KID/BLA.

c significance tests not provided in original publication

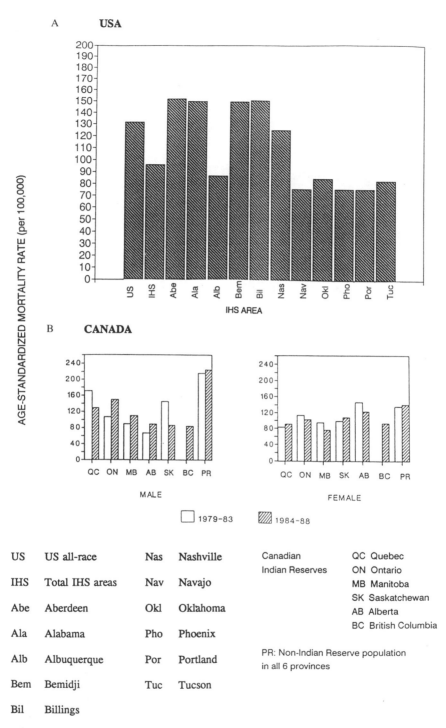

Figure 4.2. Regional variation in age-standardized mortality rate for cancer among Native Americans: (*A*) USA, 1980–87; (*B*) Canada, 1979–88.

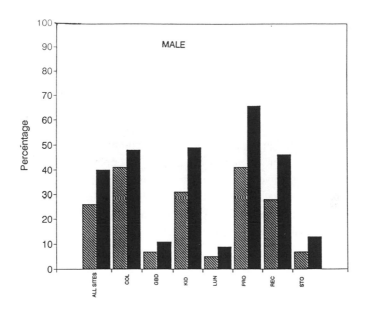

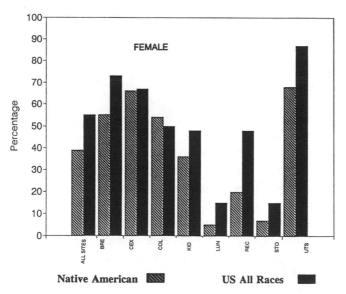

Native American ▨   **US All Races** ■

BRE Breast	**CEX** Cervix	**COL** Colon	**GBD** Gallbladder	**KID** Kidney
LUN Lung	**PRO** Prostate	**REC** Rectum	**STO** Stomach	**UTS** Uterus

Figure 4.3. Relative five-year survival rate of cancer: SEER registries, 1973–79, Native Americans and whites.

were significantly elevated for breast, cervix, lung, rectum, bladder, and non-Hodgkin's lymphoma among Native Americans (Samet et al., 1987).

Time trend data for Native Americans are available for only a few groups, particularly the Eskimo/Inuit in the Arctic regions. The small population sizes and rarity of the disease required the combination of multiple years of data to "smooth" the highly unstable rates. For many populations studied, even 5-year averages remain highly unstable.

An overall increase in cancer from all sites combined was observed among Alaskan Eskimo women between 1969 and 1983 (Lanier et al., 1989), Inuit of both sexes in the Northwest Territories between 1970 and 1984 (Gaudette et al., 1991), Indians in Saskatchewan between 1967 and 1986 (Gillis et al., 1991), and Greenlanders between 1953 and 1985 (Prener et al., 1991). Cohort analysis of Greenlanders also revealed increased cancer risk in the more recent birth cohort (Prener et al., 1991).

Much of the increase in cancer incidence among these groups is accounted for by lung cancer, particularly among women. Since the early 1970s the lung cancer incidence has increased at least twofold in these populations. In Greenland, the rate has increased at least tenfold compared to the 1950s. Schaefer noted a change in the relative proportions of the "traditional" (salivary, nasopharyngeal, esophageal) and "modern" (lung, cervix, colon, and breast) cancers between 1950–66 and 1974–80 in the central and western Canadian Arctic (Schaefer et al., 1975; Hildes and Schaefer, 1984). It should be emphasized that the risks for these traditional cancers are still very high relative to other populations in the world.

While the incidence and mortality of cancer of the cervix has been steadily declining for Canadians since 1970, the opposite trend is observed among some groups of Native women. In Saskatchewan, the ASMR among Indians rose by 52 percent between the two periods 1967–71 and 1982–86, while in the province overall there had been a 43 percent decline. The relative risk increased from 2.3 in the first period to 6.2 in the second period (Irvine et al., 1991).

Among Alaska Natives, the SIR for cervical cancer during the period 1969–83 was 2.5 for Indians and 2.1 for Eskimos (Lanier et al., 1989). However, during the earlier period from 1969–73 the SIR was only 0.5 for Indians and 0.7 for Eskimos (Lanier et al., 1980b). These had risen to 1.5 (Indians) and 1.6 (Eskimos) by 1974–78 (Lanier, Bender et al., 1982).

Greenlanders have one of the world's highest incidence of cervical cancer, with an ASIR of 64/100,000, about 4 times the rate in Denmark (Kjaer et al., 1988). The incidence has not declined, despite an improving Pap smear coverage from only 20 percent during 1976–78 to 33 percent during 1983–85 (Nielsen et al., 1988).

Etiology and Risk Factors

Despite the large number of cancers, the recognized "causes" of cancer are limited. In descending order of importance, they are tobacco, dietary factors, infectious agents, reproductive and sexual factors, occupation, alcohol, geophysical factors, pollution, medicines, and medical procedures (Doll and Peto, 1981). Some individuals, however, may also be genetically predisposed to developing certain types of cancers.

Familial aggregation of some rare cancers has been observed in Native Americans, such as hereditary nonpolyposis colorectal cancer in a Navajo family (Lynch ct al., 1985). In Alaska, not only is there family clustering of nasopharyngeal cancer, but siblings of these patients also had a higher risk of other types of cancers (Ireland et al., 1988). Investigations into HLA markers and nasopharyngeal cancer failed to demonstrate an association (Lanier et al., 1980a).

The genetics of cancer is a rapidly developing field, with the advances in DNA technologies. Current models of tumorigenesis encompass a series of genetic alterations involving oncogenes and tumor suppressor genes located on different chromosomes (Bishop, 1991).

Migrant studies (such as those involving the Japanese in Japan, Hawaii, and California) have provided useful clues to the etiology of some cancers. Conceptually such studies kept genetics "constant" while observing environmental changes. The migration of Greenlanders to Denmark in search of employment provides an opportunity to study the overall impact of rapid social and cultural change on disease patterns. Among first-generation migrants, their risk of cancer (as determined by proportionate mortality ratio) in Denmark was generally not different from that of Native Greenlanders who stayed behind, with the exception of rectal cancer, which became elevated (Prener et al., 1987). Few other Native American populations have been available for observation from the perspective of cancer incidence. The direction of research has thus mostly been on seeking explanations for temporal changes in cancer rates within the same locality.

The etiologic role of tobacco smoking in lung cancer has been firmly established, and the pursuit of this link has in fact been the main driving force in the advance of epidemiology as a discipline in the post-World War II decades. It has been estimated that 30 percent of the cancer deaths in the United States can be attributed to tobacco (Doll and Peto, 1981). Tobacco can also interact and potentiate other risk factors, for example, with asbestos and ionizing radiation in lung cancer, and with alcohol in various head and neck cancers (Saracci, 1987). The high prevalence of smoking among Native Americans has been documented in Chapter Two. Greenland offers an extreme example of the tobacco "epidemic:" the annual per capita consumption increased from about two cigarettes in 1950 to about thirteen cigarettes in 1987. This closely paralleled the dramatic increase in lung cancer rate in that population (Prener et al., 1991).

The current state of knowledge on the role of dietary factors (both causative and protective) is limited and often inconsistent [see the review by Freudenheim and Graham (1989)], although it has been estimated that as much as 35 percent of U.S. cancer deaths can be attributed to diet (Doll and Peto, 1981). Dietary fat is implicated in colorectal and breast cancer, and alcohol in cancers of the upper gastrointestinal tract (oral, pharyngeal, and esophageal) and of the breast. Potential protective factors include fiber (colon and rectum) and vitamin A or its carotenoid precursors (lung, and perhaps other epithelial tissues). Other factors, while not considered nutrients, are nonetheless related to the processing, storage, and preparation of food—examples include microbial contaminants and food additives.

"Ethnospecific" dietary factors have been sought in some cancers prevalent among Native Americans. The Inuit diet contains large amounts of nitrosable compounds, suspected carcinogens in such cancers as NPC. Whale meat is rich in secondary amines, and fish and meat kept fermenting in the ground and eaten as a delicacy may also produce N-nitroso compounds. An analysis of salivary nitrite and urinary N-nitrosoproline levels in four Inuit settlements in the Northwest Territories revealed low levels (Stich and Hornby, 1985). Analyses of fish and meat samples in Greenland also revealed generally very low levels of nitroso-di-methylamine (NDMA), with the exception of dried cod, a local staple (Poirier et al., 1987).

Of the risk factors for cervical cancer, the most important are those relating to sexual behavior, although other factors such as smoking, oral contraceptives, and diet may also be involved. Many of these factors are highly intercorrelated. More recent, multi-center case-control and cohort studies indicated that the number of sexual partners, age at first intercourse, number of pregnancies, and the number of sexual partners of the husbands were independent risk factors [reviewed by Franco (1991)]. Findings relating to "male factors" are particularly interesting since they seem to support the hypothesis that cervical cancer involves an infectious agent that is sexually transmitted.

The search for an infectious agent responsible for cervical cancer has led to a variety of candidates, such as herpes simplex virus (HSV), chlamydia, and Epstein-Barr virus (EBV). However, the sum of current epidemiologic, clinical, and laboratory evidence points to the human papillomavirus (HPV) as the prime causal agent (Reeves et al., 1989).

Despite the identification of a causal agent, cervical cancer is still a multifactorial disease since HPV is neither necessary nor sufficient for causation. There could be "fixed" cofactors that were present at the time of HPV infection, such as genetic susceptibility, diet, and sociodemographic factors. There could also be "variable" cofactors that were introduced after infection, including pregnancy, hormones, smoking, other STDs, and diet (Reeves et al., 1989).

Zur Hausen postulated that HPV was responsible for the induction of premalignant lesions. The failure of an intracellular surveillance mechanism against deleterious viral genomes that persisted from an early age in proliferating cervical cells led to carcinoma in some individuals years after initial infection. As HPV is ubiquitous, there must be cofactors that modify controlling host cell genes. It is the variation in the distribution of these cofactors rather than of HPV infection itself that likely determined geographic variation in cancer rates (zur Hausen, 1989).

Data on the prevalence of cervical cancer risk factors and HPV infection in Native populations of North America are limited. Some data on Greenlandic Eskimos (Kjaer et al., 1988) and Indians in New Mexico are available (Becker et al., 1991), and both suggested that the prevalence of HPV infection was lower than among non-Natives, despite their higher risk for cervical cancer.

What was unusual about Greenland was that the prevalence of HPV in this high cancer incidence population was low, whereas HSV infection and other risk factors such as sexual activity and smoking were very high. The prevalence odds ratio (Greenland/Denmark) for age at first intercourse under age 13 was 3.2, and for number of sexual partners > 20 it was 23.9 (Kjaer et al., 1989). Furthermore, in cross-sectional analysis, HPV infection was negatively associated with sexual activity indicators. The association of these factors with HSV infection, on the other hand, was positive and significant. There was no interaction with locality. The authors hypothesized that repeated HPV infections in highly sexually active individuals may have stimulated the immune response that results in suppression of HPV infection or even prevents further infections (Kjaer et al., 1990).

The link between hepatitis B virus (HBV) and primary hepatocellular cancer (PHC) is well established in various high-risk populations in the world. The high prevalence of HBV infection in circumpolar Eskimo/Inuit populations was discussed in Chapter 3. The actual risk of developing PHC among HBsAg carriers was 2 percent over 8–10 years among Alaskan Eskimos, a risk 300 times the expected rate in the U.S. population adjusted for age and sex (Alward et al., 1985). As indicated earlier, the risk of PHC is not uniform across all high HBV prevalence areas in the Arctic, and other factors, both promoting and preventive, may be involved. However, studies in Alaska indicated that the high risk of PHC was not due to confounding by cirrhosis of the liver, and analysis of moldy foods from high-risk families and villages failed to demonstrate the presence of aflatoxins or the fungus *Aspergillus flavus* (Lanier et al., 1987). Thus, at least among Alaskan Eskimos, HBV infection remains the only recognized risk factor.

Nasopharyngeal and salivary cancer have been linked with the Epstein-Barr virus (EBV). Serological studies in both Alaska and Greenland among Native cancer patients have shown abnormally high titers, and virus-specific DNA has been demonstrated in biopsy specimens (Lanier et al., 1981; Krishnamurthy et al., 1987; Saemundsen et al., 1982). Eskimo children from Greenland, compared to Danes, became seropositive for EBV at an early age and also showed significantly higher titers (Melbye et al., 1984a). It should be noted that EBV infection is ubiquitous and that only a small percentage of those infected in early childhood ever develop the cancer. The long latency of several decades and the low incidence of cancer suggest that EBV infection alone is not a sufficient cause of the cancer. Other risk factors may be involved, as suggested in a case-control study from Alaska, which implicated salted fish in the diet, smoking, and occupational exposure to noxious inhalants (Lanier et al., 1980a). In Greenland, high levels of the volatile nitrosamine NDMA were found in dried cod, which may act synergistically with EBV or may reactivate it to induce NPC (Poirier et al., 1987).

Although smoking is by far the most important cause of lung cancer, because of unique cultural conditions, some Native Americans are exposed to other carcinogens. Among the Navajo, the prevalence of smoking has traditionally been low, whereas a large proportion of men have been engaged in uranium mining, which has been shown to be a strong risk factor for lung cancer in this population (Samet et al., 1984). Among the Inuit, prior to the 1960s lung cancer had been primarily a disease of elderly women. This observation led to the hypothesis that exposure to the fumes and smudge containing hydrocarbons and other volatile substances while tending open-flame lamps burning seal or fish oil—a virtually round-the-clock task undertaken by women—could have been responsible (Hildes and Schaefer, 1984). There is some paleopathological evidence to support this as black pigmentation (anthracosis) has been found in the lungs of female Eskimo mummies from several centuries ago in Alaska and Greenland, far before the advent of tobacco and pollution (Zimmerman and Aufderheiden, 1984; Hansen et al., 1985).

Gallstones and gallbladder cancer tend to co-occur, and they may in fact be etiologically linked. In a study among Native Americans in the Southwest, gallstones were present in 93 percent of gallbladder cancer cases (Black et al., 1977). Among Native American patients in Arizona who underwent cholecystectomy for both benign and malignant conditions, the prevalence odds ratio for cancer was 7.4, comparing patients with large stones of 3 cm or greater diameter with those who had only small stones of less than 1 cm (Lowenfels et al., 1989). A fuller discussion of the risk factors for gallbladder disease can be found in Chapter 5. The constellation of diseases including diabetes, obesity, gallstones, and gallbladder cancer has been termed the "New World syndrome," an excessive genetic susceptibility for which is regarded as common to most Native Americans (Weiss et al., 1984b).

Few data are available for the carcinogenic role of environmental contaminants among Native Americans. Presumably Native Americans residing in particular localities would be exposed to the same occupational and environmental risk factors as other ethnic groups in the same area. No data exist to suggest that, given the same exposure, Native Americans are more likely to develop cancer than others. Exposures, however, do differ in areas where, for historical reasons, Native Americans are overrepresented in specific occupations. Apart from uranium mining among the Navajo mentioned earlier (Samet et al., 1984), there are examples of other culturally unique occupational exposures. A cluster of malignant mesothelioma in a Native pueblo in New Mexico during the mid-1980s was traced to exposure to asbestos during the manufacture of silver jewelry and the whitening of leather leggings and moccasins used in ceremonial dances. Asbestos was apparently salvaged by tribal members from insulation along an abandoned railroad and pilfered from various construction worksites (Driscoll et al., 1988).

Atmospheric nuclear testing during the 1950s and 1960s has attracted the attention of Arctic scientists because of the accumulation of such long half-life radionuclides as cesium 137 and strontium 90 in the food chain: lichens–caribou–Eskimo/Inuit. A review of exposure records and body burdens of Alaskan Eskimos revealed low maximal annual doses comparable to the natural "background" levels in many parts of the continent. Moreover, there has been no evidence of an increased risk in leukemia, breast cancer, and bone sarcoma—tumors that can potentially be induced by radiation—among Alaskan Eskimos (Stutzman et al., 1986).

Prevention and Control Strategies

Cancer may be prevented by reducing the prevalence of risk factors (primary) and by early detection (secondary). In terms of *primary prevention,* educational efforts directed at behavioral changes in smoking, alcohol consumption, sexual activity (in terms of delaying onset, limiting promiscuity, and protection from STDs), and perhaps diet (e.g., reduction in percent energy derived from fats, increase in fiber, fresh fruits and green vegetables, and maintaining energy balance) could bring about a reduced incidence of disease, although data from community preventive field trials in support of such conclusions are lacking. From a policy perspective, however, such educational efforts could not do much harm, and there may be even be effects toward reducing other non-cancer diseases as well.

A pilot intervention trial of beta-carotene was conducted among the Inuit in one community in the Northwest Territories. Rather than using cancer cases as the outcome (which would have been prohibitively costly in terms of time of follow-up and study size), the investigators studied the frequency of micronucleated cells (MNC) to quantitate the genotoxic damage in the oral mucosa of users of smokeless tobacco or snuff. The Inuit diet, which is rich in caribou and seal meat and liver but low in vegetables and fruits, results in normal serum levels of vitamin A but low levels of beta-carotene, its precursor. This study showed that a twice-weekly oral dose of beta-carotene capsules over a ten-week period was an effective inhibitor of MNC (Stich et al., 1985).

Vaccination for hepatitis B can be considered a form of primary prevention for hepatocellular cancer. The pioneering role in mass hepatitis B vaccination in the Alaska Native population was discussed in some detail in Chapter 3.

Many strategies for the early detection, or *secondary prevention*, of cancer exist, but the effectiveness of all of them has not been demonstrated (Battista and Grover, 1988). Pap smear for cervical cancer, and manual examination and mammography for breast cancer are two of the few for which the evidence of prevention is strong. The benefits of many other screening procedures are either unproven or uncertain: sigmoidoscopy, digital rectal examination, and/or stool occult blood testing for colorectal cancer; chest x-ray and sputum cytology for lung cancer; oral examination and endoscopy for oral and upper gastrointestinal cancers; urinalysis for microscopic hematuria and cytology for bladder cancer; serum acid phosphatase, digital rectal examination, and cytology for prostate cancer (Battista and Grover, 1988).

Pap Smear Screening.   While no RCTs have been done, various case-control and ecologic studies have demonstrated that screening reduces the incidence and mortality from cervical cancer, particularly in younger women. Various U.S. and Canadian national task forces have recommended schedules for Pap smear testing in terms of age range and test frequency. A Canadian task force, for example, recommended beginning screening at age 18 or onset of sexual activity, and if negative after one year, to be rescreened once every three years until age 70 (Miller et al., 1991). Conditions for a successful Pap smear screening program include a population-based registry responsible for determining eligibility to initiate screening and providing reminders for follow-up and periodic rescreening, a regionalized network of cytologic laboratories with quality control, and physical and human resources within the health care system to offer diagnostic confirmation and therapeutic interventions of those shown to be positive (Miller et al., 1991).

Some data are available on Pap smear coverage among Native American women. The SAIAN survey of 1987 of a nationally representative sample of Native American women in the United States indicated that coverage was generally lower than the all-races rate. Overall, 83 percent of Native American women over the age of 18 had had at least one Pap smear in the past (Fig. 4.4).

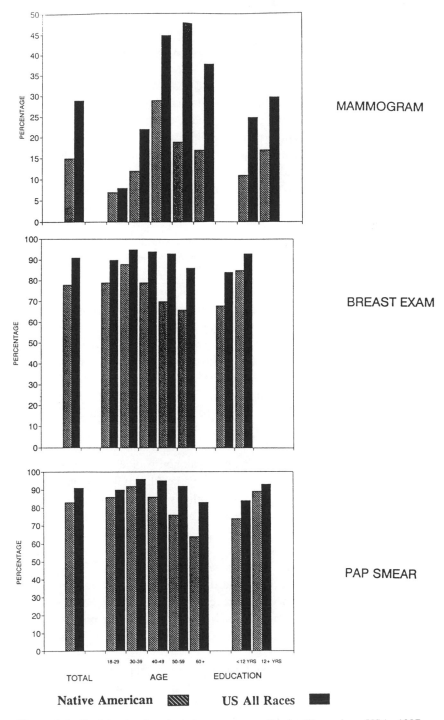

Figure 4.4. Participation in selected cancer preventive health services: USA, 1987, Native American and U.S. all-race populations.

Coverage was higher among the better educated women and peaked at age 30–39 (an inverted U-shape).

In British Columbia, where a computerized cervical cytology screening registry exists, Hislop and others (1992) performed data linkage of that registry with the official Indian Band List of 28 Indian bands, which accounted for about 15 percent of the total status Indian population in that province. They found that only 52 percent of Native women aged 13–59 were recent users (once during the past three years), about a third lower than the overall provincial coverage rate. Earlier data from Arizona and New Mexico during 1966–75 also indicated lower coverage among Native Americans, particularly those over age 50 (Jordan and Key, 1981).

While the risk of breast cancer among Native Americans is low relative to non-Natives, it is nevertheless an important cancer in terms of ranking and proportion of all cancers among Native American women. Treatment of breast cancer following detection by screening has been found to reduce mortality by as much as one-third (O'Malley and Fletcher, 1987). A variety of recommendations on the frequency and eligibility of screening have been made by different national expert panels in public health, oncology, radiology, and gynecology. The best evidence exists for screening using *clinical breast examination* (CBE) combined with *mammography,* particularly in the 50–59 age group. The effectiveness in other, younger age groups has not yet been demonstrated. The evidence supporting CBE alone or teaching women to perform breast self-examination (BSE) is not strong (O'Malley and Fletcher, 1987).

According to SAIAN (Fig. 4.4) fewer Native American women had undergone breast examination and mammography than non-Native women, conforming to a trend of lower participation in preventive health services among natives in general. It is likely that access and availability of such services, rather than deliberate decisions not to choose prevention, are responsible for the observed lower participation.

Colorectal cancer is a high ranking cancer among Native Americans but a low-risk site relative to non-Natives. The value of screening (*sigmoidoscopy* and *occult blood testing*) is controversial, and there is a divergence of opinion between the cautious stand of the U.S. Preventive Services Task Force and the Canadian Task Force for the Periodic Health Examination on the one hand, and the enthusiasm of various professional associations and cancer societies on the other (Winawer et al., 1991).

In addition to vaccination against hepatitis B, a potential strategy to prevent primary hepatocellular carcinoma—of particular importance among Alaskan Eskimos—is early diagnosis by careful clinical and serological follow-up of HbsAg carriers. The use of serial alpha-fetoprotein levels in this group may lead to early detection of cancer and successful surgical resection (Heyward et al., 1983), although as a population strategy this remains to be evaluated.

Ischemic Heart Disease

Extent and Magnitude of the Problem

Studies that compare the incidence, prevalence, and mortality of cardiovascular or circulatory diseases (CVD), particularly ischemic heart disease (IHD), among Native Americans with the national or non-Native population are summarized in Table 4.2. These include death certificate analyses, clinical record reviews, and community screening surveys. While in the context of "diseases of modernization" it is IHD that is of interest, often it is only the broader category of CVD as a whole, or "diseases of the heart," for which data are available, particularly from official sources. It should be noted that such larger groupings include a variety of pathological entities (e.g., rheumatic heart disease, heart failure, pulmonary heart disease, the cardiomyopathies, etc.) with vastly different etiologies, not all of which are necessarily associated with "lifestyle" changes (Alpert et al., 1991).

There is some consistency among studies conducted during the 1950s and 1960s in their demonstration of the rarity—but by no means absence—of IHD among Native Americans. The great majority of these were conducted among tribes and communities in the southwestern United States, particularly the Navajo and Pima. Compared to local or national groups of non-Natives, Native Americans had lower mortality/incidence rate, proportion of all deaths/hospital admissions attributed to IHD, and prevalence of electrocardiographic abnormalities. When SMR or SIR were computed, they usually ranged from 0.10 to 0.50.

Intertribal differences likely exist, but comparisons are difficult because of the different methodologies and time periods between studies. Low rates tend to be reported from the Navajos and Apaches (belonging to the Athapaskan language family), in comparison to other southwestern tribes or tribes in other parts of the United States, such as the Seminoles in Oklahoma (originally from Florida), the Chippewa in Minnesota, and the Sioux in South Dakota. Data from the U.S. Indian Health Service also indicate that there is variation in death rate due to diseases of the heart between IHS areas (Fig. 4.5A).

An estimate of self-reported CVD among Native Americans can be obtained from the Survey on American Indians and Alaska Natives (SAIAN) conducted in 1987. The age-sex-adjusted Native American prevalence was 9.8 percent, virtually identical to the U.S. all-race rate of 10.0 percent (Johnson and Taylor,

Table 4.2 Regional Studies of Cardiovascular Mortality and Morbidity among Native Americans

Authors	Years	Population[a]	Methods	Results[b]
1. Southwestern USA				
Smith (1957)	1948–52	Navajo; Navajo Indian Agency (pop: 70,000)	Death certificates (n = 178 coded to CVD and renal diseases)	SMR (compared to U.S. whites, "max. estimate") * all CVD M 0.16 F 0.21 * ASHD M 0.10 F 0.12 * stroke M 0.18 F 0.18

Streeper et al. (1960)	1950–56	Navajo; patients in Fort Defiance IHS hospital, AZ	Clinical records 4741 admissions (324 EKGs and 45 autopsies) age 30 + ; White patients in Alburquerque hospital comparison group	EKG: any abnormality—14% (cf. White 44%)
				       definite infarct—2.7%
				       probable infarct—3.0%
				 Autopsy: moderate–severe atherosclerosis 7.2%
				 IHD as proportion of all admissions:
				     Navajos 0.19% Whites 2.8%

Sievers (1966, 1967)	1957–66	Pima, Apache, Navajo, Hopi, Papago, etc; Phoenix Area IHS, AZ (pop: 48,000)	Clinical records 104,000 admissions, 1958 deaths (44% autopsied), 138 AMI cases	mean annual inicidence (age 40 +): 124/100,000
				 high (150): Pima/Papago/Chemehuevi (Uto-Aztecan)
				           Maricopa/Mohave/Yuma/Quechan, etc (Yuman)
				 low (100): Paiute/Shoshone/Ute/Washoe/Hopi (Uto-Aztecan)
				          Apache/Navajo (Athapaskan)

Clifford et al. (1963)	1957–59	Apache; Fort Apache Res. AZ (pop: 4,400)	Clinical records 147 EKGs	No evidence of IHD (e.g., MI, LBBB, 2nd/3rd degree AV block) 13% LVH, 4% RVH
Fulmer/ Roberts (1963)	1956–62	Navajo; Many Farms area, AZ (pop: 2,300)	Population survey 508 subjects age 30 +	Followed for 6 years, mean incidence 130/100,000/yr 12% EKGs abnormal SMR (cf. U.S. National) ASHD M 0.26 F 0.31 SIR (cf. Framingham, aged 30–60 only) M 0.11 no F cases

Study	Years	Population	Methods	Findings
Ingelfinger et al. (1976)	1965–73	Pima; Gila River Res. AZ (pop: 6,000)	Population survey (n = 701) age 40 +, Autopsy series (n = 120)	EKG: major Q wave changes M 2.4% F 0.6% Prevalence about half of Tecumseh Study Autopsy M 15% F 8% evidence of myocardial infarction
Davis/Kunitz (1978)	1972	Navajo; Navajo Res. AZ (pop: 123,000)	Clinical records (hospital discharge diagnoses)	Discharge rate for CVD among Navajos 36/10,000 (cf. U.S. rate 189/10,000, standardized ratio 0.37)
Sievers/Fisher (1979)	1975–78	SW Indians, 18 tribes; Phoenix Area IHS (pop: 58,000)	Clinical records EKG and autopsies 67 AMI cases age 30 +	Compared with 1957–66, rate doubled (greater increase in F) Athapaskans still lower than other SW Indians, although rates have also increased 3 times
Coulehan et al. (1986), Klain et al. (1988)	1976–86	Navajo; Navajo Reservation AZ and NM (pop: 150,000)	Clinical records EKG and enzyme criteria for acute myocardial infarction	ASIR for AMI age 35 +

Coulehan et al. / Klain et al. — ASIR for AMI age 35 +

	1976–79	1980–83	1984–86
Male: (/100,000)	84	79	203
Female: (/100,000)	12	54	62

Ratio Navajo/US national: age 15–44 = 0.33; 45–64 = 0.14; 64+ = 0.19 (both sexes)

Study	Years	Population	Methods	Findings
Becker et al. 1988	1958–82	Indians in NM	Death certificates	ASMR for IHD

Becker et al. — ASMR for IHD

	1958–62	1963–67	1968–72	1973–77	1978–82
M (/100,000)	95	74	102	98	77
F (/100,000)	45	63	59	39	28

Study	Years	Population	Methods	Findings
Sievers et al. (1990)	1975–84	Pima; Gila River Reservation, AZ	Death certificates and clinical records (n = 677)	Heart disease: ASMR 213, Pima/US ratio 0.6 Stroke: ASMR 99, Pima/U.S. ratio 1.3 Ratio Indians/U.S. whites consistently 0.2 (M,F) all periods

2. Other USA

Study	Years	Population	Methods	Findings
Mayberry/Lindeman (1963)	1950–59	Seminole; Seminole County, OK (pop: 2,400)	Death certificates (n = 206), age 25 +	Mean annual mortality rate

Mayberry/Lindeman — mortality

	% all deaths	Mean annual mortality rate
All CVD	M 45% F 31%	M 450/100,000 F 240/100,000
IHD	M 16% F 11%	M 155/100,000 F 84/100,000
Stroke	M 14% F 8%	M 140/100,000 F 60/100,000

Rates and proportions < whites living in same county

continued

Table 4.2 Regional Studies of Cardiovascular Mortality and Morbidity among Native Americans (continued)

Authors	Years	Population[a]	Methods	Results[b]
Pinkerton/ Badke (1974)	1956–69	Crow, Cheyenne; 2 res. in MT (pop: 5,200 Crow, 2,400 Cheyenne)	Clinical records (n = 39 AMI age 30–74) EKG and enzyme criteria	ASIR of AMI (14–years): M 4.7% (Crow), 1.9% (Cheyenne), 5.4% Framingham whites F 3.7% (Crow), 3.0% (Cheyenne), 1.0% Framingham whites
Minnesota Health Dept (1980) cited in Gillum et al. (1984)	1968–73	Indians in Minnesota (predominantly Chippewa)	Death certificates (1100 Indian deaths)	Heart disease and stroke cause of death (26%) ASMR among Indians: 449/100,000 (cf. 455 all races) Urban Indians slightly higher than rural

Mahoney et al. (1989d)	1955–84	Seneca; 2 reservations and nearby counties in western NY (pop: 3,262)	Death certificates, fixed cohort followed from 1955 to 1984, all ages	SMR All CVD M 0.84 F 0.79
				        AMI M 0.64 F 0.73
				        Stroke M 0.88 F 0.73

Hrabovsky et al. (1989)	1983–85	Sioux; 2 reservations in SD (pop: 13,000)	Clinical records and death certificates (n = 64 AMI cases) EKG and enzyme criteria	Age-specific incidence: M similar to Framingham, F higher M > F under age 55, F > M age 55 + 35 + rate: M 690/100,000, F 400/100,000 M rate 3 × higher and F rate 6 × higher than Navajos
3. Canadian Indians				
Abu-Zeid et al. (1978)	1960–62	Indians in Manitoba	Death certificates (n = 38 IHD deaths among Indians)	SMR for IHD, M = 0.34, F not significantly different from 1.0 (part of larger study of IHD in various ethnic groups in Manitoba)

continued

Reference	Years	Population	Data source	Findings
Young (1982)	1972–81	Cree and Ojibwa, northwestern Ontario	Clinical records (n = 668 deaths from all causes)	PMR for circulatory diseases 14% (cf. 48% all Canada) SMR 0.6 circulatory diseases (0.7 for heart diseases and 0.8 for stroke)
Millar (1982)	1974–76	Indians in Alberta	Death certificates (n = 826 all causes)	PMR for circulatory diseases M 18.3% (cf. Alberta 43.8%), F 15.3% (cf. Alberta 46.5%), and both sexes 17.1% (cf. Alberta 44.8%)
Robinson (1985)	1975–82	Cree in James Bay, northern Quebec	Clinical records (n = 310 all causes)	SMR (cf. with Canada) 0.77 for circulatory diseases PMR 22%
Robinson (1988)	1981–84	Cree in James Bay, northern Quebec	Health insurance, hospitalization database	Age-standardized hospitalization rate for CVD: M Cree 9.2/1000 ratio 0.6—(Cree/all Quebec) F Cree 14.0/1000 ratio 1.3
Mao et al. (1986)	1977–82	Residents of Indian reserves in 7 provinces	Death certificates; National Mortality Database, age 1–69 only	ASMR Indians Canada IHD M 104.5 F 41.6 M 116.1 F 33.4 stroke M 22.9 F 24.0 M 16.6 F 12.1

4. Eskimos/Inuit

Reference	Years	Population	Data source	Findings
Maynard (1967)	1955–65	Alaska Natives	Death certificates (n = 1806 all causes, 378 deaths from CVD)	Lower rates in all age-sex groups than USA. Regional/ethnic differences within state, Eskimos < Indians and Aleuts
Kroman/Green (1980)	1950–74	Greenland: Upernavik District (pop 1800)	Clinical records (hospital-based registry)	3 cases of AMI (40 cases expected based on Danish rate)
Clausen (1974)	1960–69	Greenland	Death certificates (n = 226 IHD deaths)	Mortality rate from IHD < in Denmark; but age 65 + not significantly different in F; higher in M among Greenlanders

Table 4.2 Regional Studies of Cardiovascular Mortality and Morbidity among Native Americans (continued)

Authors	Years	Population[a]	Methods	Results[b]
Schaefer, et al. (1980a)	1976–78	NWT: Arctic Bay and Inuvik	Population survey (n = 176)	ECGS: RVH and RBBB common; IHD present in 1/72 Arctic Bay and 4/35 Inuvik residents
Colbert et al. (1978)	1968–72	Alaska: 4 villages in NW and SW	Population survey (n = 90, age 40+)	ECGs: lower rate than Tecumseh, Michigan, but higher than Masai in East Africa in all age-sex groups
Maynard (1976)		Alaska	Population survey (n = 2356, age 15+)	ECGs: evidence of prior MI absent under age 50; lower rate of abnormalities than U.S. population
Bjerregaard Dyerberg (1988)	1968–83	Greenland	Death certificates (n = 5285 all causes 737 CVD deaths)	SMR total CVD M:1.0, F:1.4; IHD M:0.6, F:0.9. IHD mortality rate in towns > small settlements. Time trend: decline from 1968–72 to 1979–83. Stroke: Greenland > Denmark; M > F, no decline with time
Middaugh (1990)	1980–86	Alaska	Death certificates (n = 3526 total Native 292 IHD, 123 stroke)	Native/non-Native IHD RR 0.63 (M = F), significant. Stroke RR (M 1.13, F 1.03), not significant

[a]States/Provinces/Territories: *USA—AZ*, Arizona; MN, Minnesota; MT, Montana; NM, New Mexico; NY, New York; OK, Oklahoma; SD, South Dakota. *Canada*: NWT, Northwest Territories.

[b]AMI, acute myocardial infarction; ASHD, atherosclerotic heart disease; ASIR, age-standardized incidence rate; ASMR, age-standardized mortality rate; AV, atrioventricular; CHD, coronary heart disease; CVD, cardiovascular disease; ECG, electrocardiographs; IHD, ischemic heart disease; IHS, Indian Health Service; LBBB, left bundle branch block; LVH, left ventricular hypertrophy; NCHS, National Center for Health Statistics; PMR, proportionate mortality rate; RBBB, right bundle branch block; RVH, right ventricular hypertrophy; SMR, standardized mortality ratio; SIR, standardized incidence ratio. Abbreviations: n = study size; pop = population; M = male; F = female; res = reservation.

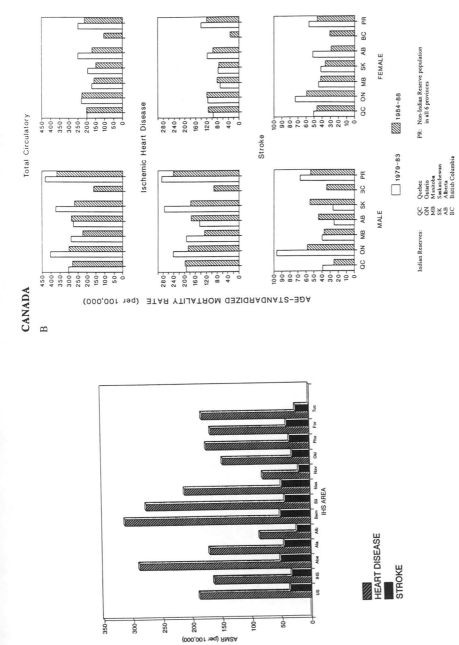

Figure 4.5. Regional variation in age-standardized mortality rate for diseases of heart and stroke among Native Americans: (A) USA, 1980–87;(B) Canada, 1979–88.

1991). It should be noted that such prevalence data can only include survivors at one point in time, and they are more useful as indicator of health service needs than the frequency of occurrence of disease.

An important effort to ascertain the burden of CVD mortality and morbidity and prevalence of risk factors among Native Americans was launched in the early 1990s. Using standardized methods, the Strong Heart Study (Lee et al., 1990) covered twelve tribes in the Southwest, Oklahoma, and North and South Dakota.

Evidence for the increasing rates of CVD among American Indians is conflicting. Sievers and Fisher (1979) showed an increase among southwestern Indians between the period 1957–66 and 1975–78. The increase was least among the Navajos and Apaches. Coulehan and others (1986) studied acute myocardial infarction on the Navajo Reservation—one of the largest reservations in the United States, with a population of some 150,000—showed little change among men between 1976–79 and 1980–83. However, when data collection was extended to 1986, an upward trend was observed among both men and women, but particularly among men (Klain et al., 1988).

The most complete trend data for any regional group of Native Americans were provided by Becker and others (1988), covering age-standardized mortality rates for IHD in New Mexico during the periods 1958–62, 1963–67, 1968–72, 1973–77, and 1978–82. They found a pattern similar to that observed for the United States nationally. Among male Native Americans, there was an increase until about 1970, when a decline began. Among women, the peak occurred in the mid 1960s. A cohort analysis confirmed the rise-and-fall pattern in age-specific mortality. In terms of the ratio of age-standardized mortality rates between Native Americans in that state and U.S. whites nationally, the ratio remained consistent at around 0.2, in both men and women (Becker et al., 1988).

Gillum (1988) reviewed national data on Native American ischemic heart disease from two periods 1969–71 and 1979–81. A decline of about 30 percent was actually observed in the crude death rate, while the proportionate mortality rate did not change. The age-standardized mortality rate for IHD similarly declined from 132/100,000 in the first period to 94/100,000 a decade later.

Trend data are available from the U.S. IHS for "diseases of the heart." In the mid-1960s, the age-adjusted Native American mortality rate was about 200/100,000, a ratio of 0.7 compared to the U.S. all-race rate of the same period (Hill and Spector, 1971). Since that time, both the Native American and U.S. rates have declined. The mean Native American rate for 1970–75 was 167 (U.S. DHEW, 1978a) and 1980–85 was 150 (U.S. DHHS, 1988), with the Native/all-race ratio remaining relatively constant at around 0.8.

Among Native Canadians, data from Indian reserves in seven provinces showed that, for Indians under age 70, the female IHD and stroke rate was higher than for all Canadians, while among men, the stroke rate but not the IHD rate was higher (Mao et al., 1986). Most other regional studies, using the standard-ized mortality ratio (SMR) for all ages, generally showed an Indian deficit in cardiovascular diseases (Young, 1983; Robinson, 1988; Abu-Zeid et al., 1978). When SMR is computed based on the mortality experience of all ages, the all-Canada Indian male and female IHD SMRs are still significantly less than unity (Fig. 4.5B). A clear regional variation in the IHD mortality among Indians is not demonstrated in Canada.

The low incidence of CVD among the Inuit has been recognized for some time. Several autopsy series among Alaskan Eskimos and Canadian Inuit (Ar-thaud, 1970; Lederman et al., 1962) during the 1950s and 1960s indicate that cases of atherosclerosis, while not an important cause of death, were by no means absent. An analysis of death certificates in Alaska during 1955–65 showed that the mortality rate of heart diseases among Eskimos was much lower than in the U.S. population, even after age standardization (Maynard et al., 1967). An update covering the period 1980–86 showed that Alaska Natives (which include both Eskimos and Indians) still had significant reduced risk of mortality from IHD, with a relative risk of 0.63 compared to non-Natives in the state (Middaugh, 1990).

Similarly low rates have also been reported from Greenland (Clausen, 1974; Kroman and Green, 1980). The most comprehensive review of Eskimo deaths in Greenland based on the Danish national death registry from 1968–83 showed that the risk of IHD was lower among Eskimos when compared to Danes (Bjer-regaard and Dyerberg, 1988).

Electrocardiogram surveys conducted in both the Northwest Territories (Schaefer et al., 1980a) and Alaska (Maynard, 1976; Colbert et al., 1978) gen-erally showed low rates of abnormalities, particularly ischemic changes.

Etiology and Risk Factors

Many large-scale epidemiological studies have concluded that cigarette smoking, hypertension, and elevated serum cholesterol levels are major independent risk factors for ischemic heart disease. Other risk factors include diabetes, physical inactivity, obesity, stress, and personality characteristics (Fraser, 1986). Because the major risk factors can be modified, ischemic heart disease is largely a pre-ventable disease.

In this chapter, data relating to serum lipids and hypertension among Native Americans are reviewed. Smoking, as a risk factor for a variety of diseases, was discussed in Chapter 2. Diabetes and obesity are covered in Chapter 5. It should be noted that these conditions, while risk factors for IHD and stroke, can be considered "diseases" in their own right with their own risk factors.

It should be recognized that IHD is the clinical "endpoint" of atherosclerosis, a pathologic process that may begin early in life. Unlike IHD, atherosclerosis is much harder to study in a population setting, because its presence can be determined only by autopsy and, among the living, by the highly invasive procedure of angiography. The ability of portable ultrasonography to detect atherosclerotic plaques in peripheral arteries offers a noninvasive means to ascertain the prevalence of atherosclerosis in a free-living population. A study of 61 Greenland Eskimos from the remote northwest, compared with age-sex-matched Danes in Copenhagen, showed that Greenlanders had almost the same degree and extent of atherosclerosis in the carotid and femoral arteries, and by extrapolation, in other arteries of the body as well (Hansen et al., 1990).

A considerable literature has been accumulated on social and cultural influences in cardiovascular diseases, conducted in a variety of ethnic groups around the world [see the review by Dressler (1984)]. Little research has been conducted among Native Americans beyond establishing the presence of a differential in disease burden or, at most, explaining the differential in terms of the prevalence of classical risk factors. How and why those social and cultural factors that constitute Native Americans as a distinct ethnic group affect IHD incidence has not been explored.

Stroke

Magnitude and Extent of the Problem

Table 4.2 includes data on stroke provided by studies on CVD mortality and morbidity in various Native American populations. In the United States the age-standardized mortality rate for stroke appeared to have declined from over 65/100,000 in the mid-1960s (Hill and Spector, 1971) to below 50/100,000 during the 1970s (U.S. DHEW, 1978a). This has further been reduced to around 25/100,000 during 1980–85 (U.S. DHHS, 1988). Throughout these years, the Native American rate has consistently been lower than the U.S. all-race rate.

Among Native Canadians, data from Indian reserves in seven provinces showed that, for Indians under age 70, the stroke mortality rate was higher than for all Canadians in both males and females (Mao et al., 1986). When SMR is computed based on the mortality experience of all ages, the Canadian Indian male stroke SMR was significantly less than unity, whereas the female stroke SMR was not significantly different from unity (Fig. 4.5B). The age-standardized mortality rate for stroke did not show a clear east-west gradient.

The risk of stroke mortality among Alaska Natives was not significantly different from non-Natives in that state (Middaugh, 1990). Greenlandic Eskimos are at higher risk than Danes (Kroman and Green, 1980; Bjerregaard and Dyerberg, 1988), both for bleeding intracranial aneurysms and for other forms of stroke.

Etiology and Risk Factors

An extensive literature exists on the risk factors for stroke (Ostfield and Wilk, 1990). The more established ones include hypertension, diabetes, and a history of previous transient ischemic attacks, strokes, IHD, arrhythmias, or left ventricular hypertrophy. More recent studies have implicated alcohol, an elevated hematocrit, oral contraceptives, physical inactivity, and obesity. It should be recognized that stroke is the clinical manifestation of different disease processes, the two main types being thromboembolism and hemorrhage. Risk factors may have opposite effects depending on the type of "endpoints." Thus moderate or heavy alcohol consumption has been found to be associated with hemorrhagic stroke, whereas for thromboembolic stroke, the relationship is less clear and may even be inverse. Similarly, there seems to be an inverse relationship between serum cholesterol level and hemorrhagic stroke but a positive association with nonhemorrhagic stroke (Ostfield and Wilk, 1990).

The high risk of intracranial aneurysms among Greenlandic Eskimos has been attributed to different connective tissue properties (Ostergaard Kristensen, 1983). The reduced platelet aggregability demonstrated in Greenland (Dyerberg and Bang, 1975) should lead on the one hand to reduced thrombosis and on the other to increased bleeding tendency, which may account for the low risk for acute myocardial infarction and the high risk for cerebral hemorrhage.

Hypertension

Magnitude and Extent of the Problem

The prevalence of hypertension and distribution of blood pressure levels have often been determined in conjunction with health and nutrition surveys among North American Indians, many of which involved mainly small populations in a few communities.

The 1987 SAIAN national survey provided an estimate of self-reported hypertension in a representative sample of adult Native Americans (Johnson and Taylor, 1991). The age-sex-adjusted prevalence of 23 percent in Native Americans was identical to the U.S. all-race rate. The only substantial difference was among those aged 65 and above, where the Native American rate was 37 percent, compared to the U.S. national rate of 49 percent (Fig. 4.6).

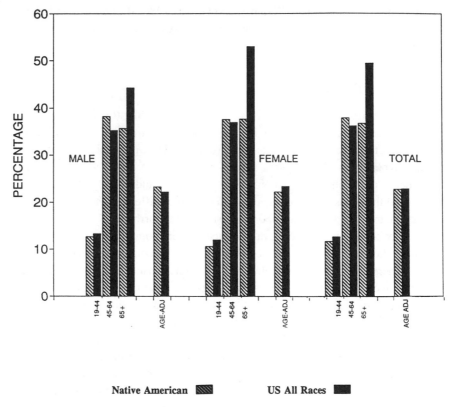

Figure 4.6. Prevalence of self-reported hypertension: USA, 1987, Native American and U.S. all-race populations.

Several studies done in the 1950s and 1960s generally showed a low prevalence of hypertension in the Southwest, with some exceptions such as the Apaches (Table 4.3). By the mid-1970s a trend toward an increased prevalence was noted by Sievers (1977) among all southwestern tribes.

A screening program on the Navajo Reservation revealed a lower prevalence of hypertension than for either U.S. whites or blacks (DeStefano et al. 1979). Gillum and colleagues (1980) measured Indian children attending grades 1–3 in Minneapolis, Minnesota, and reported slightly higher SBP but lower DBP than either black or white children. Elsewhere in the United States, studies among the Seminoles in Oklahoma (Mayberry and Lindeman, 1963) and the Penobscot in Maine (Deprez et al., 1985) showed comparable rates to non-Natives in the same states.

In Canada a survey among the Ojibwa and Cree in the 1980s showed higher mean DBP in all age-sex groups compared to Canadians nationally, while for systolic blood pressure, the Indians' level was lower above the age of 45 (Young, 1991).

In Alaska, a survey of Eskimo National Guardsmen in the 1950s (Mann et al., 1962), studies under the International Biological Program in the 1970s (Colbert et al., 1978), as well as a large cardiovascular risk factor survey among 2356 male adult Alaskan Eskimos in the mid 1970s (Maynard, 1976), found that blood pressure levels were still generally low, and the prevalence of hypertension lower than in the U.S. population. A pocket of high hypertension prevalence, however, existed among the Aleuts, distant relatives of the Eskimos (Torrey, 1979). The prevalence of hypertension was reported to be low among Greenland Eskimos (Bjerager et al., 1982).

Much interest has been shown in whether blood pressure rises with age among Eskimos, a phenomenon not demonstrated by some preindustrial populations around the world. In Igloolik, Northwest Territories, a survey of 400 subjects in 1969–70 showed a low mean blood pressure but no rise with age (Hildes and Schaefer, 1973). Later surveys showed an age-dependent increase in blood pressure in both sexes in Inuvik, a large town, but not among men in remote Arctic Bay (Schaefer et al., 1980b). No present Native American populations can be considered "primitive" or "preindustrial." The multinational INTERSALT study, however, included two remote, relatively unacculturated Amazonian Indian populations from Brazil. These populations not only had the lowest mean blood pressure measurements among the fifty-two sites but also there was no rise with age (Carvalho et al., 1989).

Etiology and Risk Factors

The etiology of hypertension is closely linked with that of other chronic diseases such as obesity, atherosclerosis, and dyslipidemia, and current thinking points to insulin resistance as the key, underlying metabolic "cause." This is discussed further in Chapter 5. As in other chronic diseases, there is an important role for genetic factors, as evidenced from family aggregation and twin studies (Havlik and Feinleib, 1982).

Of the environmental risk factors, the role of salt appears well established, with consistent evidence from both between-population and within-population studies, clinical, and laboratory studies. This risk appears to be continuous. Moreover, a reduction of salt intake can be expected to lead to improved outcome (Joossens and Geboers, 1987). Amazonian Indians who took part in the INTER-SALT study had one of the lowest daily salt intakes, as measured by 24-hour urinary sodium excretion. On a between-population basis, the low level of salt

Table 4.3 Regional Studies of Hypertension Prevalence among Native Americans

Authors	Years	Population	Methods	Results
1. Indians in USA				
Fulmer/ Roberts (1963)	1956–62	Navajo: (pop: 2,300) Many Farms, AZ	Population survey asge 30+ (n = 413)	>160/95: M 6.2%; F 3.4%; total 4.7%
Darby et al. (1956)	1955	Navajo: 2 communities within Navajo Res. AZ	Population survey (n = 785)	>140/90: 7.1% in Ganado; 4.2% in Pinon Higher prevalence among obese Increase with age among adults of both sexes Above age 45, prevalence higher in females
Clifford et al. (1963)	1958	Apache: Fort Apache Res. AZ (pop: 4,400)	Population survey (n = 327) Casual readings	DBP>100: M 26%; F 23% (cf. U.S. blacks: M 5%; F 23%) >160/95: higher prevalence in younger age groups, esp. males
Ingelfinger et al. (1976)	1970s	Pima: Gila river Res. AZ	Population survey (n = 701) age 40+	Mean BP increases with age in both sexes Higher BP among diabetics than nondiabetics
Mayberry/ Lindeman (1963)	1960s	Seminole; Seminole County, OK (pop: 2,400)	Population survey (n = 302)	Mean BP comparable to whites in same county >160/100: 10.9% among Indians (cf. 12.3% in whites)
DeStefano et al. (1979)	1977	Navajo; Fort Defiance IHS (pop 15,000)	Population survey (n = 640, age 20+)	DBP ≥ 90: M24%; F 11%; total 17%; DBP ≥ 95: M 11%; F 5%; total 7% Lower BP and previous HPT than blacks and whites Risk factors: obesity in both sexes, alcohol use in males Small increase with age Acculturation index not a risk factor
Gillum et al. (1980)	1978	Minneapolis school children (grades 1–3)	Population survey (n = 307, age 6–9) random-zero BP	Indian children slightly higher mean SBP than blacks/whites but lower DBP Obesity (BMI) significant determinant of excess in SBP but not deficit in DBP
Gillum et al. (1984)	1980s	Urban Indians in Minneapolis (public housing project + visitors to Indian festival)	Population survey (n = 242, age 16–84)	Compared with whites in Minnesota Heart Survey self-reported HPT: housing project 23%, others 25%, whites 27% SBP ≥ 140: Indian (15% housing project, 11% others) whites (14%) DBP: Indians (14% housing project, 11% others) >whites (7%) Increase with age; mean BP M > F

Deprez et al. (1985)	1981	Penobscot Reservation, Maine	Population survey (n = 100, age 18+)	prevalence of HPT (DBP ≥ 90 or on treatment): age-sex adjusted 23%, similar to Maine Statewide Survey
2. Canadian Indians				
McIntyre/ Shah (1986)	1983	Ojibwa;, 3 communities in NW Ontario	Population survey (n = 668 age 15+)	estimated prevalence 13% (previously diagnosed + new) increase with age in both sexes, but DBP decline after age 50 ≤3% ≥ 140/90 re-examined 6 months later still hypertensive
Young (1991)	1986–87	Cree and Ojibwa; 6 communities in northern Ontario and Manitoba	Population survey (n = 704 age 20–64)	Prevalence M 43% F 27% (previously diagnosed + new >140/90) cf Canada Health Survey, DBP higher in Indians in all age-sex SBP: Indians lower beyond age 45
3. Eskimos/Inuit				
Ehrstrom (1951)	1948–49	Greenland: Umanak District	Population survey (n = 1071 all ages)	BP levels comparable to Finns; 7.4% SBP > 165
Bjerager (1982)	1977	Greenland: Uppernavik and Scorebysund Districts	Population survey (n = 410)	M = F; SBP correlates with age in both sexes, DBP corr. with age only in Scoresbysund District BP levels comparable to Copenhagen
Mann et al. (1962)	1958	Alaska: members of National Guard + villagers	Population survey (n = 713 M guardsmen, 805 villagers, M/F)	Low prevalence of hypertension, rise of BP with age
Colbert et al. (1978)	1968–72	Alaska: 4 villages in NW and SW	Population survey (n = 251, aged 18–74)	Prevalence of hypertension generally lower than USA except for females in southwest
Hildes/ Schaefer (1973)	1969 1971	Igloolik, NWT	Population survey (n = 422, 130 adults)	Low mean BP, no rise with age; 1971 mean higher than 1969 in all groups except middle-aged hunters
Schaefer et al. (1980b)	1976	Arctic Bay and Inuvik, NWT	Population survey (n = 503 all ages)	BP rise with age in both sexes in Inuvik but not Arctic Bay
Torrey et al. (1979)	1966 1976	Aleuts in 1 village, Pribilof Islands (pop: 450)	Population survey (n = 159 in 1966, 231 in 1976)	Prevalence of hypertension (>160/95) higher than USA

intake correlated well with their low mean blood pressure (Carvalho et al., 1989). There is little information on salt intake and hypertension among North American Indians. A study among the Papagos in Arizona investigated the health effects of exposure to drinking water with a high salt content. No consistent association between sodium intake (whether estimated from food and water or from urinary excretion) and blood pressure on multivariate analysis. Interestingly, the overall intake was higher among the Papagos as a group, compared to white and Hispanic subjects served by the same water supply (Welty et al., 1986).

In the Navajo survey mentioned earlier, the risk factors were obesity in both sexes, alcohol use in men, but not the degree of acculturation (DeStefano et al., 1979). In Minneapolis, Gillum (1980) found that among children attending grades 1–3 the increase in SBP among Native Americans could be accounted for by their higher body mass index.

In a survey of over 700 Cree and Ojibwa Indians in northern Canada, Young (1991) found that age, male sex, unemployment, body mass index, total cholesterol, positive family history, and single marital status were independent predictors of hypertensive status on multivariate analysis.

Studies in other populations have suggested that migrants from rural to urban, or "traditional" to "modern," societies tend to have increased prevalence of hypertension. Only one study on the effect of migration on blood pressure levels among Native Americans has been reported. Alfred (1970) compared three groups of Navajo men: (a) those who participated in an earlier blood pressure survey on the reservation [reported in Fulmer and Roberts (1963)]; (b) applicants for relocation assistance from the Bureau of Indian Affairs; and (c) urban residents. Comparison of groups (a) and (b) indicated that they did not differ in mean systolic blood pressure, whereas for diastolic blood pressure, group (b) was greater than (a). Comparing group (c) and (b), both systolic and diagnostic blood pressure were higher in the former. In group (c), some participants had earlier belonged to group (b) and had records of pre-migration blood pressure measurements. For such individuals the blood pressure was significantly higher after migration. No correlation, however, was found between the length of urban residence and the change in blood pressure (Alfred, 1970).

The role of "acculturative stress" was explored among Navajos aged 65 and above by Kunitz and Levy (1986). They found that the prevalence of previously diagnosed hypertension was associated with various measures of acculturation among women but not among men. When their data were reanalyzed to generate odds ratios, the risk of hypertension was found to be 4.0 for those women with nine or more years of education, 3.2 for those who had attended off-reservation schools, 1.8 for those who had lived off reservation for more than a year, 1.6 for those who spoke fluent English, and 1.5 for those who did not adhere to a traditional religion. When an "isolation-integration" index was constructed (composed of marital status, camp size, presence of children and visitors), those who were the most isolated had 4.6 times the risk of being hypertensive. There also appeared to be interaction between education and isolation, such that the "protective" effect of low education and low isolation were synergistic when both were present.

At the other end of the age spectrum, a survey of Navajo adolescents attending high schools in towns and living in dormitories failed to demonstrate an independent effect of "acculturation score" on either systolic or diastolic blood pressure when other risk factors have been controlled for. The acculturation score was based on language, religion, source of family income, and type and location of home. This study, however, did show that among women, poor personal adjustment (covering such attributes as school difficulties, delinquent behaviors, and personal feelings of loneliness, anger, and trust) was a predictor of systolic blood pressure (Coulehan et al., 1990).

Dyslipidemia

Magnitude and Extent of the Problem

The epidemiologic, clinical, and laboratory literature on serum lipids and apolipoproteins has increased exponentially over the past several decades. A joint statement of the American Heart Association and the National Heart, Lung and Blood Institute concluded that there was a continuous and positive association between serum cholesterol levels and the risk of IHD (La Rosa et al., 1990).

Epidemiologic data on population levels of serum cholesterol and other lipids in Native Americans are patchy. Among most U.S. groups studied, particularly those from the Southwest, serum cholesterol levels were lower than comparison groups of whites or the national population (Table 4.4). Due to the different laboratory methods used, actual mean values are not of critical importance; rather, it is their relative ranking between tribes (if done in the same study), or vis à vis whites, which is of interest.

The Seminoles in Oklahoma had mean serum cholesterol levels similar to those of whites in the same county (Mayberry and Lindeman, 1963), while among urban Indians in Minneapolis the levels were not significantly different from whites under age 55, but were lower above the age of 55 (Gillum et al., 1984).

Fractions of cholesterol were studied to a lesser extent in Native American groups. In a small metabolic ward study (involving subjects from three tribes) the rates of synthesis of apo-LDL, plasma LDL, and apo-LDL were all lower

Table 4.4 Regional Studies of Serum Lipids among Native Americans

Authors	Years	Population	Methods	Results[a]
1. Indians in USA				
Page et al. (1956)	1950s	Navajos; in-patients Fort Defiance IHS hospital, AZ	Clinical study (n = 36), age 17–85	TCH lower than Cleveland Clinic "control" sample No increase with age
Abraham/ Miller (1959)	1955–56	Pueblos, NM; Crows, MT; Apaches, AZ; Sioux, SD; Chippewa, WI	5-reservation survey household interveiw and examination (n = 258)	TCH lower than Cleveland Clinic controls Little difference between tribes Females have lower levels than males
Darby et al. (1956)	1955	Navajo: 2 communities within Navajo Res., AZ	Population survey (n = 785)	TCH higher than reported in Page et al. (1956) but not significantly different from Cleveland Clinic controls
Fulmer/ Roberts (1963)	1956–62	Navajo: Many Farms, AZ (pop: 2,300)	Population survey age 30 + (n = 202)	Lower TCH compared to Framingham at all age-sex groups
Clifford et al. (1963)	1958	Apache: Fort Apache Res., AZ (pop: 4,400)	Population survey age 20 + (n = 188)	TCH lower than Framingham; percent ≥ 210 mg/dl: M 30% (cf. Framingham 66%) F 53% (cf. Framingham 73%)
Kositchek et al. (1961)	1950s	Navajo: Fort Defiance, AZ + Indian prisoners	Clinical study (n = 30)	TCH low
Sievers (1968b)	1963–65	Various southwestern tribes: in-patients Phoenix IHS hospital, AZ	Hospital survey (n = 746 SW Indians, 70 non-SW Indians, 163 white hospital staff)	Age-adjusted mean TCH white > non-SW > SW Indians No increase with age No association with obesity

Author (year)	Location	Study type	Findings
Mayberry/ Lindeman (1963)	Seminole; Seminole County, OK (pop: 2,400)	Population survey (n = 302)	Mean TCH similar to whites in same county; percent > 260 mg/dl: M 9% (cf. whites 16%) F 5% (cf. whites 9%)
Savage et al. (1976)	Pima: Gila River Res., AZ	Population survey (n = 2281); longitudinal and cross-sectional	Comparison with Tecumseh Study: cord blood at birth—no difference. age 5–16: 20–30 mg/dl lower; adults: 50–60 mg/cl lower; age 17–25: increase with age; trend corroborated by longitudinal data; low association with height, weight, glucose tolerance, and serum creatinine (as a muscle mass index)
Garnick et al. (1979)	Pima, Navajo, Hopi	Clinical study (n = 10 Indians, 5 whites)	Lower LDL, apo-LDL, higher HDL Reduced rate of apo-LDL synthesis rather than difference in fractional catabolic rates
Ingelfinger et al. (1976)	Pima: Gila River Res., AZ	Population survey 85% participation rate (n = 701) age 40 +	Low TCH (higher among diabetics) No change with age
Howard et al. (1983)	Pima: Gila River Res., AZ	Population survey (n = 1391)	TCH, HDL, LDL lower than whites (both sexes) TRG greater than whites (among males <35 and females <55)
Gillum et al. (1984)	Indians in Minneapolis, MN	Population survey (n = 213)	Compared with Minnesota Heart Study: <55, Indians = whites; >55, Indians lower than whites; HDL among males: Indians = whites; female: Indians < whites

2. Canadian Indians

Author (year)	Location	Study type	Findings
Desai/Lee (1971)	Nootka and Chilcotin reserves, BC	Population survey (n = 372)	Percent > 300 mg/dl 18% in Ahousat, 9% in Anaham > 200 mg/dl, about 75% in both communities, F > M
Desai/Lee (1974)	2 Athapaskan communities, Yukon	Population survey	Lower TCH than BC study; percent > 300 mg/dl almost zero percent > 200 mg/dl 20% in Upper Liard and 30% in Ross River
Reeder et al. (1988)	4 Cree-Ojibwa communities (pop = 800) in NW Ontario	Population survey (n = 316, of which 193 fasting)	HDL, TRG: M = F, no increase with age; LDL, TCH: M > F, rise with age; higher TRG, TCH and LDL among obese

continued

Table 4.4 Regional Studies of Serum Lipids among Native Americans (continued)

Authors	Years	Population	Methods	Results[a]
3. Eskimos/Inuit				
Scott et al. (1958)	1958	Members of National Guard (M); villagers (both sexes)	Population survey (n = 842, aged 17–53)	Little difference from USA data; inter-village variations
Canada DNHW (1975a)	1972	4 communities, NWT	Population survey (n = 355)	8% at "high risk;" 5% >95th percentile of national sample
Verdier et al. (1987)	1976 1978 1980	Arctic Bay, NWT	Population survery (n = 300 in 1976; 91 in 1978; 287 in 1980)	Change in prevalence between 1976, 1978, and 1980: 5%, 6%, 14% ("high risk" using Nutrition Canada criteria); 3%, 4%, 8% (>95th percentile of national sample)
Bang/ Dyerberg (1972), Dyerberg et al. (1975, 1977)	1970–82	Umanak district Greenland 5 separate surveys	Population survey (n = 130 age 30–83 in first survey)	TCH, TRG, and LDL < Danes in all age-sex groups; HDL higher in Greenlanders among males aged 41 + but not in F; fatty acids (linoleic, linolenic) lower among Greenlanders but long-chain fatty acids (EPA) of marine mammal origin higher

[a]TCH, total cholesterol; TRG, triglycerides; HDL, high-density lipoprotein cholesterol; LDL, low-density lipoprotein cholesterol. For abbreviations of states, provinces, and territories, see Table 4.1 and Table 4.2.

among Indians while the plasma HDL level was higher (Garnick et al., 1979). This is in conflict with larger survey of Pimas where the HDL levels were low in both sexes (Howard et al., 1983). In the Minneapolis study HDL levels were similar between Indian and white males, but lower among Indian females (Gillum et al., 1984).

In Canada, the Nutrition Canada Survey during the early 1970s (Canada DNHW, 1975c) provided some data on serum cholesterol, which showed that the proportion of people at "high" risk, using the age-dependent criteria from the Framingham Study, was lower among Indians than the national sample. With the exception of triglycerides in Indian women, the distribution of these lipids among Indians tended to be shifted to the left when compared with Canadians nationally (Fig. 4.7).

There has been a long tradition of studies on lipid metabolism among the Eskimos dating back to pre-World War II days, in an attempt to discover the causes of the low incidence of ischemic heart disease in that population (Corcoran et al., 1937; Wilber and Levine, 1950; Scott et al., 1958). The Nutrition Canada Survey in the early 1970s still showed generally low levels of serum cholesterol among Canadian Inuit, particularly men (Canada DNHW, 1975a). Studies in northwestern Alaska (Feldman et al., 1972) and northwestern Greenland (Bang and Dyerberg, 1972) further revealed low levels of very low-density lipoprotein cholesterol among the Eskimos compared to whites.

Etiology and Risk Factors

There are both genetic and environmental determinants of serum cholesterol levels. While there are familial dyslipidemia syndromes that are transmitted by single genes, the serum cholesterol level of most individuals is probably controlled by multiple genes. Studies have been conducted using various "candidate" genes believed to be involved in different aspects of lipid metabolism. Alleles at the apolipoprotein E locus have been found to have a significant effect on cholesterol and apo B levels. While LDL receptor defects have been detected, studies on DNA markers of apolipoprotein loci associated with dyslipidemia and IHD have not been consistent (Motulsky, 1987).

Among the Dogrib Indians in the Northwest Territories, where IHD is still very rare, genotype-associated quantitative lipoprotein variation can still be demonstrated in the absence of disease. Fasting triglyceride levels in women varied significantly with the XmnI locus of the apolipoprotein A-I/C-III/A-IV gene cluster (Cole et al., 1989). The extent to which observed lipoprotein gene frequency differences between Native and non-Native populations contributes to the differences in CVD frequency remains to be investigated.

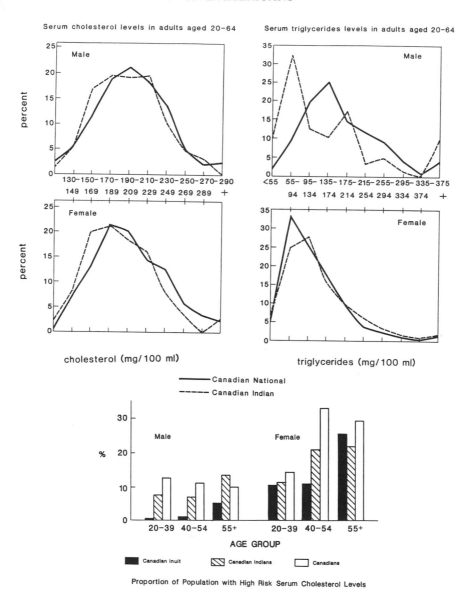

Figure 4.7. Serum lipids (total cholesterol and triglycerides): Canada, 1972, Indians and all Canadians.

Of the environmental factors, dietary cholesterol has been shown to be strongly associated with serum cholesterol (La Rosa et al., 1990). Even short-term dietary change has been shown to have an impact on serum cholesterol, lipoproteins, triglycerides, and weight gain in a study among the Tarahumara Indians of Mexico. This "unacculturated" group, who are known to have a low risk for IHD and whose traditional low-fat, high-fiber diet on the average consists of only 2,700 kcal per day, were subjected to five weeks of a 4100-kcal diet high in total fat, saturated fat, and cholesterol (McMurtry et al., 1991).

The different extent of dietary acculturation has been suggested to account for an observed geographic gradient in serum cholesterol levels in Alaska (Draper, 1976). In the Northwest Territories, health surveys in two Arctic communities also revealed higher serum cholesterol levels in the more "acculturated" group (Schaefer et al., 1980b).

Through a series of dietary, metabolic, and hemostatic studies conducted during five medical expeditions to the Umanak District of Greenland in the 1970s and early 1980s, Bang, Dyerberg, and colleagues proposed an elegant hypothesis linking dietary fatty acids, serum lipids, prostaglandin synthesis, and platelet aggregability in the development of IHD. Of critical importance in the underlying biological mechanism is the role played by omega-3 fatty acids (particularly eicosapentaenoic acid, or EPA) found in fish and marine mammals common in the Eskimo diet. EPA and other polyunsaturated fatty acids inhibit platelet aggregation and reduce plasma triglycerides and VLDL cholesterol [For a review of the Greenlandic studies, see Dyerberg (1989)]. Chemical analyses of adipose tissues in various Eskimo foods have also been done in the Canadian Arctic. Innis and Kuhnlein (1987) found substantial quantities of long-chain omega-3 fatty acids in land-based caribou.

A study of Tsimshian Indians on Vancouver Island found that 50 percent of calories in the "traditional" diet were derived from salmon, rich in EPA and docosahexaenoic (DHA) acid, another in the class of omega-3 fatty acids (Bates et al., 1985). They also had low levels of arachidonic acid (AA), an omega-6 fatty acid, which remain unchanged among those who had abandoned the traditional diet, Horrobin (1987) suggested that the low AA levels among Eskimos and Tsimshian Indians may be due to a genetically determined enzymatic deficiency or reduced activity. As AA is prothrombotic, its low level should reduce the risk of IHD. There is thus another example of the interaction of genetic and environmental factors in the etiology of chronic diseases.

Prevention and Control of Cardiovascular Diseases

Primary Prevention

Most public health authorities advocate primary prevention to reduce the prevalence of multiple risk factors. While smoking cessation, cholesterol reduction, control of hypertension, maintenance of ideal body weight, and regular exercise all appear to reduce the risk of IHD substantially, the efficacy of available strategies to modify personal risk behavior and lifestyle is variable, ranging from unknown to poor to fair for most factors, and good in the case of hypertension control and cholesterol reduction (Manson et al., 1992).

There are two basic approaches to the prevention of chronic diseases such as cardiovascular diseases—the population approach and the high-risk approach (Rose, 1985). The former aims at shifting the distribution of a particular risk factor (e.g., blood pressure, serum cholesterol) in the total population to a lower level. The latter is directed only at those individuals at the upper end of the distribution, who are selected for intervention. Although high-risk individuals can be identified, a greater proportion of all diseases in fact may occur among individuals not recognized as being at high risk. The population approach may thus have a greater impact on reducing the overall burden of disease.

Several large-scale, population-based demonstration projects have been tried in both North America and Europe, with varying degrees of success. Notable examples include the North Karelia (Finland), Stanford Five-Cities (California), Minnesota, and Pawtucket (Rhode Island) projects. These were primarily educational projects that used different communication strategies directed at the entire population (Blackburn, 1983). While there are scattered efforts by health professionals in individual communities to influence lifestyle, no large-scale, systematic primary prevention trial has yet been attempted and evaluated in a Native American population.

Changes in the diet are often included in health-promotion "packages." Several national bodies in both the United States and Canada have reviewed the extensive literature linking diet and health and have made recommendations for healthful diets. The U.S. Surgeon General suggested that the consumption of fats should be decreased, especially saturated fat and cholesterol; complex carbohydrates and fiber should be increased, and sodium decreased; and alcohol should be consumed in only moderate quantities (U.S. DHHS, Surgeon General's Report, 1988). The Canadian Government's recommendation was more specific; not more than 30 percent of energy from fat, and not more than 10 percent from saturated fats; and 55 percent from carbohydrates (Canada, DNHW, 1990). Both bodies emphasized the importance of adequate intake of energy and essential nutrients, and the maintenance of body weight. Dietary change is a matter of both personal choice and larger societal pressures. Effective strategies for behavioral change, particularly in ethnic groups such as Native Americans, must be directed at both the individual level through education and at the social level through such actions as protecting traditional subsistence activities, ensuring the availability of foods at affordable prices, and promoting the marketing of appropriate foods.

Efforts directed at adults may, in fact, have "missed the boat." While adults in any population carry the heaviest burden of IHD, there is considerable evidence from different populations to indicate that changes in risk factor levels such as blood pressure and serum cholesterol, as well as the atherosclerotic process itself, begin in childhood (Labarthe et al., 1991). Little research among Native American children directed at percursors of chronic diseases has been done. A survey of Onondaga school children (aged 5–16) in New York showed that 85 percent of the children had three or more cardiovascular risk factors (Botash et al., 1991). It would be prudent, even before definitive research data become available, to launch primary prevention programs directed at younger age groups, as recommended by such bodies as the World Health Organization (1990).

Secondary Prevention

The impact of some cardiovascular risk factors can be reduced through early detection and treatment. For hypertension, the benefit of early detection is well established. The Joint National Committee on Detection, Evaluation and Treatment of High Blood Pressure (1988) recommended blood pressure measurement at least once every one or two years. For those whose levels exceed established criteria, protocols exist to guide the clinician in retesting, additional laboratory evaluation, and a stepped-care approach to treatment, which may begin with behavioral and non-pharmacologic means. The SAIAN survey indicated that Native Americans did not differ substantially from the U.S. national population in terms of the frequency of blood pressure measurement. Generally the frequency increased with age, and was higher among women and among the better educated (Johnson and Taylor, 1991).

Cultural factors must be recognized (and reconciled) by health professionals within the Western biomedical tradition. Ethnographic studies of cultural knowledge of hypertension in some communities have provided important data on Native American concepts of disease causation, manifestation, and treatment. For example, in an Ojibwa community in southern Manitoba, Garro (1988) found that the cultural model can be at odds with the prevalent biomedical view on the chronicity of the illness and the importance of "compliance" with treatment. Hypertension is conceived by the Ojibwa as episodic in nature, accompanied by perceptible symptoms, and treatment is needed only when symptoms are present.

While the link between serum cholesterol and IHD appears strongly established, there is controversy over how best to reduce serum cholesterol levels in the general population. Some expert bodies have advocated population-wide screening, followed by dietary or drug interventions of selected positive screenees. A critical review by the Toronto Working Group on Cholesterol Policy recommended against this approach, since a substantial proportion of the population would be monitored and put on drug therapy, with dubious net gain for the individual or the health care system (Naylor et al., 1990).

5

Emergence of Chronic Diseases (II)

Obesity

Definition and Measurement of Obesity

Simply defined, obesity is the excess of body fat. While fat or adipose tissue is essential for a variety of physiological functions, its excess can lead to significant health problems. Many of the chronic diseases discussed in this and the previous chapter are associated with obesity: ischemic heart disease, hypertension, diabetes, gallbladder disease, and certain cancers. Obesity is associated with an increase in the size of fat cells (i.e., hypertrophy), and in cases of extreme obesity, an increase in the number of fat cells, or hyperplasia (National Institutes of Health Consensus Development Panel, 1985).

It has been recognized that the regional distribution of body fat and not simply overall obesity has important health implications. Fat cells around the waist and in the abdomen are more active metabolically than those in the thighs and buttocks, and a surfeit of the former—called *central, centripetal,* or *truncal* obesity—has emerged as an important risk factor for many chronic diseases, either in addition to, or instead of, overall obesity (Stern and Haffner, 1986).

A variety of methods are used to measure obesity (Gibson, 1990; Shephard, 1991). Physiological measures based on body density and isotope studies, often considered the "gold standard" of obesity measures, are cumbersome and so are not suitable for large population surveys. Indices based on height and weight are attractive because of their ease of measurement and reproducibility, but they do not measure fat directly, as muscle, bone, and edema all contribute to body weight. The body mass index (BMI), or Quetelet's index, is widely used in epidemiology. In most populations it correlates only minimally with height and thus is not affected by the "non-fat" component of body weight. On the other hand it correlates well with weight and body density measures. The correlation of BMI with such body composition indices as percent fat, fat mass, and fat-free mass was demonstrated in the Pima (Knowler et al., 1991).

Skinfold thicknesses provide more direct measures of body fat than height-and-weight-based indices, although they are technically more demanding and more liable to interobserver variation. There is also considerable variation in fat tissue deposits in different body sites. Skinfolds have also been shown to be highly correlated with densitometric indices of body fat.

Commonly used measures of regional fat patterning are the ratio of waist to hip circumference (WHR) and the ratio of subscapular to triceps skinfolds (STR). Studies have shown that these two indices are not highly correlated and are independent predictors of various measures of glucose and lipid metabolism (Haffner et al., 1987; Young and Sevenhuysen, 1989).

There are no universally accepted criteria for obesity, although various investigators have proposed guidelines based on risks of complications. For BMI, values of 25–30 have been defined as "overweight" and those over 30 as "obese." For WHR, the cut-off points for males and females are 0.9 and 0.8 (Bray, 1989).

Extent and Magnitude of the Problem

Ethnographic observations, clinical impressions, and limited survey data all support the conclusion that obesity is widespread among many groups of North American Indians (e.g., Gillum et al., 1980, 1984; Clifford et al., 1963; Terry and Bass, 1984; McIntyre and Shah, 1986; Young and Sevenhuysen, 1989; Broussard et al., 1991; Knowler et al., 1991). One study of the Navajos in the 1960s, however, showed a lower prevalence of obesity (Fulmer and Roberts, 1963), but more recently an increase in the prevalence in this population was also reported (Hall et al., 1991). In Canada, as recently as the 1940s, two surveys in Subarctic communities in the James Bay region and northern Manitoba revealed an Indian population hovering on the brink of starvation, with deficient energy and nutrient intakes (Vivian et al., 1948; Moore et al., 1946). By the 1970s, the Nutrition Canada (Canada DNHW, 1980) survey showed that Canadian Indians generally had much higher weight-for-age compared to Canadians nationally (Fig. 5.1).

Among the Pimas, the mean BMI by age has increased in successive periods between 1965 and 1988 in both adult men and women. In children, comparison of weight-for-height with data collected by the anthropologist Hrdlicka in the early 1900s also showed a temporal increase (Knowler et al., 1991).

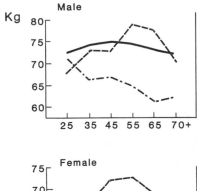

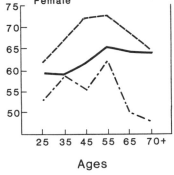

Kg

Male

————— Canadian national
—————— Canadian Indian
— · —— · Canadian Inuit

Figure 5.1. Mean weight-for-age: Canada, 1972, Indians, Inuit, and all Canadians.

Many of the tribes with a high prevalence of diabetes (discussed in the following section) also have a high prevalence of obesity.

In the United States, the Survey of American Indians and Alaska Natives (SAIAN) provided self-reported data on heights and weights in a nationally representative sample of adult Native Americans. The 85th and 95th percentile of the NHANES II reference for men and women age 20–29 yr were used as the criteria for overweight and obesity, respectively. [These correspond to BMI values of 27.8 in men and 27.3 in women for overweight, and 31.1 in men and 32.3 in women for obesity]. The prevalence of overweight and obesity in Native Americans exceeded that of U.S. all races in all age-sex groups (Fig. 5.2). Overall, the prevalence of overweight was 34 percent in Native men and 40 percent in Native women, compared to U.S. all-races rates of 24 percent (M) and 25 percent (F). Data from other sources indicated that the prevalence of overweight among both Native children and Native adolescents was also higher than the respective rates for U.S. all-races combined (Broussard et al., 1991).

Among the Inuit, a large number of anthropometric data were collected as part

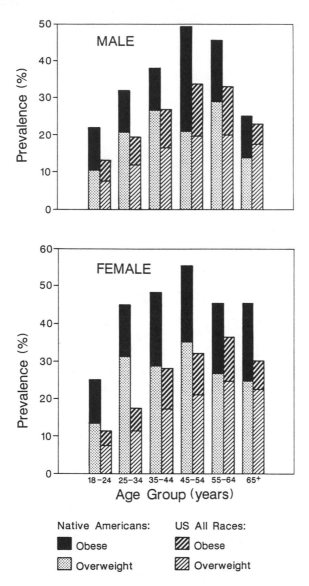

Figure 5.2. Prevalence of obesity: USA, 1987, Native American and U.S. all-race populations. NOTE: "Overweight" and "obese" categories are based on the 85th and 95th percentile of NHANES II reference for men and women age 20–29 years. These correspond to BMIs of 27.8 in males and 27.3 in females for "overweight" and 31.1 in males and 32.3 in females for "obese."

of the International Biological Program's Human Adaptability studies (Auger et al., 1980). In the Nutrition Canada survey, the Inuit sample showed that adults in all age groups and of both sexes were less heavy than either Canadian Indians or Canadians nationally (Canada DNHW, 1980). Schaefer's skinfold thickness data on over 1,000 Inuit in various parts of the central and eastern Arctic during the 1960s (Schaefer, 1977) also supported the general observation that obesity was less prevalent among the Inuit, which set them apart from the vast majority of Indians in North America.

Few data on fat distribution are available for Native American populations. Among the Cree-Ojibwa, overall, 38 percent of men had waist/hip ratio (WHR) greater than 0.99, compared to only 11 percent among women. If this were taken as the cut-off point for "central" obesity, then among men with BMI of over 30, 75 percent were of the central type, while among men with BMI between 26 and 30, 46 percent were of the central type. Central obesity was much less evident among women, where only 18 percent of those with BMI over 30 and 13 percent of those with BMI between 26 and 30 could be considered centrally obese (Young and Sevenhuysen, 1989). Among the Navajo, the mean WHR was quite high, even among nondiabetics: 0.96 among men and 0.89 among women (Hall et al., 1991).

Obesity is associated with higher risks of mortality from all causes, a fact well established in actuarial studies from large cohorts of enrollees in life insurance plans. Among Native Americans, data from the Pima indicated that below a BMI of 40, there was little variation in the age-adjusted mortality rate among males, which ranged from 17 to 25 deaths per 1000 person-years. The rate, however, increased substantially to 65/1000 if the BMI exceeded 40. Among females, the rate ranged from 9 to 14 per 1000 person-years and it varied little with increasing BMI (Pettitt et al., 1982).

Etiology and Risk Factors

Obesity can be regarded simplistically as an imbalance between caloric intake and energy expenditure. An excess of the former and/or a reduction in the latter, such as through physical inactivity, could lead to obesity. The precise relationship, particularly temporal sequence, is not always easily established. Few longitudinal studies that observe the development of obesity in a nonobese cohort and correlate its occurrence with different dietary patterns and physical activity levels have been conducted. The pathophysiological mechanisms of obesity are complex, involving a variety of regulatory hormones and intracellular enzymes and the actions of the autonomic nervous system. Among Native Americans, extensive metabolic studies have been conducted in only one tribe, the Pima, covering such aspects as fat cell morphology, glucose transport, lipid metabolism, and associated enzymes (Howard et al., 1991).

Accumulating evidence from a variety of twin, family, and adoption studies indicates that obesity is also to some extent genetically determined. Except for some rare syndromes, obesity is not inherited in mendelian fashion. It is typical of a multifactorial phenotype whose expression may be altered by many environmental factors. Genetic studies of obesity are complicated by the fact that there are different types of obesity in physiological terms and different methods of measurement. In their review, Bouchard and Pérusse (1988) estimated that when BMI was used as the measure, less than 10 percent of the variation could be attributed to genetic effect. The "heritability" of obesity was around 25 percent if one used measures of body fat, fat mass, and fat patterning.

In a small clinical study involving elaborate procedures of underwater weighing to determine body composition and needle biopsy to determine fat cell size, Abbott and Foley (1987) found that lean, prepubertal Pima children had larger abdominal, but not gluteal, adipocytes than whites. The large cell size was also associated with fasting glucose and insulin level but independent of BMI and percent body fat. The enlargement of abdominal fat cells may represent an early stage in the development of obesity and diabetes in this population.

That obesity in childhood predicts obesity in adulthood has not been demonstrated consistently, and depends on the age of onset of obesity and the type of indicators used (Johnston, 1985). What is not in dispute is that obesity in childhood is prevalent among Native Americans, as demonstrated in surveys among the Cherokees in North Carolina (Story et al., 1986), urban Natives in Minneapolis (Johnston et al., 1978), the Pima (Knowler et al., 1991) and the Navajo (Sugarman et al., 1990b). Among the Navajo, a secular increase was also observed compared to an earlier survey in 1955.

Maternal diabetes is an important determinant of obesity in the offspring. The offspring of women who were diabetic during pregnancy, regardless of the degree of maternal obesity, were more likely to be heavier at birth and to develop obesity during childhood and young adulthood than those born to nondiabetic or "prediabetic" women. (The unique longitudinal design of the Pima study allows such a designation for women who were not diabetic during the index pregnancy but subsequently developed diabetes.) Even if the birth weight was normal for gestational age, offspring of diabetic women still became heavier eventually (Pettitt et al., 1987).

A study of weight gain among the Pima showed that low 24-hour energy expenditure (which incorporates the metabolic rate at rest, the thermogenic effect of food, and the caloric cost of physical activity) increased fourfold the risk of gaining at least 7.5 kg over 2 years (Ravussin et al., 1988). There was also familial aggregation of low energy expenditure, which may contribute to the observed familial aggregation of obesity.

Prevention and Control Strategies

While clinical treatment of obesity is available (including such drastic measures as surgery), the control of the problem requires a public health approach. Education programs emphasizing behavioral change can be directed at individuals, families, schools, or other groups. Usually dietary change is the objective, which may be coupled with exercise or other multiple risk factor interventions. At the societal level, economic changes affecting food availability and food purchasing power may have favorable impact on the prevalence of obesity. While intuitively attractive, few of these approaches have been evaluated. Of eighteen intervention studies reviewed by Jackson and others (1991), only one study involved a Native American community. The program consisted of aerobic exercises and comprehensive health education from kindergarten to grade 12. The Zuni Diabetes Project, discussed in further detail later in this chapter, while directed at diabetes patients, is open to community members. It is also an exercise-based program aimed at weight control (Heath et al., 1991).

A prerequisite for any successful control program is the recognition of the existence of the problem and motivation for behavioral change. Although some societies in the past may have regarded obesity as a sign of wealth and honor, there is some evidence to suggest that overweight is now recognized by Native Americans as a health problem and that most obese persons do want to reduce weight. In a survey of Eastern Cherokee women, Terry and Bass (1984) found that over 70 percent of the respondents perceived themselves as overweight, and the majority of those were dissatisfied with their current weight. A similarly high proportion (75%) of women had engaged in weight reduction activities in the past, evenly distributed between self-prescribed diet, medically prescribed diet, drugs, and exercise.

Diabetes

Extent and Magnitude of the Problem

The prevalence of diabetes is known to vary widely between populations belonging to different geographical, cultural, and socioeconomic groups. As a population undergoes urbanization, modernization, or lifestyle changes, the prevalence of diabetes generally tends to increase (Jarrett, 1989). In 1974, the late

Dr. Kelly West, who can be considered the father of diabetes epidemiology, reviewed exhaustively the literature on diabetes among North American Indians as well as aboriginal populations in other parts of the world (West, 1974). Since that time the problem has received the attention of many researchers, and the literature on diabetes among North American Indians has grown substantially. While intensive epidemiologic and metabolic studies have been conducted in some tribes, particularly the Pima in the southwestern United States (Bennett et al., 1976; Knowler et al., 1990), nationwide surveys of the burden and impact of the disease have demonstrated wide geographical variation (Sievers and Fisher, 1985; Gohdes, 1986; Young et al., 1990b). Although the factors that contribute to these differences are not well understood, they probably reflect the differential effects of genetic susceptibility, overall level of "acculturation," and the contributions of specific risk factors such as physical activity, diet, and obesity.

Diabetes among North American Indians is overwhelmingly of the non-insulin-dependent type (NIDDM), previously called maturity-onset or type 2 diabetes, as distinct from the insulin-dependent type (IDDM). Among the Pimas, even among young diabetics under the age of 25, detailed clinical and laboratory studies have characterized them as NIDDM cases not associated with pancreatic islet cell antibodies, ketoacidosis, and dependence on insulin for survival (Knowler et al., 1979). While many NIDDM patients are treated with insulin, few are truly insulin-dependent. In Manitoba, a trend toward earlier onset of NIDDM during the young teen years has been observed (Dean et al., 1992). Although exceedingly rare, confirmed cases of IDDM have been reported in the aboriginal population (e.g., Dean and Carson, 1989). Unless otherwise specified, all discussion on diabetes in this chapter refers to NIDDM.

Table 5.1 summarizes the regionally based studies on physician-diagnosed diabetes in North America. It should be emphasized that the methodologies used in these studies varied widely, and that no single set of diagnostic criteria was uniformly applied.

In these studies, the comparative group was most often the national, all-race, or white USA/Canada population. Some studies provided local non-native "controls." For example, in southwestern Ontario, the age-adjusted prevalence rate among Indians was 6.7 times that of whites using the same clinic (Evers et al., 1987). The Pimas in Arizona have the world's highest documented frequency of diabetes, with an age-sex-adjusted prevalence 13 times and an incidence 19 times that of the predominantly white population of Rochester, Minnesota (Knowler et al., 1978).

A national estimate of the prevalence of self-reported diabetes among Native Americans can be obtained from the Survey of American Indians and Alaska

Table 5.1 Regional Studies of Diabetes Prevalence among Native Americans[a]

Authors	Years	Methods[b]	Location/Tribe[c]	Crude Prevalence (%)
A. Arctic				
Mouratoff et al. (1967, 1973)	1962	Survey: 2 hr OGT 100 gm load (n = 705, age 20+)	10 Eskimo villages, western Alaska (2167)	2-hr BG $\geq$ 8.3 mmol/L 1962: M (0.7) F (7.2)
	1972	(n = 320, adults)	6 villages retested	1972: M (5.0) F (9.4)
Dippe et al. (1976)	1970s	Survey: 2 hr OGT 75 gm load (n = 335, age 10+)	Aleuts Pribilof Islands, AK	Known cases + 2-hr PG $\geq$ 11.1 mmol/L Age 10+ (7.2), 40+ (16.4)
Schraer et al. (1988)	1985	Case registry	Eskimos in Alaska (39308) Aleuts in Alaska (9314)	*Total* *0–34* *35–64* *65+* 0.5 0.04 1.2 3.6 1.5 0.15 3.5 12.4
Young et al. (1992)	1987	Case registry	Inuit in NT (18733)	*Total* *25–44* *45–64* *65+* 0.3 0.3 0.7 1.0
B. Subarctic				
Mouratoff et al. (1969)	1962	Survey: 2 hr OGT 100 gm load (n = 360, age 20+)	Athapaskans, various tribes 7 villages, AK	Known cases + 2-hr BG $\geq$ 8.3 mmol/L Age 20+ (1.3)
Szathmary/ Holt (1983)	1979	Survey: 2 hr OGT 100 gm load (n = 157, age 20+)	Dogrib in 3 villages, NWT	No known clinical case 2-hr PG $\geq$ 11.1 mmol/L Age 20+ (9.6)
Young et al. (1985)	1983	Case registry	30 Cree/Ojibwa communities northern ON/MB (14000)	*Total* *0–24* *25–64* *65+* 2.8 0.2 7.6 9.6
Schraer et al. (1988)	1985	Case registry	Athapaskans in Interior Service Unit, AK (8522)	All ages (0.9)

continued

Table 5.1 Regional Studies of Diabetes Prevalence among Native Americans[a] (continued)

Authors	Years	Methods[b]	Location/Tribe[c]	Crude Prevalence (%)			
				Total	*25–44*	*45–64*	*65+*
Young et al. (1992)	1987	Case registry	Athapaskans, various tribes				
			NWT (11194)	0.6	1.1	1.2	1.6
			YT (4249)	0.7	0.5	1.6	6.4
Young et al. (1990b)	1987	Case registry	Algonkians	All ages:		*Population*	*Prevalence*
			N. Ojibwa/Saulteaux, ON,MB			15774	3.3
			Woods/Swampy Cree, ON,MB,SK			32980	2.1
			Attikamek, QC			3178	2.3
			Montagnais, QC			7842	3.1
			Athapaskans				
			Chipewyan, MB,SK,AB,NT			8308	0.6
			Beaver/Sekani, BC,AB			2128	0.3
			Carrier/Chilcotin/Tahltan, BC			6163	0.4

C. Northwest Coast

Authors	Years	Methods[b]	Location/Tribe[c]	Crude Prevalence (%)			
Schraer et al. (1988)	1985	Case registry	Tlingit, Tsimshian, Haida in 2 Service Units, Alaska	All ages (1.6)			
Freeman et al. (1989)	1987	Case registry	3 reservations WA (5175) Makah/Quinault/Lummi	All ages: Makah (2.6), Quinault (2.8), Lummi (2.1)			
Young et al. (1990b)	1987	Case registry	Indian reserves in BC:	All ages:		*Population*	*Prevalence*
			Wakashans: Haisla/Heiltsuk/Kwakiutl/Nootka			6217	0.9
			Tsimshians: Gitksan/Niska/Tsimshian			6129	1.1
			Haidans: Haida			864	0.9
			Salishans: Comox/Bella Coola Cowichan/ Puntlatch/Songish/Semiahmoo/Squamish/ Seechelt			9971	1.1

D. Plateau

				Population	Prevalence
Freeman et al. (1989)	1987	Case registry	5 reservations WA, OR, ID: Spokane, Colville, Yakima, Nez Perce, Umatilla (15696)		
			All ages: Spokane (3.2), Colville (3.5), Yakima (3.8), Nez Perce (7.6), Umatilla (3.7)	8854	0.9
Young et al. (1990b)	1987	Case registry	Indian reserves in BC: Salishans: Lillooet/Shuswap Ntlakyapamuk/ Okanagan; Kootenaians: Kootenay	372	1.3

E. Plains

				Population	Prevalence
West (1974)	Early 1970s	Case registry	Oklahoma various IHS units: Cheyenne-Arapaho (1000); Age 35+ (19.5)		
West (1974)	Early 1970s	Survey: 2 hr OGT 75 gm load (age 30+)	Oklahoma various IHS units: Kiowa/Comanche (n = 80); Age 30+ (14.0) 2 hr PG $\geq$ 9.4 mmol/L		
Brosseau et al. (1979)	1978	Case registry	Fort Berthold, ND (3719) (1682 full-blood) Three affiliated tribes; < 35 (0.7); 35+ (22.3) [full-blood]; Age 35+ Mandan (39.0), Arickara (22.8), Hidatsa (21.2)		
Lang (1985)	1983	Case registry	Sioux reservation, ND (657 age 35+); Age 35+ (24)		
Young et al. (1990b)	1987	Case registry	Athapaskans: Sarcee, AB — All ages:	704	3.4
			Siouans: Dakota, AB,SK,MB	6223	2.8
			Assinboin, SK	1818	2.1
			Algonkians: Blackfoot, AB	9231	2.1
			Plains Cree, AB,SK	31127	1.6
			Plains Ojibwa, MB,SK	7392	2.6

continued

Table 5.1 Regional Studies of Diabetes Prevalence among Native Americans[a] (continued)

Authors	Years	Methods[b]	Location/Tribe[c]	Crude Prevalence (%)
F. Northeast				
Doeblin et al. (1969)	1967	Survey: 1 hr OGT 75 gm load (n = 209, age 25 +)	Seneca Cattaraugus res. NY	Known cases + 1 hr PG ≥ 11.1 mmol/L age 25+ (33.5)
West (1974)	Early 1970s	Case registry	Oklahoma various IHS units: Kickapoo (520) Sauk/Fox	All ages (5.4) Age 30 + (16) Age 30 + (16.0)
Montour/ Macaulay (1985)	1981	Case registry	Mohawks, Kahnawake, QC (Total 5163, age 45–64, 544)	Age 45–64 (12.0)
Evers et al. (1987)	1985	Case registry	2 southwest ON communities Oneida, Chippewa, Delaware (1179)	All ages (9.8) Age 35–64 (range 15–45) Age 65 + (>35)
Young et al. (1990b)	1987	Case registry	Iroquoians: Huron, QC Mohawk, ON Oneida, ON Six Nations res. ON Algonkians: Algonquins, QC Malecite/Micmac, NB,PE,NS Ojibwa/Ottawa/Delaware, ON	*All ages* *Population* *Prevalence* 772 2.1 6051 4.0 1495 6.2 7199 4.0 3639 4.3 12912 3.6 12756 4.9
G. Great Basin				
Bartha et al. (1973)	1970	Survey: 2 hr OGT 75 gm load (n = 243 age (15 +)	2 Washoe communities NV, CA Paiute, Fort McDermitt, NV	Known cases + 2 hr PG ≥ 11.1 mmol/L Washoe 15–34(2.2) 35 + (12.1) Paiute 15–34(1.3) 35 + (22.2

Reference	Year(s)	Method	Location (n)	Results
Bennett et al. (1976)	1960s	Survey: 2-hr OGT 75 gm load	Washoe (n = 66) Paiute (n = 54)	Age 35+, 2hr PG ≥ 8.9 mmol/L Washoe (16.9), Paiute (25.9)
Freeman et al. (1989)	1987	Case registry	2 reservations ID and OR Shoshone-Bannock (4973) Northern Paiute (3110)	All ages: Shoshone-Bannock (4.9), Northern Paiute (3.3)

H. Southeast

Reference	Year(s)	Method	Location (n)	Results
Johnson/ McNutt (1964)	1960–63	Survey: 2 hr OGT 100 gm load (n = 171, all ages)	Alabama-Coushatta res., TX (600)	Known cases + 2 hr BG ≥ 6.7 mmol/L All ages (9.7)
Mayberry/ Lindeman (1963)	1960	Survey: 2 hr OGT (n = 302, age 15+)	Seminole County, OK	Known cases + 2 hr BG ≥ 7.2 mmol/L Age 15+ (9.0)
Elston et al. (1974)	1964–66	Survey: 1 hr OGT 75 gm load (n = 471, age 6+)	Seminole 2 reservations, FL 1 county, OK	Known cases + 1 hr PG ≥ 11.1 mmol/L Florida (16.1), Oklahoma (25.8)
Westfall/ Rosenbloom (1971)	1969	Survey: 2 hr OGT 1.75 gm/kg body wt (n = 118, age 2+)	Seminole Big Cypress res. FL	Known cases + 2 hr BG ≥ 7.8 mmol/L Age 2+ (13.2)
Stein et al. (1965)	1964	Survey: 2 hr OGT 1 gm/kg body wt (n = 448, age 35+)	Cherokee res., NC (1225)	Known cases + 2 hr BG ≥ 8.3 mmol/L Age 35+ (29.0), 35–64 (28.2), 65+ (33.8)
West (1974)	1960s 1970s	Survey: 2 hr OGT 75 gm load or 1 gm/kg body wt (age 30+)	Oklahoma various IHS unit Cherokee (n = 124) Seminole/Creek (n = 89)	Age 30+ (20.2) 2 hr BG ≥ 150 mg/100 ml (19.0) 1 hr PG ≥ 200 mg/100 ml
West (1974)	1960s 1970s	Case registry	Oklahoma various IHS units: Chickasaw (2300) Cherokee (4000) Choctaw (2900) Shawnee	Age 35+ (13.5) Age 35+ (13.3) Age 35+ (17.2) Age 30+ (19.0)

continued

Table 5.1 Regional Studies of Diabetes Prevalence among Native Americans[a] (continued)

Authors	Years	Methods[b]	Location/Tribe[c]	Crude Prevalence (%)
I. Southwest				
Henry et al. (1969)	1960s	Survey: 2 hr OGT 75 gm load (n = 182, age 5+)	Cocopahs, Yuma County, AZ	Known cases + 2 hr PG ≥ 11.1 mmol/L Age 5+ (12.1)
Prosnitz/ Mandell (1967)	1965	Case registry	Tuba City IHS unit, AZ Navajo (15000), Hopi (3000)	All ages: Navajo (0.5), Hopi (0.8)
Bennett et al. (1976)	1971	Survey: 2 hr OGT 75 gm load	Apache/White River (n = 268) Apache/San Carlos (n = 317) Navajo (n = 55) Upland Yumans (n = 313) Cocopah (n = 79) Papago (n = 365) Pima (n = 898) Zuni (n = 292)	Age 35+, 2 hr PG ≥ 8.9 mmol/L (11.0) (24.8) (12.8) (29.9) (33.3) (42.3) (49.6) (31.3) 2 hr PG ≥ 10.0 mmol/L
Knowler et al. (1978, 1990)	1965–88	Survey: 2 hr OGT 75 gm load (n = 3733, age 5+)	Pima, Gila River Res., AZ 3 periods 1965/72, 1973/80, 1981–88	Total age 5+ (13.7), 5–34 (3.2) Age 35–64 (42.4), 65+ (41.1) Most recent period, age 55+ (>60)
Long (1978)	1975–76	Case registry	Zuni Res., NM (6305)	All ages (4.3) <25 (0.1) 25–44 (6.0) 45–64 (23.9) 65+ (26.0)

				All ages	<35	35+
Carter et al. (1989)	1985	Case registry	20 tribes in NM:			
			Rio Grand Pueblos (15747)	5.7	0.5	21.3
			Zuni (7057)	8.0	1.3	28.2
			Apache/Jicarilla (2176)	3.0	0.7	9.8
			Apache/Mescalero (2256)	4.4	0.5	16.4
			Navajo/Alamo (1408)	4.6	0.7	16.5
Sugarman/ Percy (1989)	1986–87	Survey: RBG + FBG (n = 494, age 20–74)	Navajo Res., AZ	20–44 (9.9) 45–54 (8.5) 55–64 (12.8) 65–74 (17.7)		
Sugarman et al. (1990a)	1986–87	Case registry	Navajo Res., AZ (176321)	All ages (3.2), 45 + (16.9)		

[a]Based on published studies only; studies based on random blood sugar or urine tests only excluded; only population-based prevalence included, data presented as proportion of hospital admissions excluded; some recalculations performed; where sufficient data were presented, prevalence was readjusted using WHO (1985) criteria

[b]All glucose values in SI units: 6.7 mmol/L = 120 mg/100 ml; 7.2 = 130; 7.8 = 140; 8.3 = 150; 8.9 = 160; 9.4 = 170; 10.0 = 180; 11.1 = 200; 12.2 = 220. M, male; F, female; OGT, oral glucose tolerance test; BG, whole blood glucose; PG, plasma/serum glucose. *U.S. states:* AZ, Arizona; AK, Alaska; CA, California; FL, Florida; ID, Idaho; NM, New Mexico; NV, Nevada; OK, Oklahoma; OR, Oregon; TX, Texas. *Canadian provinces/territories:* AB, Alberta; BC, British Columbia; MB, Manitoba; NB, New Brunswick; NT, Northwest Territories; NS, Nova Scotia; ON, Ontario; PE, Prince Edward Island; QC, Quebec; SK, Saskatchewan; YT, Yukon Territory.

[c]Figures in parentheses refer to population, total or age-specific

Native (SAIAN) of 1987 (Fig. 5.3). Overall, the prevalence was higher than the U.S. all-race rate (Johnson and Taylor, 1991).

To determine the true prevalence of diabetes, oral glucose tolerance surveys are necessary. According to the National Health and Nutrition Examination Survey in the United States during 1976–80, it was found that for every known case of diabetes, there was at least one undiagnosed case (Harris et al., 1987). Table 5.1 also summarizes these screening studies in a variety of tribes. Again, differences in survey methods—for example, the amount of glucose load used and the diagnostic cut-off points—make comparisons over time and between studies difficult to interpret. With the evolution and international acceptance of criteria such as those proposed by the World Health Organization (1985), the definition and classification of diabetes and impaired glucose tolerance has become standardized.

Studies during the 1960s and 1970s suggested that the Eskimo/Inuit appeared to have been "spared" the diabetes "epidemic" (Scott and Griffith, 1957; Mouratoff et al., 1967; Mouratoff and Scott, 1973; Sagild et al., 1966). Surveys during the 1980s indicated that, while the prevalence was still low relative to other Amerindian groups, it had nonetheless increased when compared to the prevalence two decades earlier (Schraer et al., 1988).

Clinical studies among hospitalized Inuit patients showed that while one-half

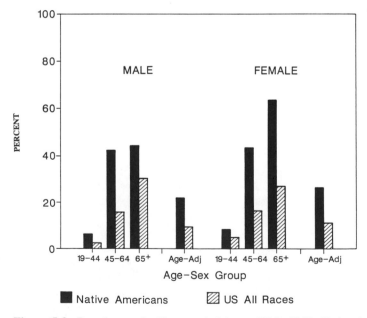

Figure 5.3. Prevalence of self-reported diabetes: USA, 1987, Native American and U.S. all-race populations.

reacted abnormally to oral glucose tolerance testing, all responded normally to an intravenous glucose load (Schaefer, 1968). Schaefer hypothesized that the release of insulin following carbohydrate ingestion in anticipation of a rise in blood glucose level was lacking in a high proportion of Inuit not adapted to a high carbohydrate diet. By preceding the oral glucose tolerance test with a protein meal, the blood sugar and serum insulin response became normal (Schaefer, 1968; Schaefer et al., 1972). This finding has important implications for any screening survey for diabetes among the Inuit and other Native peoples with similar diets.

Regional variation in the burden of diabetes among Native Americans is evident in the United States, whether ASMR, prevalence, or incidence is used as the indicator (Fig. 5.4). In general, the Alaska, Navajo, and Portland IHS areas showed the lowest rates, whereas the Aberdeen, Tucson, and Phoenix areas showed the highest. This is in keeping with the observations that Eskimos and Athapaskan Indians are at the lowest risk of diabetes compared to other tribes. In the Portland Area, covering Washington, Oregon, and Idaho, the age-adjusted prevalence was significantly different among tribes belonging to the Northwest Coast (4.5%), Plateau (7.2%), and Great Basin (8.8%) culture areas (Freeman et al., 1989). Within Alaska, which overall has the lowest prevalence, intertribal differences could be observed as well. The prevalence among the Aleuts (2.7%) was higher than among the Indians (2.2%), whose prevalence was higher than the Eskimos (0.9%). Among the Indians, tribes in southeastern Alaska, belonging to the Northwest Coast culture, had rates higher than subarctic Athapaskans. Among the Eskimos, rates also differed between Inupiaq and Yupik areas (Schraer et al., 1988).

The extent of geographical variation in diabetes prevalence among Native Canadians was also demonstrated in a national review of diagnosed cases undertaken in 1987 (Young et al., 1990b). The age-sex adjusted rate varied among the Indians from a low of 0.8 percent in the Northwest Territories to a high of 8.7 percent in the Atlantic region. Among the Inuit, the prevalence was only 0.4 percent. Most cases occurred in middle-aged or older individuals.

In comparison to non-Natives, the age-sex adjusted prevalence of diabetes in Native Canadians was higher in all but three regions (Fig. 5.5). The 1978 Canada Health Survey and the 1985 General Social Survey gave self-reported rates of diabetes (for all ages) as 1.7 percent and 2.4 percent, respectively. Only in British Columbia, the Yukon, and the Northwest Territories were Native diabetes rates lower than these. In other regions, Native Canadian rates were 2 to 5 times higher than in all other Canadians.

Prevalence rates also varied according to language family, culture area, latitude, longitude, and geographical isolation. An ecologic analysis was performed with the crude prevalence of individual communities regressed upon independent

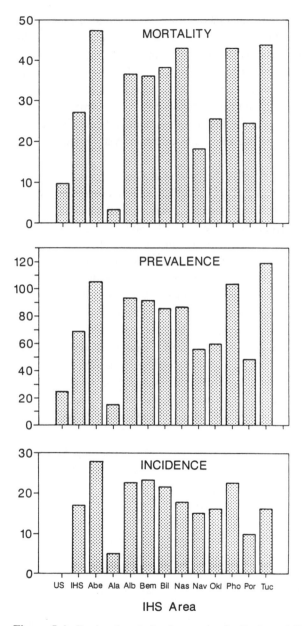

Figure 5.4. Regional variation in age-standardized mortality, prevalence and incidence of diabetes among Native Americans, USA, 1980–1987. NOTE: ASMR expressed as per 100,000; prevalence and incidence rates expressed as per 1,000.

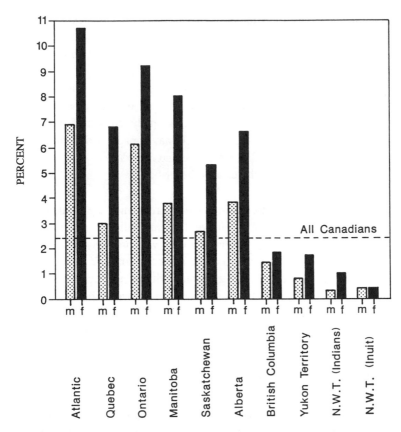

Figure 5.5. Regional variation in age-standardized prevalence of diabetes among Native Americans, Canada, 1987.

variables that included longitude, latitude, geographic isolation, and composite language phylum-culture area predictors. Six predictors ranked in decreasing order of importance, explained 48 percent of the variation in diabetes prevalence: latitude, Northeast-Algonkian, Northeast-Iroquoian, Subarctic-Algonkian, Plains-Siouan, and Plains-Algonkian. All these groups had rates significantly greater than that found in the reference group of Arctic-Eskimoan in the multiple regression analysis. The findings from this national survey support the conclusion that the distribution of diabetes among Native Canadians is influenced by both genetic and environmental factors.

From a continental perspective, the large number of tribes for which prevalence estimates are available (summarized in Table 5.1) can be grouped into three categories, as follows:

1. A low-prevalence group can be defined as those in which the all-age prevalence is <1 percent or adult (age 35+) prevalence is <5 percent, using a

registry of known cases, or adult prevalence is <10 percent using OGTT screening. Included in this group are the Eskimo/Inuit, various subarctic Athapaskans, the Aleut, various Northwest Coast tribes in British Columbia and Alaska, and the Navajo in the 1960s.

2. A high-prevalence group includes those in which the all-age prevalence is >5 percent and the adult prevalence >15 percent, using registry data, or adult prevalence >30 percent using OGTT screening. Included in this group are various tribes in the Southwest such as the Pima, Papago, Cocopah, Zuni, and Yuma, and the Iroquoian tribes Cherokee and Seneca.

3. A medium-prevalence group includes all other tribes.

Statistical data indicating time trends in diabetes prevalence are limited since few groups have been continuously monitored longitudinally for any length of time. The observation by West (1974) that diabetes was probably unknown or extremely rare among North American Indians prior to World War II seems to be correct, even allowing for changes in the availability of, and accessibility to, health services. Among the Pima, an increase in prevalence in both sexes has been observed between 1981–88, 1973–80, and 1965–72 (Knowler et al., 1990). A review of various studies done since the 1930s among the Navajos showed that, even among this group, which has generally lower prevalence than other tribes in the Southwest, the prevalence of diabetes has also increased (Sugarman et al., 1990a). The only national trend data available are those relating to diabetes mortality (Fig. 5.6).

Some indirect evidence supports the suggestion that diabetes is a health problem of relatively recent origin. The mean duration of disease among Mohawk diabetics was less than 7 years (Montour et al., 1989). Among the Cree-Ojibwa about half of all existing and still-living cases have been diagnosed in the last 5 years of a 25-year period (Young et al., 1985). Prevalence, as a function of both incidence and survival, can be expected to increase over time in nonlethal, chronic illnesses of long duration. Among the Pima, one of the few populations (Native or non-Native) where the incidence of diabetes has been estimated, a temporal trend was also observed. The incidence of diabetes during 1975–85 was 1.5 times that in 1965–75, controlling for age and sex (Knowler et al., 1990).

An estimate of the *incidence* of diabetes in all IHS areas during 1987 was obtained by counting unduplicated individuals who had an outpatient visit associated with a diabetes diagnosis but no similar diagnosis in the previous three years. The total age-adjusted incidence was 17.1 for all age groups and 21.7/ 1000 for all persons aged 15 and older (Valway et al., unpublished data, 1989). Among the Navajos, a group known for its low prevalence relative to other Southwestern tribes, the incidence in the late 1980s was estimated to be 9.9/

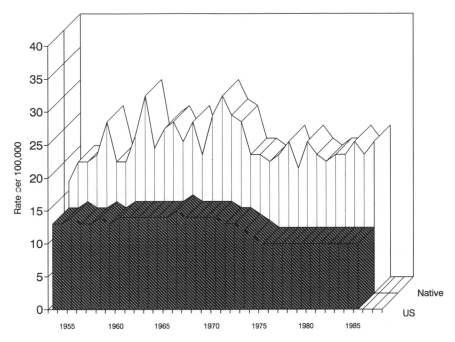

Figure 5.6. Age-standardized mortality rate for diabetes: USA, 1955–87, Native American and U.S. all-race populations.

1000 person-years age 20 and above (Sugarman et al., 1992). The only comparable U.S. all-race data are based on self-reports in the annual National Health Interview Surveys. For 1987, the incidence rate was estimated to be 2.9/1000, all ages and both sexes combined (CDC Division of Diabetes Translation, 1990).

Etiology and Risk Factors

Diabetes is an example of a chronic disease with a multifactorial etiology. The older literature has been summarized in West's monograph (1978), and more recent studies have also been reviewed (Jarrett, 1989). To date, epidemiological evidence of varying consistency has implicated heredity, obesity, physical activity, diet, and metabolic factors as potential risk factors.

Despite the large number of descriptive studies, whether based on physician-diagnosed cases or oral glucose tolerance surveys, relatively little is known about the risk factors for diabetes among Amerindians, with the exception of the Pimas in Arizona (Knowler et al., 1990).

Native Americans are genetically heterogeneous, and they live in diverse physical and sociocultural environments. The frequencies of genes involved in predisposition to diabetes may vary not just within, but also between, Native populations. Studies in the United States comparing Indians with non-Indians have shown that Indian ancestry is an important risk factor. Some have even suggested that the degree of Indian admixture has a dose-response relationship to the presence of diabetes. Among Mexican-Americans in Texas, the amount of Amerindian genetic admixture estimated from skin color (measured by light reflectance using a portable spectrophotometer) correlated with diabetes prevalence (Gardner et al., 1984). In one reservation in North Dakota inhabited by the Three Affiliated Tribes—Mandan, Arikara and Hidatsa—a gradation in the prevalence of diagnosed diabetes was demonstrated between full-blooded Indians (22%), those with between ⅛ and ⅝ Indian heritage (15%), and those with ⅛ or less (4%) (Brosseau et al. 1979). Among the Pima, those with full heritage (based on self-report) had an age-adjusted prevalence of 36 percent, compared to 29 percent among those with half heritage. When European admixture was estimated with the haplotype $Gm^{3;5,13,14}$, a strong inverse association with diabetes was observed (Knowler et al., 1988). However, among Mexican-Americans in Starr County, Texas, individual Amerindian admixture estimates based on sixteen markers (including such loci as ABO, MNS, and Rh) did not correlate with the prevalence of diabetes (Hanis et al., 1986).

The mode of inheritance of diabetes is complex, and has been likened to a "nightmare" by James Neel, a noted geneticist. A large body of data exists [see the reviews by O'Rahilly et al. (1988) and Granner and O'Brien (1992)]. The evidence for a genetic role in diabetes in a variety of populations can be found in studies of concordance in twins, familial aggregation, and the association with genetic markers. It should be noted that familial aggregation by itself does not necessarily require a genetic explanation; common exposure to environmental factors such as diet and infections during childhood may have been responsible.

Among the Pima, the risk of diabetes was 2.3 times as high among those with one diabetic parent, and 3.9 times as high among those with two diabetic parents, compared to those with neither parent diabetic, adjusting for age and obesity (Knowler et al., 1981). The age at which diabetes developed in the parents is also important. The prevalence of diabetes was highest among those whose parents both developed diabetes before age 45 ("early"), followed by those with one parent "early," either parent "late" (i.e., after age 45), and least of all, both parents nondiabetic (Knowler et al., 1990). In the Pimas, familial aggregation of insulin resistance, believed to be the underlying metabolic defect in NIDDM, has also been demonstrated (Lillioja et al., 1987). Among Indians in Oklahoma, the prevalence of diabetes among siblings was higher in families with parental diabetes than in those where neither parents were diabetic. There was, however, no difference between those with only one parent and those with both parents diabetic (Lee et al., 1985).

The bimodality of fasting and two-hour glucose found in the Pima and other extreme-high-prevalence populations has been explained on the basis that the second peak was the result of a major gene effect (Knowler et al., 1990). Pedigree analyses in the Oklahoma Seminole and Pima populations appeared to support the autosomal dominance mode of transmission (Elston et al., 1974; Yamashita et al., 1984). In most other Native American populations, glucose levels are unimodal, and pedigree analysis in some tribes—for example, the Dogrib— did not support the existence of a major gene but suggested that action of many genes, some of which were dominant, and that their action was enhanced by intragenerational environmental effects (Szathmary, 1985).

While certain HLA markers (such as DR3 and DR4) have been found to be associated with IDDM (Thomson, 1988), no specific markers have been identified for NIDDM which are common for different ethnic groups. Scattered reports from a variety of populations have implicated markers on four human chromosomes: Rh on chromosome 1, Gc on 4, HLA and GLO on 6, and Hp and PGP on 16. If these associations were real, then either polygenic inheritance or genetic heterogeneity of NIDDM is indicated. In the Pima, diabetics had 2.2 times the prevalence of the HLA-A2 marker compared to nondiabetics (Williams et al., 1981). Positive associations have also been found for the red cell enzyme phosphoglycolate phosphatase (PGP) in the Pima (Cadien et al., 1979) and Dogrib (Szathmary, 1985). Another locus on the same chromosome, haptoglobin (Hp), has been associated with Mexican Americans, perhaps reflecting their Amerindian ancestry (Stern et al., 1986).

Recent advances in molecular biology permit the identification of genes at the DNA level that may be involved in the development of NIDDM. Various candidate genes, while not themselves believed to be the cause of diabetes, are nevertheless closely related to the regulation of some aspect of carbohydrate metabolism (Granner and O'Brien, 1992). Examples include the insulin gene, insulin receptor gene, glucose transporter gene, and genes for various neuropeptides within the endocrine pancreas. Research to date among the Pima, however, has not shown an association of diabetes with polymorphic alleles at the insulin gene (Knowler et al., 1984). Direct sequencing of the insulin receptor from cells obtained from Pimas also found no difference between diabetics and nondiabetics (Moller et al., 1989).

In most descriptive studies of diabetes, the prevalence tends to increase with age. The sex ratio varies from population to population, with a preponderance of female cases in most North American Indian tribes studied (Sievers and Fisher, 1985). The incidence of diabetes also varies with age. In the Pimas, the incidence rate tends to peak in late middle age and decline in the older age groups (Knowler et al., 1990). Various explanations can be posited for such a pattern. It is likely that older people had not been subjected to the intense exposure to those environmental risk factors that had only become prevalent in the post-

World War II era. Another explanation is that age operates as a cofactor or promoting factor for the other risk factors of diabetes in early life only. Yet a third possibility is that the pool of susceptible persons among those who had not already become diabetic rapidly shrinks with rising age.

Among the potential environmental risk factors for diabetes established from various large-scale epidemiological studies, obesity is considered the strongest. The high prevalence of obesity in many North American Indian populations was reviewed in the previous section.

In a review of diabetes and obesity, Barrett-Connor (1989) pointed out the complexity of the relationship and listed several issues that remain to be clarified: the existence of a threshold effect; the relative importance of current versus previous obesity, childhood versus adult-onset obesity, and degree versus duration of obesity; the independent contributions of overall obesity and regional fat distribution; and the role of weight loss in reducing the risk of diabetes and its complications. Data on North American Indians are limited, and few of these issues have been resolved. With the exception of the Pima, much of the current evidence is cross-sectional rather than longitudinal, and thus deals with factors associated with *being* diabetic rather than with *becoming* diabetic.

The Pima study demonstrated a continuous increase in risk with increasing body mass index. While *incidence* of diabetes was strongly related to preceding obesity, the *prevalence* of diabetes was not associated with concurrent obesity. It should be noted that even among Pimas with low BMI (20–25), the age-sex-adjusted incidence rate of diabetes was still 8 times that of whites. Obesity also interacted with parental diabetes such that the effect of obesity on diabetes incidence was strongest when both parents were diabetic, compared to those with only one parent and neither parent diabetic (Knowler et al., 1981).

Among the Cree-Ojibwa, several factors have been found to be associated with diabetic status or high plasma glucose levels (as measured by fasting plasma glucose and glycosylated hemoglobin) on multivariate analyses. While age, triglycerides, and BMI were predictive of diabetic status, fasting plasma glucose, and glycosylated hemoglobin levels, education, and waist/hip ratio were associated with elevated glycosylated hemoglobin levels only (Young et al., 1990a).

The independent role of fat distribution, particularly "central" or "centripetal" fat, in predicting diabetes or glucose intolerance has been demonstrated in a variety of populations, including the Dogrib Indians in the Northwest Territories (Szathmary and Holt, 1983). In a matched case-control study among the Oneida and Ojibwa in southwestern Ontario, central obesity was also found to be associated with diabetes, but among men only (Evers et al., 1989). Among the Navajos, those belonging to the highest of three categories of central obesity (based on the waist/hip ratio) had 3.6 times the odds of being diabetic compared to those at the lowest, and those at the medium level had a 2.2 times higher risk than those at the lowest, age and body mass index having been adjusted for (Hall et al., 1991).

The etiologic role of dietary factors in the development of diabetes is not clearly defined from the epidemiological literature (West, 1978). Specific nutrients such as carbohydrates, sucrose, fat, and lack of fiber have been implicated, as well as total caloric intake. Studies examining the relationships between diet and disease are complex and need to surmount potential methodological problems in terms of data collection, analysis, and interpretation (Willett, 1990).

Patterns of dietary change, particularly the substitution of "modern" for "traditional" diets, have been demonstrated in many Native populations (discussed in Chapter 1), and these can be correlated with the prevalence of diabetes in cross-sectional, between-population studies. However, one would prefer to confirm the diet-diabetes association in within-population, prospective cohort studies. To date, only the Pima study has offered this type of data. Of 187 nondiabetic women age 25–44 at baseline, significantly higher rates of diabetes developed in those who initially consumed more total carbohydrates and starch (Bennett et al., 1984). It should be cautioned that strong correlations exist between individual nutrients, as well as between specific nutrients and overall caloric intake. Various methods have been proposed to disentangle these intercorrelations, such as the determination of "calorie-adjusted" nutrient intakes (Willett, 1990).

Among Canadian Natives, the Cree-Ojibwa study of diabetics showed a "paradoxically" higher intake of calorie-adjusted proteins and lower carbohydrates than nondiabetics. As a cross-sectional survey, it was impossible to determine if such dietary differences preceded the onset of diabetes or were the consequences of the disease process and its management. Energy intake per unit body weight, however, was lower among diabetics, reflecting their lower physical activity level (Young et al., 1990a). Among the Dogribs, dietary differences between villages at different levels of acculturation were demonstrated, but they had little influence on the plasma glucose levels (Szathmary et al., 1987).

While the physiologic effect of exercise on glucose and insulin metabolism has been well demonstrated, the epidemiologic evidence supporting the role of physical inactivity as a risk factor for diabetes is sparse and inconsistent, and much of it is based on cross-sectional and ecologic studies (Jarrett, 1989). The most convincing prospective study, conducted among male alumni of an American university followed for 14 years, showed a protective effect for leisure-time physical activity, independent of obesity, hypertension, and parental history of diabetes (Helmrich et al., 1991). Among Native Americans, research on physical activity has been hampered by the lack of a culturally appropriate survey instrument, although one such instrument has been developed and validated in the Pima (Kriska et al., 1990). In the Northwest Territories, the 1985 Health Promotion Survey reported that Inuit and Indians were less likely than non-Natives to exercise more than fifteen minutes per day at least three times per week, the respective proportions being 43 percent, 38 percent and 51 percent (Imrie and Warren, 1988). However, the need for "leisure-time" physical activity may be much lower in a population where a substantial proportion of people are still engaged in physically demanding tasks such as hunting and trapping.

The prenatal environment is an important determinant of subsequent diabetes and obesity in the offspring (Pettitt et al., 1987, 1988). At age 20–24, the prevalence of diabetes was 45 percent among those whose mothers were diabetic during pregnancy, compared to 9 percent among those whose mothers were "prediabetic," and only 1.4 percent among those whose mothers were nondiabetic. On multivariate analysis, maternal diabetes was an independent predictor even after adjustment for paternal diabetes, the age of diabetes onset in the parents, and degree of obesity in the offspring (Pettitt et al., 1988). Genetic susceptibility cannot account entirely for this phenomenon, and the intrauterine environment, perhaps related to glucose and insulin metabolism, to which the fetus has been exposed probably also plays a role.

The WHO criteria allow an intermediate category between diabetes and normality termed "impaired glucose tolerance" (IGT). Studies on the Pimas indicated that IGT is itself a risk factor or precursor of NIDDM. Among subjects with IGT followed for 11 years, 31 percent developed NIDDM, 26 percent remained in the IGT state, while 43 percent reverted to normal. Compared to nondiabetics, Pimas with IGT had 6.3 times the risk of developing NIDDM (Saad et al., 1988). During the transition from normality to IGT, the fasting and two-hour insulin levels increase, and from IGT to NIDDM, there is a further increase in fasting insulin but no longer an increased insulin response to glucose stimulation (Saad et al., 1989).

Even among subjects who did not have IGT or NIDDM, a higher level of fasting or two-hour plasma glucose and insulin is predictive of future development of NIDDM. A measure of insulin response is the ratio of the two-hr to fasting insulin level. In multivariate models, the insulin response can be substituted for fasting and two-hr insulin and emerges as an independent predictor (Saad et al., 1988).

The role of hyperinsulinemia and insulin resistance as the underlying metabolic defect of not only diabetes but other conditions such as obesity, hypertension, dyslipidemia, and atherosclerosis is discussed in more detail later in this chapter.

In the national survey of Native Canadian diabetes (Young et al., 1990b), the joint role of genetic and environmental factors in determining the distribution of diabetes was implicated, using relatively crude "proxy" measures such as language family, culture area, geographical coordinates, and degree of isolation.

Further research in this field—particularly longitudinal studies—is needed to investigate a full range of biological and sociocultural variables.

Complications of Diabetes

Diabetes is of public health importance primarily because of its association with various acute and chronic long-term complications such as coronary and peripheral vascular disease, retinopathy, nephropathy, and peripheral neuropathy, all of which may lead to premature mortality. Earlier reports from the 1960s, which suggested that Native American diabetics were somehow spared the risk of complications (Prosnitz and Mandell, 1967) and that the disease was a rather "benign chemical abnormality" (Saiki and Rimoin, 1968), have been proved incorrect. Cross-sectional studies among the Hopi and Navajo (Rate et al., 1983) and in Oklahoma (West et al., 1980) revealed the presence of retinopathy in 50%–70% of diabetic cases and proteinuria in 30%–50% of cases.

In terms of mortality, both Canadian and U.S. national surveys have demonstrated an increased risk of death from diabetes among Native Americans. In a study of mortality on Indian reserves in seven provinces during 1977–82, the risk of death from diabetes was 2.2 times higher among Native men and 4.1 times higher among Native women than Canadian men and women in general (Mao et al., 1986). An excess in diabetes mortality among Native Americans compared to the U.S. all-races population has been observed from the mid 1950s onward (Fig. 5.6). Compared to nondiabetics, Pima diabetics had an elevated risk of mortality, adjusted for age and BMI, among females but not males (Pettit et al., 1982).

In a national survey of end-stage renal disease (ESRD), using data from the Canadian Renal Failure Registry, the overall risk of ESRD from all causes among Native Canadians was 2.5 to 4 times higher, and the risk of ESRD due to diabetes specifically was at least 3 times higher (Young et al., 1989). U.S. national Medicare data also indicated that the Native ESRD incidence was 3 times higher than that of whites, and that the incidence of ESRD due to diabetes was 6 times higher than for whites (Newman et al., 1990). Among the Navajos, the age-adjusted incidence of ESRD from all causes was 4 times that of U.S. whites, while that for ESRD due to diabetes was 9.6 times higher (Megill et al., 1988).

Studies among the Pimas indicated that the diabetic nephropathy observed in that population did not differ clinically or pathologically from that observed in whites; it only occurred more frequently. Diabetic Pimas developed ESRD at the rate of 9.4/1000 person-years. Compared with U.S. national data, the rate of ESRD due to diabetes among the Pimas was not substantially different under the age of 45 but was more than 10 times as frequent over the age of 45. Comparing diabetics with nondiabetics, the risk of ESRD was 62 times higher, controlling for age and sex. The presence of hypertension and duration of diabetes were independent risk factors for ESRD (Nelson et al., 1988). The risk of heavy proteinuria was much higher than ESRD, at 37/1000 person-years in 10–15 years and 106/1000 person-years in 15–20 years. The severity of diabetes, in addition to its duration and the presence of hypertension, were determinants of proteinuria (Kunzelman et al., 1989).

Diabetics in general suffer from a higher risk of lower-extremity amputations. Among the Pimas, the age-sex-adjusted incidence rate was 24/1000 person-years, almost 4 times the rate in six U.S. states from which population-based estimates have been obtained. The risk was higher in men than in women, and was positively associated with the duration of diabetes and the degree of hyperglycemia (Nelson et al., 1988).

Among Cree-Ojibwa diabetics, the duration of illness and coexisting hypertension were associated with the prevalence of complications, whereas the initial glucose level and weight status were not (Young et al., 1985). Among Mohawk diabetics, over 60 percent had at least one major complication (such as ischemic heart disease, stroke, or peripheral vascular disease). The risk for having such complications was 6 times that experienced by nondiabetics in the same community, even after adjusting for differences in age, sex, and the level of smoking, hypertension, and obesity (Macaulay et al., 1988).

Diabetics also suffer from characteristic microvascular changes in the retina which if untreated may lead to blindness. The only longitudinal observational study of retinopathy reported to date from an Amerindian group is, once again, the Pima. On multivariate analysis, the incidence of retinopathy was positively associated with duration of diabetes and age, but not sex. When these three variables had been controlled for, hypertension, hypercholesterolemia, and insulin treatment were found to be independent predictors (Nelson et al., 1989). That insulin use among NIDDM patients may be harmful in the long run has important policy implications.

In Canada a study of diabetic retinopathy in southern Alberta, which included a substantial Native sample, identified a high prevalence of serious and untreated diabetic retinopathy in both insulin-using and non-insulin-using Native diabetics. Also, Natives have a high prevalence of both microalbuminuria and macroalbuminuria. Both these abnormalities indicate eventual serious hypertension and renal failure. Over 80 percent of insulin-using Native diabetics have adequate endogenous production of insulin compared to 40 percent of non-Native insulin-users. The data to date further suggest that insulin use may be a prominent risk factor for vascular complications in NIDDM patients who take insulin (Ross and Fick, 1990, 1991).

Prevention and Control Strategies

As diabetes is a "new" disease that has rapidly increased in magnitude and extent in aboriginal populations with little previous collective experience of it, an understanding of how the people interpret their illness experience and respond to treatment regimens rooted in Western scientific traditions has both theoretical and practical importance. While medical anthropologists can make considerable contributions to such understandings, research in this field is limited (Hagey, 1984; Garro and Lang, 1993).

The high prevalence of diabetes among certain Native groups has important implications for their health care. Health professionals who serve Native peoples are confronted with the need to adapt their treatment regimen and education programs to the culture and social environment of their patients. Furthermore, many Native communities are located in geographically remote areas poorly served by specialists in diabetes.

Innovative education programs can be found in scattered localities in Canada and the United States (Macaulay and Hanusaik, 1988; Lang, 1985). In the United States, the Indian Health Service instituted model programs in several reservations. Of these, the program in the Zuni reservation has been evaluated. The Zuni project, initiated in 1983, was a community-based exercise and weight-control program offered to both diabetes patients and the general public. After two years of follow-up, compared to diabetic nonparticipants, participants were found to experience weight loss, decline in fasting glucose values, and reduction in the use of hypoglycemic drugs. Age, duration of diabetes, and BMI did not influence the effect of participation on the metabolic outcome. In addition, a more limited, ten-week weight loss competition was also held, and was successful in achieving completion and substantial weight loss (>2.3 kg) in 45 percent of participants (Heath et al., 1991).

Current education programs are mostly directed at diabetic patients with established disease, to help them manage their illness better and prevent complications, and such programs should thus be considered as "tertiary" prevention efforts.

While primary prevention—the reduction of risk factors in the population to reduce the incidence of disease—is advocated as potentially promising for diabetes (King and Dowd, 1990; Stern, 1991) community intervention trials are needed to identify and evaluate effective strategies. Because of the high burden of disease, Native American communities would be ideal demonstration sites.

Secondary prevention, the use of screening to detect disease at an early stage, is not considered appropriate for diabetes, as the link between improving glucose control and reduction in complications is weak. However, the demonstration of abnormal chemical values may prove to be an incentive toward weight control in an obese person (Singer et al., 1988).

Genetic counseling is not a realizable goal for diabetes at the present stage of knowledge, but the search for the diabetes susceptibility gene does have practical applications. Stern (1991) suggested that if genetically susceptible individuals could be identified, the development of the phenotype (i.e., clinical disease) may be averted through lifestyle alterations. Even a linked marker, while not the gene itself, can serve as a screening tool.

Gallbladder Disease

Extent and Magnitude of the Problem

Native Americans have been recognized as suffering from a higher burden of diseases of the gallbladder (GBD) and biliary tract, particularly gallstones (cholelithiasis) and acute and chronic cholecystitis. [Cancer of the gallbladder was considered in Chapter 4, together with cancers in other sites]. This is evident from several case series of hospitalized patients and autopsies during the 1960s, particularly from the Southwest (Brown and Christensen, 1967; Sievers and Marquis, 1962). Since then population-based prevalence surveys based on registries of known, physician-diagnosed cases and radiographic screening have been conducted in a few tribes, such as the Chippewa in Minnesota (Thistle et al., 1971), the Micmac in Nova Scotia (Williams et al., 1977), and the Pima in Arizona (Comess et al., 1967; Sampliner et al., 1970). The Pima occupy the extreme high end of the spectrum, similar to their position with regard to diabetes, with prevalence exceeding 70 percent among women over age 25.

The Survey of American Indians and Alaska Natives (SAIAN) showed that the self-reported rates of GBD was higher among Native Americans than in the U.S. population at large (Fig. 5.7). The excess, while present in all age groups, was more prominent among women than men.

It is noteworthy that Hispanics in New Mexico and Texas, who have substantial Amerindian admixture, also have high rates of GBD (Samet et al., 1988; Hanis et al., 1985; Diehl et al., 1987).

Another indication of the high prevalence of GBD among Native Canadians is their high rate of cholecystectomy. In a province-wide study in Manitoba covering the period 1972–84, the age-adjusted cholecystectomy rates for Native women were higher than for non-Natives, with the peak rate occurring some 20–30 years earlier at age 30–39. The rates for females were three times higher than in males, which did not differ between Natives and non-Natives. Native patients were 1.5 times more likely to be readmitted to hospital for surgical complica-

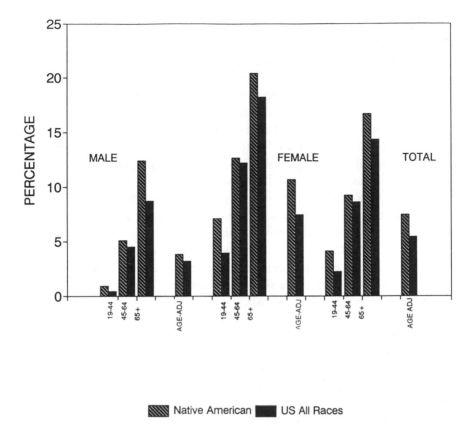

Figure 5.7. Prevalence of self-reported gallbladder disease: USA, 1987, Native American and U.S. all-race populations.

tions, even after controlling for age, sex, rural/urban residence, hospital type, simple/complicated surgery, and presence of multiple diagnoses (Cohen et al., 1989). While differences in medical care practices in the Native and non-Native populations may account in part for the difference in surgical rates, the excessive disease burden in Native women is the more likely explanation.

Etiology and Risk Factors

Studies in various populations have implicated age, sex, obesity, central fat distribution, parity, and serum lipids as risk factors for GBD. These risk factors generally refer to cholesterol or mixed stones, which constitute over 75 percent of gallstones in North America. The other type of gallstones, pigment stones, are uncommon among Native Americans and are clinically, morphologically, and epidemiologically distinct from cholesterol stones. Pigment stones are associated with chronic hemolytic states, biliary tract infections, cirrhosis, and alcoholism (Diehl, 1991).

Most epidemiological studies on Native American populations have been cross-sectional, which often cannot confirm a temporal sequence between exposure and outcome. (This is important in the case of serum lipids, which may well be altered subsequent to the diagnosis of the disease). Another problem is that different results are obtained depending on the way disease status is determined. Studies utilizing "clinical" GBD differ from those where GBD cases are detected in normal, nonsymptomatic people by radiographic or ultrasonographic screening procedures.

That GBD is primarily a disease of older women is well demonstrated in most populations, although among Native American women the age of onset is generally earlier. The high parity among Native women was discussed in Chapter 2. According to the Canada Census of 1981, on the average, 4.8 children were born to ever-married Native women, compared to 2.5 for all Canadian women; 35 percent of Indian women had six or more children, compared to only 8 percent in the country as a whole (Statistics Canada, 1984).

The high prevalence of obesity was discussed earlier in this chapter. The high overall levels of obesity among women in most Indian populations may indeed obscure the association between obesity and the presence of GBD. Among the Pima, obesity has not been shown to be a risk factor (Sampliner et al., 1970). Among the Cree-Ojibwa in northern Ontario and Manitoba, neither body mass index nor waist/hip ratio remained as independent predictors on multivariate analysis (Young and Roche, 1990).

In the Cree-Ojibwa study, increased serum triglycerides and reduced total cholesterol were independently associated with GBD (Young and Roche, 1990). A lower total cholesterol was also observed among Mexican-American GBD cases in Texas (Hanis et al., 1985). It is possible that cholecystectomy itself may affect cholesterol metabolism. Alternatively, patients diagnosed with GBD may alter their diet. The metabolic basis of GBD has been studied in some American Indian tribes, where a highly saturated bile was demonstrated (Grundy et al., 1972; Thistle and Schoenfield, 1971). The early appearance of this "lithogenic bile" during puberty among Pima girls suggests that it may be the precursor of gallstone disease in later life (Bennion et al., 1979).

An association between GBD and diabetes has been suspected for some time, although the evidence is inconsistent. Among the Cree-Ojibwa, diabetic status was not an independent predictor of GBD (Young and Roche, 1990). Among Mexican-Americans in Texas, clinical GBD (based on self-reports) was associated with diabetes even after adjusting for BMI and body fat distribution (Haffner et al., 1990). The association is intriguing, and particularly relevant for Native Americans where both diabetes and GBD are prevalent. Several mechanisms may be responsible: diabetic bile may be supersaturated with cholesterol, gall-bladder emptying may be impaired in diabetics, and the hyperinsulinemia associated with diabetes is also responsible for GBD (Diehl, 1991).

There are other minor risk factors for GBD (Diehl, 1991). Moderate alcohol use has been found to be protective for cholesterol stones, while alcoholism and cirrhosis are risk factors for pigment stones. Smoking and oral contraceptive use may confer a small risk for GBD. Little consensus has emerged on the role of specific dietary constituents in gallstone induction (Diehl, 1991).

Prevention and Control Strategies

In terms of primary prevention, the commonality of risk factors for the various chronic diseases suggests that there is no need for a specific GBD prevention strategy. Programs dealing with diet, physical activity, and weight control suggested for diabetes, obesity, and cardiovascular diseases would also be beneficial for controlling of GBD.

Screening for gallstones, even in a high-risk population such as Native Americans, requires careful weighing of risks and benefits. While a noninvasive and relatively portable procedure such as ultrasonography is available and can be used as a population screening tool, there is no surgical consensus as to whether "silent" gallstones should be operated on, with all the attendant complication risks of surgery and anesthesia. Medical decision analyses on "prophylactic" cholecystectomy compared to "expectant" management of silent gallstones indicated little advantage in terms of survival (Ransohoff et al., 1983).

A variety of new technologies that are less invasive than conventional cholecystectomy have become available, including oral medications or locally instilled contact solutions to dissolve stones, extracorporeal shock wave lithotripsy, and other methods of stone fragmentation, as well as laparoscopic cholecystectomy (Parish et al., 1991). While these procedures may offer clinical advantages, the resource implications for the health care system need to be assessed prior to advocating them as part of any population-based GBD control strategy.

Insulin Resistance: A Common Metabolic Defect?

There is increasing evidence to suggest that insulin resistance may be the key metabolic defect that leads to such related disorders as obesity, hypertension, diabetes, dyslipidemia, and atherosclerosis (DeFronzo and Ferrannini, 1991). As has been shown in this and the previous chapter, obesity, diabetes, and hypertension are serious health problems in the majority of Native populations studied.

The interrelationships between insulin resistance and the pentad of metabolic disorders can be represented by a "metabolic cascade," an example of which was presented by DeFronzo and Ferrannini (1991). Figure 5.8 is a modification of this model, which by necessity has to simplify very complex relationships and interactions. Although genetic susceptibility is indicated in Figure 5.8, as contributing to insulin resistance, such a genotype generally remains unexpressed. DeFronzo and Ferrannini (1991) hypothesized that in the presence of other susceptibility genes (for hypertension, atherosclerosis, diabetes, dyslipidemia, or obesity) the phenotypic expression of the insulin resistance gene assumes the clinical characteristics of the latter.

Controversy exists as to which comes first—insulin resistance or hyperinsulinemia (Zimmet, 1992). Whatever the initial lesion, a vicious cycle develops between insulin resistance and hyperinsulinemia among those who are genetically susceptible in an attempt to maintain glucose homeostasis. Downregulation of insulin receptors results in hyperglycemia and compensatory beta-cell stimulation, which further exacerbates hyperinsulinemia and insulin resistance. Ultimately beta-cell exhaustion occurs and NIDDM ensues (Zimmet, 1992). A two-stage model is subscribed to by some, wherein insulin resistance is the main determinant of the transition from normality to IGT, and beta-cell dysfunction is responsible for the worsening of IGT to NIDDM (Saad et al., 1991a; DeFronzo et al., 1992).

Whether a model of metabolic cascade holds true for all populations (or in fact, any population) remains to be tested. For the Pima at least, the relationship

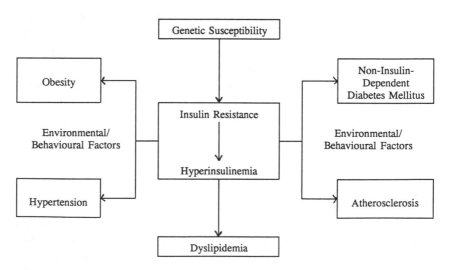

Figure 5.8. Interrelationship of insulin resistance/hyperinsulinemia and obesity, diabetes, hypertension, dyslipidemia, and atherosclerosis.

between insulin resistance, hyperinsulinemia, and hypertension has been found to differ from that observed in Caucasians. After adjusting for age, sex, body weight, and percent body fat, the mean blood pressure (1/3 systolic + 2/3 diastolic) correlated with fasting insulin and rate of glucose disposal in whites but not in Pimas (Saad et al., 1991b), suggesting that yet other or stronger factors may operate in regulating blood pressure.

Studies from such high prevalence populations as the Pima (Aronoff et al., 1977; Nagulesparan et al., 1982), the Naruans in the South Pacific (Zimmet et al., 1990), and Mexican Americans in Texas (Haffner et al., 1986) showed that fasting and post-challenge serum insulin levels were elevated even among the nondiabetics when compared to Caucasians. In Canada, the only group for which data on serum insulin levels are available is the Dogrib in the Northwest Territories. Fasting hyperinsulinemia, however, is not present in the Dogrib. There are, however, significant differences in fasting levels by Gc genotypes (a serum protein used as a genetic marker) among nondiabetic individuals (Szathmary, 1987). The "universality" of hyperinsulinemia among different Native American populations along the full spectrum of disease risk needs to be demonstrated.

Chronic Diseases: An Evolutionary Perspective

Why is diabetes so prevalent in many North American Indian populations, and why has there been an increase compared to half a century ago? Certainly these populations have been exposed to an increasingly high prevalence of environmental risk factors that have been demonstrated to play a role. It is also clear that, if there were a diabetes-susceptibility genotype, it must have been present when the ancestors of Amerindians crossed the Bering land bridge and was somehow sustained in the population in the ensuing tens of thousands of years. The evolutionary forces (e.g., founder effect, natural selection) at work remain to be clarified, and several theories exist (Neel, 1982; Weiss et al., 1984a,b; Ritenbaugh and Goodby, 1989; Szathmary, 1990).

Neel first proposed the "thrifty genotype" hypothesis in 1962 and revised it in 1982. Neel noted that, for it to persist over time, the diabetic genotype must have conferred survival advantage under previously prevailing "feast-or-famine" environmental conditions. The thrifty gene enabled an individual to produce insulin rapidly in response to rising blood glucose levels (the "quick insulin trigger"), which facilitates the storage of glucose in the form of triglycerides in fat cells. In times of food scarcity, such individuals would have fat stores from which to derive energy. However, with sedentarization, the development of agricultural societies, and the assurance of a continuous and ample food supply, the quick insulin trigger would result in too much insulin, hyperglycemia, obesity, and diabetes.

Weiss and others (1984b) noted the high prevalence and co-occurrence of gall-bladder disease, obesity, and NIDDM in diverse Native American populations, and referred to them collectively as the "New World" syndrome. They postulated the existence of genes involved in the metabolism of lipids.

Szathmary (1990) noted that the thrifty gene model assumed a nutritional environment in which carbohydrate intake exceeded daily energy requirements. This was not the situation when the ancestors of modern Native Americans first occupied the continent, where the diet was one based predominantly on meat and fat. Survival advantage in a low carbohydrate, Arctic/Subarctic environment was provided by having an efficient formation of endogenous glucose through gluconeogenesis, efficient use of free fatty acids to provide for the energy needs of non-glucose-dependent tissues, and the efficient use of ketone bodies as fuel. Under such conditions, selection should have favored individuals in whom gluconeogenesis and free fatty acid release and use were enhanced.

Ritenbaugh and Goodby (1989) also emphasized the physiologic consequences of the northern hunting lifestyle: low carbohydrate availability, intermittent lipid storage, protein sufficiency, and high energy demands for activity and body warmth. With the transition to agriculturally based subsistence systems and modern industrial societies, genetically controlled modifications could have occurred in several enzymatically mediated pathways in lipid and glucose metabolism to "spare" glucose.

Wendorf and Goldfine (1991) attempted to "validate" the thrifty genotype hypothesis with archeological evidence for big-game hunting (primarily bison) among ancestral Indian groups who had migrated into temperate North America between 12,000 and 11,000 years ago. Despite the drastic environmental changes, these groups continued to practice the food-gathering strategy more suited to the Arctic environment. They were thus subject to an unpredictable food supply, for which a thrifty genotype would offer some selective advantage. Subscribing to the theory that Asiatic peoples migrated to North America in three separate waves (see Chapter 1), these authors believed that the Na-Dene and Eskimos, who migrated around 10,000 and 5,000 years ago, respectively, much later than the Paleo-Indians (20,000–25,000 years ago), did not develop the thrifty genotype. This accounted for their still much lower prevalence of diabetes. Wendorff and Goldfine offered a physiological explanation of the thrifty genotype, which operates through insulin resistance in peripheral muscles. This blunts the hypoglycemia from periods of fasting but allows energy storage in fat and the liver during periods of feasts. Among those who subsequently changed to a sedentary lifestyle, and constant food supply results in obesity and insulin resistance in fat and the liver, chronic hyperglycemia and reduced circulating insulin, and ultimately NIDDM (Wendorf and Goldfine, 1991).

All these theories and models highlight the importance of integrating data from a variety of disciplines and approaches in understanding the distribution and etiology of diseases of significance to Native Americans. That the level of enquiry ranges from DNA to populations, and from the present to remote prehistoric times only serves to highlight the excitement and attraction of an epidemiology that is bioculturally based.

6

Injuries and the Social Pathologies

Among the most serious health problems affecting Native Americans in the decades since the end of the Second World War are injuries due to accidents and violence. In the younger age groups injuries are by far the most important causes of mortality and morbidity, and overall, they may account for as much as 25%–40% of all deaths.

Injuries can be broadly classified according to whether they are intentional or unintentional (or "accidents"). Within the "intentional" category, injuries may be interpersonal or self-inflicted. The ICD-9 employs two systems for coding injuries: one is according to the type of injury and body parts affected—e.g., fracture of skull, fracture of femur, burns, amputations, etc.; the other system, the so-called "E-codes," codes injuries according to the "external cause"—e.g., drowning, falls, fires, motor vehicle accidents, suicides, homicides, etc. From the perspective of prevention and control, the E-codes are far more informative and useful (Smith et al., 1990).

While injury mortality data are usually readily available, not all injuries result in death. To estimate the incidence of injuries, it is necessary to combine different data sources, including vital statistics, hospital care (in-patient, out-patient, and emergency room), and physician office visits. A study on the Hopi reservation in New Mexico combined mortality and hospital admission data from 1979–80 and estimated the incidence of injuries to be 12/1000 per year, with the highest risk group being those age 85 and above (Simpson et al., 1983). Studies in non-Native populations estimated that for every injury death among adolescents, there were 40 injury hospitalizations and 1100 cases treated in emergency rooms (Runyan and Gerken, 1989). Minor injuries, which do not result in any contact with the health care system, can only be ascertained by a population-based survey. For nonfatal injuries, varying degrees of disability may result, often associated with serious medical and social sequelae. Regardless of their source, injury statistics among Native Americans are often unreliable. Under-reporting and misclassification of particular types of injuries (e.g., suicides) may result from cultural bias of the investigator, community and family reticence in furnishing information, and the lack of supporting circumstantial evidence to allow the accurate assigning of a cause.

The study of injury epidemiology and control has undergone a conceptual shift since the 1970s, owing in particular to the theoretical and empirical contributions of such researchers as Haddon and Baker (Haddon, 1980; Baker et al., 1992). The term "accidents" is no longer considered adequate or appropriate, as it obscures the existence of preventable causes. From a preoccupation with indi-vidual behavior or susceptibility, research studies have emphasized the larger role played by the physical and social environments. The definition of injury has been broadened to include any damage sustained by the human body as a result of energy exchange. The forms of energy are familiar to students of physics: mechanical (e.g., car crash, fall), thermal (e.g., burn), chemical (drug over-dose), electrical (e.g., electrocution), or ionizing radiation.

Analytical studies of the risk factors for injuries in Native American commu-nities are relatively few compared to descriptive studies, and formal evaluations of prevention strategies are even more scarce. Many studies purporting to ex-amine risk factors are case series without internal or external comparison groups. Opinions and anecdotes often substitute for rigorously collected epidemiological data. In comparison to cross-sectional and case-control studies, cohort studies are seldom conducted, and are usually not of sufficiently long duration to allow for a "developmental" perspective.

In this chapter, Native American injuries will be considered under the sub-headings of unintentional injuries, and suicides, homicides and violence. Be-cause alcohol and substance abuse is strongly implicated as an underlying cause of many injuries among Native Americans, and since it is a serious health prob-lem in its own right, it is discussed in a separate section.

Unintentional Injuries

Extent and Magnitude of the Problem

The much higher risk of mortality from unintentional injuries among Native Americans relative to the national population can be demonstrated in both Can-ada and the United States. Figure 6.1 compares the age-standardized mortality

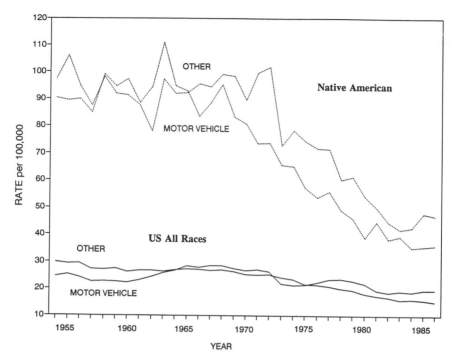

Figure 6.1. Age-standardized mortality rate for unintentional injuries: USA, 1955–87, Native American and U.S. all-race populations.

rate from motor vehicle accidents and other accidents among Native Americans in the United States from 1955 to 1987. A declining trend is also evident.

Such national data often obscure regional and tribal differences (Fig. 6.2A, USA, and Fig. 6.2B, Canada). Table 6.1 summarizes the various regional studies where estimates of relative risks were provided. The higher risks of injury mortality are demonstrated not just relative to the national all-race population, but within regions, the highest rates are usually reported from Native Americans among the various ethnic groups, for example, in New Mexico (Sewell et al., 1989) and Alaska (Kraus and Buffler, 1979).

Children and adolescents are at greater risk of mortality from some types of injuries than those in the older age groups. Two national studies that examined childhood injuries in Canada (MacWilliams et al., 1987) and the USA (Waller et al., 1989), and that provided data on Native Americans, are summarized in Table 6.2. Regional studies of childhood injury mortality, for example in New Mexico, fit the national picture of an excess among Native Americans. Over the period of surveillance, from 1958–1982, mortality rates for most causes of injury among Native Americans peaked around the early 1970s and began to show a decline in the most recent 5-year period (Olson et al., 1990).

National data on the age-specific mortality rates from motor vehicle and other unintentional injuries are shown in Figure 6.3. It is evident that the great excess of mortality among Native Americans occurred in different age groups from different types of injuries: young adults for motor vehicle accidents, drowning, and firearm accidents, and the elderly for falls and housefires.

Among Canadian Indian infants from five provinces between 1976 and 1983, the SMR for all injuries was 6 in the neonatal period and 3.8 in the postneonatal period. The specific causes of injury such as motor vehicle accidents, fires, and suffocation, the SMRs in the postneonatal period were 3.5, 8.2, and 4.4 respectively (Morrison et al., 1986).

Fewer data are available for the *incidence* of unintentional injuries compared to mortality. A study of all medical care records on the Navajo Reservation during 1966–67 indicated a different age-sex pattern. While injuries among men still outnumbered women by about 2:1, the age differential was less marked, ranging from a low of 34/1000/yr among the 55–64 age group to a high of 47/1000/yr in the 65 and older group (Brown et al., 1970).

While Native Americans are at higher risk for sustaining various injuries, the extent and severity of injuries are also greater than for non-Natives. In a case series of burns, patients treated in a referral hospital in Alberta during 1977–86, Callegari and associates (1989) found that Native patients suffered larger total body surface area burns and were hospitalized on average 17 days longer than non-Native patients, although overall case-fatality rates were similar (4%–5%).

Etiology and Risk Factors

The excess mortality from unintentional injuries has often been attributed, on the "macro" level, to the prevailing economic conditions and social stress that Native Americans experience. Alcohol abuse is believed to play a major role in most violent and accidental deaths. The medical examiner's office in many jurisdictions often provides important data from toxicological, pathological, and police investigations into the causes and circumstances surrounding violent and accidental deaths, particularly if they are drug or alcohol related (Trott et al., 1981). Detailed sociological inquiries have provided further information on the circumstances surrounding many "accidental" deaths, many of which are associated with alcohol intoxication (Jarvis and Boldt, 1982).

The relative importance of the different causes of injury deaths in both U.S. and Canadian Natives is summarized in Table 6.3.

USA

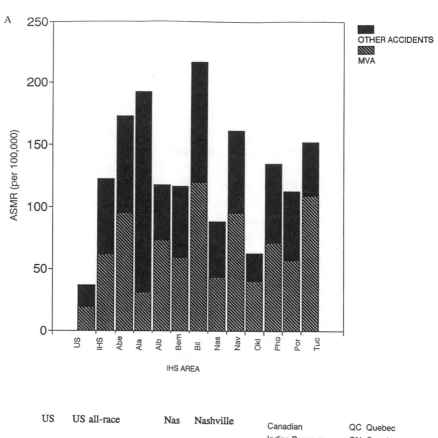

US	US all-race	Nas	Nashville
IHS	Total IHS areas	Nav	Navajo
Abe	Aberdeen	Okl	Oklahoma
Ala	Alabama	Pho	Phoenix
Alb	Albuquerque	Por	Portland
Bem	Bemidji	Tuc	Tucson
Bil	Billings		

Canadian
Indian Reserves

QC Quebec
ON Ontario
MB Manitoba
SK Saskatchewan
AB Alberta
BC British Columbia

PR: Non-Indian Reserve population
in all 6 provinces

Figure 6.2. Regional variation in age-standardized mortality rate for unintentional injuries among Native Americans: (*A*) USA, 1980–87; (*B*) Canada, 1979–88.

Total Injuries

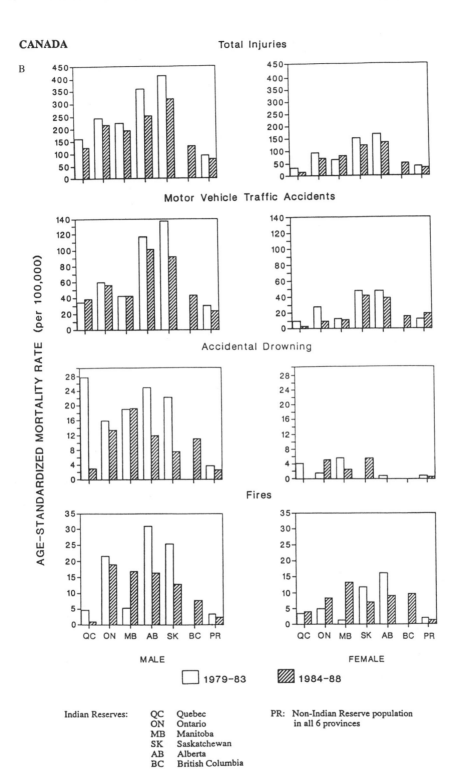

Motor Vehicle Traffic Accidents

Accidental Drowning

Fires

AGE-STANDARDIZED MORTALITY RATE (per 100,000)

MALE

FEMALE

☐ 1979-83   ▨ 1984-88

Indian Reserves: QC   Quebec   PR: Non-Indian Reserve population
                   ON   Ontario   in all 6 provinces
                   MB   Manitoba
                   SK   Saskatchewan
                   AB   Alberta
                   BC   British Columbia

Table 6.1 Regional Studies of Injury Mortality among Native Americans

Region/ Population[a]	Years	Authors	Sex	Standardized Mortality Ratio[b]										
				Inj	MVTA	RaWa	WaTA	Pois	Falls	Fires	Drow	FArm	Suic	Homi
Canada: 7 provinces	1977–82	Mao et al. (1986)	M	3.2	2.3				2.4	5.6	5.6		2.7	7.8
			F	3.7	2.7				2.3	6.9	2.4		2.7	5.8
ON: Cree/ Ojibwa	1972–81	Young (1983)	M/F	4.5	1.0	57.0	54.7		1.0	10.8	6.5	21.9	1.8	9.4
QC: James Bay Cree	1975–81	Robinson (1988)	M/F	2.0							10.0			
BC: All Indians	1953–78	Hislop et al. (1987)	M		2.7	19.3		2.4	2.0	9.4	6.0		1.9	10.5
			F		4.2	52.0		4.4	2.3	11.7	7.8		1.6	9.8
NY: Seneca	1955–84	Mahoney et al. (1989d)	M	4.0	4.1								1.8	1.9
			F	2.7	2.4								2.0	6.3
AZ: Pima	1975–84	Sievers et al. (1990)	M/F	5.9	6.9								4.3	7.4
NM: Apache/ Navajo/ Pueblo	1957–68	Van Winkle/ May (1986)	M/F									Apache Navajo Pueblo	3.4 0.8 1.7	
	1969–79		M/F									Apache Navajo Pueblo	4.9 1.7 3.2	

[a] States and provinces: AZ, Arizona; BC, British Columbia; NM, New Mexico; NY, New York; ON, Ontario; QC, Quebec.
[b] Inj, all injuries; MVTA, motor vehicle traffic accidents; RaWA, railway accidents; WaTA, water transport accidents; Pois, poisoning; Drow, Drowning; FArm, firearms accidents; Suic, suicide; homi, homicide.

Table 6.2 Mortality Risk of Non-intentional Injuries among Native American Children
(< 15 years) Relative to the National Populations of Canada and the United States

Cause of Injury	USA (1980–85)	Canada (1977–82)
All injuries	1.8	3.2
Motor vehicle	—	1.6
occupant	2.2	—
pedestrian traffic	1.5	—
pedestrian non-traffic	3.9	—
Drowning	1.7	4.4
Fires	1.4	6.1
Falls	1.5	2.5
Poisoning	3.5	2.5
Aspiration	2.6	—

Source: Waller et al. (1989) and MacWilliams et al. (1987).

Transportation Accidents.   Motor vehicle accidents (MVAs) are the single most important cause of injury deaths, accounting for just under 40 percent of all injury mortality among Native Americans in the United States during 1980–86 (Baker et al., 1992). Among Native Canadians, MVAs accounted for a smaller proportion—less than 30 percent—of all injury deaths. MVAs have been observed to occur more frequently in areas of low per capita income and in rural areas in North America (Baker et al., 1987), and most Native American communities qualify on both counts. The inverse correlation with population density may reflect greater driving distances. Most rural roads, particularly those in Indian reservations, are poorly paved, lit, and maintained. The mechanical condition of cars is often poor, the number of passengers excessive, and few people wear seat belts even when they are available. The greater distances also hinder access to major trauma centers. While distance may not affect the incidence of accidents, it reduces the probability of surviving a crash. In New York State, 74 percent of Native victims of fatal motor vehicle accident died before reaching a medical care facility (Mahoney, 1991).

In New Mexico, where Native Americans had three times the risk of death from all unintentional injuries during 1980–89, the relative risk for pedestrian-motor vehicle collisions was 7.5 and for hypothermia 30.5. Analysis of alcohol levels and site of occurrence indicated that death occurred most frequently on the road leading to the reservation or in border towns adjacent to the reservation. As alcohol was prohibited on reservations, drinkers who had consumed alcohol outside the reservation usually walked back in the late evening or early morning, where they ran the risk of being struck by motor vehicles or suffer from hypothermia as a result of intoxication and exposure (Gallaher et al., 1992). In New York, pedestrian-motor vehicle collisions were also the most important cause of fatal motor vehicle accidents. Among victims who were tested, 77 percent had detectable levels of blood alcohol (Mahoney, 1991).

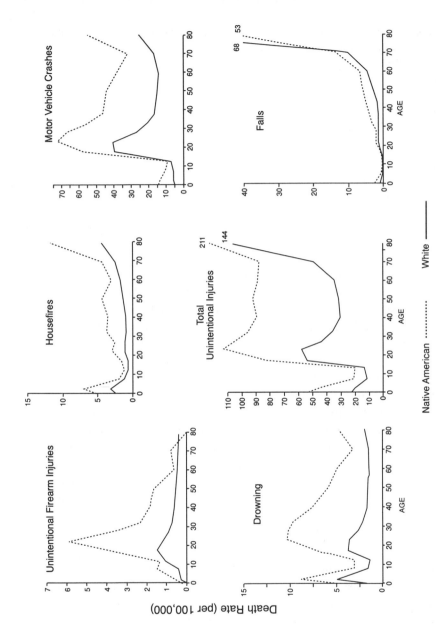

Figure 6.3. Age-specific mortality rate for unintentional injuries: USA, 1980–86, Native Americans and whites.

Native American ·········   White ———

Table 6.3 Distribution of Injury Mortality by External Cause among Native Americans in the United States 1980–86 and Canada 1979–88, All Ages and Both Sexes Combined

Cause (ICD Code)	USA (%)	Canada (%)
Motor vehicle traffic (E810-9)	39	29
Drowning (E910)	5	6
Poisoning (E850-869)	3	3
Falls (E880-8)	3	3
Fires and burns (E890-9)	4	8
Suicide (E950-9)	12	21
Homicide (E960-9)	13	9
Other	21	21
Total	100	100

Source: USA data from Baker et al. (1992). Canadian data from unpublished tables from the Canadian Mortality Database (rounded).

In many remote Native communities where roads and motor vehicles are few, the risk of mortality from motor vehicle accidents is comparable to or even lower than that of the national population. On the other hand, the risk of death from other transport accidents (e.g., railway and boats), where these are the chief means of transportation, is extremely high, as though in compensation for the relative lack of cars. [See for example, data from British Columbia and northwestern Ontario in Table 6.1.] In the Navajo Reservation, falls from horses were an important cause of non-fatal injuries (Brown et al., 1970).

In recent years injuries associated with off-road recreational vehicles have become increasingly of public health concern (Postl et al., 1987). Motorbikes, snowmobiles, and all-terrain vehicles are essential means of transportation in many rural and remote communities. In Labrador the circumstances under which snowmobile accidents occurred suggested the importance of human factors: bad weather and mechanical failure were far less important than drivers who had no drivers' license, were not wearing helmets, drove on roads, or were under the influence of alcohol (Hamby et al., 1988).

Fires and Burns.   Fires and burns accounted for 4 percent of all Native American injury deaths in the United States during 1980–86 (Baker et al., 1992) and 8 percent in Canada during 1979–88. On Canadian Indian reserves, the number of fires increased linearly throughout the 1970s and 1980s: the mean annual number of fires increased 70 percent between 1970–79 and 1980–89. On the other hand, the mortality from fires has been declining steadily at about 5 percent per year during these two decades. The causes of these fires were heating equipment (18%), arson (14%), electrical installation (13%), child-related (11%), smoking (7%), and burning grass and trash (6%) (Young et al., 1991:11,63).

Friesen (1985) conducted one of the more detailed investigations of housefires among Indians in Manitoba during 1976–82. Inspired by "Haddon's matrix" (a tool for the analysis of injury causation) he categorized the factors associated with fatal fires into those of the host, agent, and the physical and social environment. Such a scheme facilitates the identification of potential preventive strategies. Thus host factors included personal behaviors such as smoking, drinking, leaving children unattended, and having suicidal intent. Various agents or vehicles responsible for the fires included candles, oil burners, electrical appliances, and faulty wiring in the dwelling. The presence in the physical environment of unsecured combustible materials, buildings with blocked exits, nonfunctional fire extinguishers, inflammable clothing and mattresses, and the lack of piped water in the homes contributed to injuries from fires. The social environment encompassed poverty, which led to disconnected electricity due to non-payment, alcoholism, lack of fire protection service in the community, non-adherence to building codes, lack of child care, and lack of mental health programs.

Different patterns of housefires could be observed in different regions. In the Southwest, fire-related fatalities rarely resulted from cigarettes because there is a low prevalence of smoking. Heating sources include kerosene lanterns and fires built in metal cans or drums (Olson et al., 1990). While the actual sources of ignition differed from Native communities in northern Canada, underlying poverty contributed to the use of unsafe heating and lighting sources, and the failure to use smoke detectors.

The role of alcohol as a risk factor in fire-related injuries has been the subject of much investigation, although most studies merely reported on the proportion of the victims who had been drinking. A few studies, none of which were conducted among Native Americans, generated relative risk estimates. In their review, Howland and Hingson (1987) found that the risk of death from fires, death from fires due to smoking, and injuries from fires was elevated among those exposed to alcohol compared to controls.

Drowning.   The drowning rate, indicative of the geographical proximity to large bodies of water of many Native communities and the dependence on boats for basic transportation, also suggests faulty boat safety practices and inadequate safety instruction. Yet, surprisingly, in a "desert" state like New Mexico, the drowning rate among children was still highest among Native Americans, and the state's overall rate was higher than the national average (Olson et al., 1990). It was suggested that Native children lacked access to organized and supervised swimming activities, and often fell victim to drowning in unguarded rivers and irrigation canals. It would appear that in drowning deaths among children, social factors can override the ecological.

Accidents, violence, and alcohol and substance abuse have been referred to collectively as the "social pathologies" (e.g., Levy and Kunitz, 1971). The sociocultural explanation of their occurrence in Native communities in North America is discussed in greater detail at the end of this chapter.

Prevention and Control Strategies

A systematic approach to the prevention and control of injuries has been proposed by Haddon (1980). His ten strategies are basic to and theoretically available in all situations. As a guide to policy they ensure that consideration is given to all possible control measures, regardless of the extent of current knowledge of causation. These ten strategies are:

1. To prevent the creation of the hazard in the first place
2. To reduce the amount of hazard brought into being
3. To prevent the release of the hazard that already exists
4. To modify the rate or spatial distribution of release of the hazard from its source
5. To separate, in time or space, the hazard and that which is to be protected
6. To separate the hazard and that which is to be protected by interposition of a material barrier
7. To modify relevant basic qualities of the hazard
8. To make what is to be protected more resistant to damage from the hazard
9. To begin to counter the damage already done by the environmental hazard
10. To stabilize, repair, and rehabilitate the object of the damage

Haddon also proposed a three-phase approach to injury prevention, which Friesen (1985) applied to the case of housefires in Manitoba. Strategies directed at the *pre-event phase* may include programs that modify the host's behavior with respect to drinking and smoking, substitute safer forms of heating and lighting than woodstoves and candles, and prohibit alcohol in the community. Strategies that operate at the *event phase* may include safety education on proper procedures during a fire, installation of smoke detectors and fire extinguishers at home, improvement of community water supply, and formation of a volunteer fire brigade. During the *post-event phase* first-aid treatment for burns and medical evacuation of the critically injured, if instituted, could reduce the extent and severity of injury and improve the outcome in terms of survival and rehabilitation.

These are only potential strategies. They need to be prioritized according to the prevalence of the problem and the effectiveness of the intervention. Generally, emphasis on individual education to change behavior alone is not adequate ("active" measures); it must be combined with "passive" measures relating to product modification, environmental redesign, and legislative action.

An epidemiological investigation of motor vehicle accidents in an Apache reservation in Arizona resulted in a local intervention program operated jointly by IHS, the tribal government, and the state department of transport. This program emphasized such environmental redesign as funding for street lights along the route where pedestrians were most frequently injured, legislating the penning of livestock and penalizing owners whose animals strayed onto roads, the widening of a two-lane road to four-lanes, and the installation of traffic lights (CDC MMWR, 1989;38:589).

The awareness of safety precautions may be influenced by socioeconomic status and cultural practices. Using the Framingham Safety Survey sponsored by the American Academy of Pediatrics' Injury Prevention Program, Hsu and Williams (1991) studied families with children under 5 years of age in Salt Lake City, Utah. It was found that Native American families were less likely to keep small objects, household products, and medicines out of the reach of children, and to possess and understand the use of ipecac, a substance used to induce vomiting after certain poisonous substances have been ingested.

A substantial gap also exists in safety practices among the age group at the highest risk for motor vehicle-related injuries. Of the over 13,000 Native American students from grades 7–12 who took part in the Adolescent Health Survey, which covered over eight IHS Service Areas, 44 percent said they rarely or never wear seatbelts. Of those who were drinkers, 40 percent admitted to having driven after drinking. Just under a quarter of the respondents said they often or sometimes ride with a driver who had been drinking (Blum et al., 1992).

Compared to the Canadian National Health Knowledge Survey, Native junior high school students from seven Alberta Indian reserves scored lower in their knowledge of first aid for burns and stopping bleeding but higher in terms of knowledge of fire safety measures (McKinnon et al., 1991).

The U.S. Indian Health Service initiated community injury control programs in 1982, primarily consisting of public education. In an evaluation of such programs in 54 service units three years afterwards, it was found that there had been substantial declines in hospitalization rates for falls, motor vehicle accidents, and assaults. Multivariate analysis indicated that for falls, the reduction in hospitalizations was associated with the extent of coverage of training in general safety, recreational safety, and first aid. The benefits of other types of training and injury prevention activity were less clear cut (Robertson, 1986).

The IHS also began in 1987 an Injury Control Fellowship program to upgrade baccalaureate-level health workers in the epidemiology and prevention of injuries. The intent was to increase the quantity and level of knowledge and skills of these designated injury control officers, and ultimately reduce the incidence of injuries in Native communities (Smith, 1988).

Suicide, Homicide, and Violence

Extent and Magnitude of the Problem

Suicide and homicide are extreme (and lethal) outcomes of violent behavior, whether inflicted on oneself or directed at others. The excessive mortality and morbidity associated with these conditions among Native Americans, in comparison to non-Native populations in North America, are almost universal across tribes and regions.

Acts of violence are intimately related to the mental health of individuals and the "social" health of the community. A review of the voluminous literature on Native American mental health is beyond the scope of this volume [see, for example, the bibliography by Kelso and Attneave (1981) and reviews by Shore and Manson (1983) and O'Nell (1989)]. In this chapter, suicide, homicide, and nonfatal violence are considered mainly within the context of the epidemiology of injuries. Mental health issues will be discussed where they are pertinent as risk factors or in the design of prevention programs.

Epidemiological data on Native American suicides and homicides are very variable in quality. Many studies (particularly those reported in the clinical journals), based on single communities with very small populations and followed for only one or two years, purported to show "epidemics." Often, these inadequate descriptive studies formed the basis for the generation of etiologic hypotheses or the evaluation of subsequent prevention programs.

The much higher risk of suicide and homicide among Native Americans is evident from national U.S. and Canadian data. Figure 6.4 compares the age-standardized mortality rate between Native Americans and the U.S. all-races population from 1955 to 1987. A continuing decline was evident from the mid-1970s on.

Considerable regional and tribal differences exist (Fig. 6.5A, USA, and Fig. 6.5B, Canada). Table 6.1 also summarizes the various regional studies where estimates of relative risks (to the national, all-races, or white populations) are provided. Even within a single state such as New Mexico, tribal differences—between Apache, Pueblo, and Navajo—can also be demonstrated (Van Winkle and May, 1986). Many researchers tried to dispel the fallacy of the stereotypical "suicidal Indian" and emphasized the diversity and cultural specificity of suicidal rates (Shore, 1975). In Alaska, the Athapaskan Indians, who inhabit the interior, and the Inupiat Eskimos of the North Slope experienced the largest

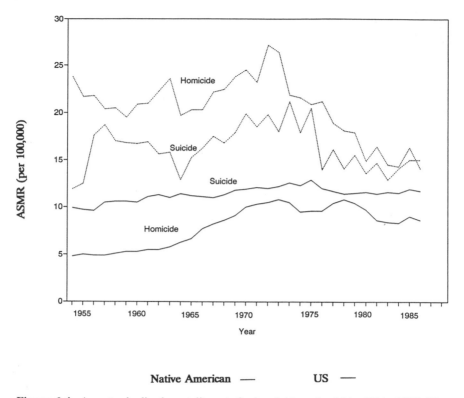

Figure 6.4. Age-standardized mortality rate for homicide and suicide: USA, 1955–87, Native American and U.S. all-race population.

increase in suicide rate during the 1960s and 1970s. These were the groups most affected by the economic boom associated with oil and related activities (Kraus and Buffler, 1979). In Manitoba between 1973 and 1982, the suicide rate was 2.6 times higher in southern communities, compared to the remote, northern ones. Tribal differences were also pronounced: the mean annual rate for Northern Ojibwa was 5/100,000, Chipewyan 13, Cree 22, Saulteaux 48, and Sioux 80/ 100,000. This correlated well with their degree of isolation; the more isolated and more northerly located the tribe, the lower was the rate (Garro, 1988). The direction of the north-south gradient, however, was reversed in Alberta, where the rate in northern reserves was 2.3 times that of southern ones. In addition to northerly latitudes, the suicide rate was also positively correlated with a lower per capita income and longer distance from an urban center (Bagley et al., 1990).

The age-specific rates are depicted in Figure 6.6. Compared to the U.S. all-races population, the excess in suicide and homicide among Native Americans was almost entirely among males. For homicide, the excess was observed in all ages, whereas for suicide, Native Americans in fact had a lower risk beyond age

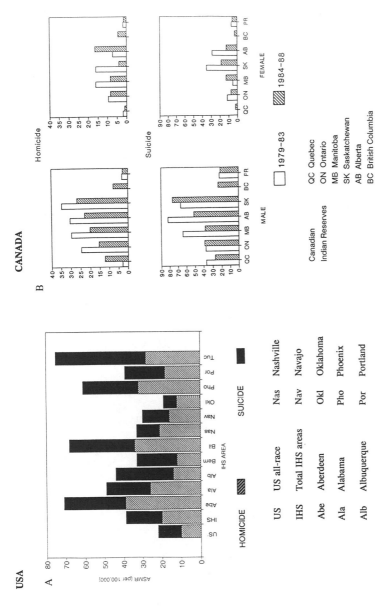

Figure 6.5. Regional variation in age-standardized mortality rate for homicide and suicide among Native Americans: (*A*) USA, 1980–87; (*B*) Canada, 1979–88.

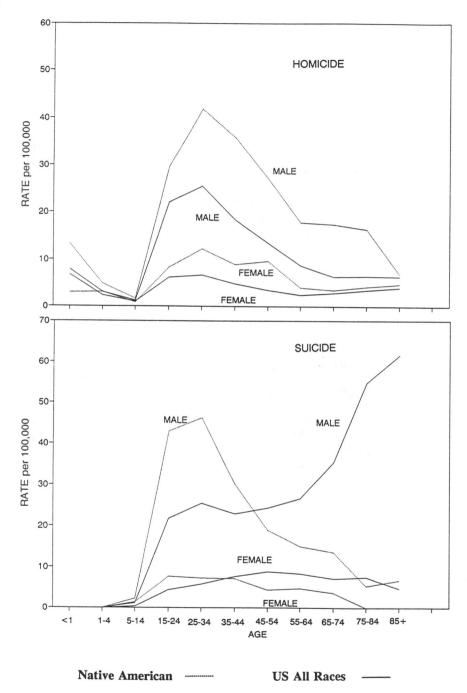

Figure 6.6. Age-specific mortality rate for homicide and suicide: USA, 1980–86, Native American and U.S. all-race populations.

45. Since the 1960s the trend appeared to be one of increasingly earlier onset. This trend, however, began to be reversed in the 1980s, for both suicide and homicide (Fig. 6.7). One characteristic of adolescent suicides is their tendency to occur in epidemics, or space-time clusters (e.g., Ward and Fox, 1977; Ross and Davis, 1986).

The methods used in suicide varied regionally among Native Americans, and between Native Americans and other ethnic groups. In the United States between 1980 and 1986, firearms were used in 55 percent of suicides, hanging 28 percent, and poisoning 9 percent (Baker et al., 1992). This is quite similar to the distribution among Indian suicides in Manitoba during 1973–82 (Garro, 1988). In Alaska, however, firearms wcrc considerably more important, constituting 80 percent of all Native suicides between 1979 and 1984, compared to a U.S. all-race national figure of 59 percent. Hanging and poisoning accounted for 9 per-

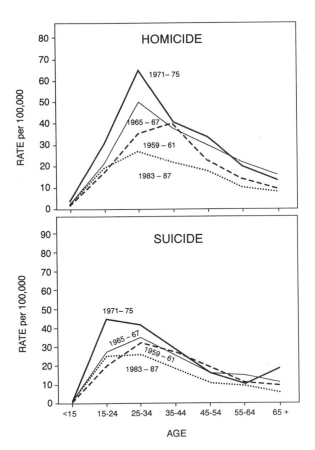

Figure 6.7. Change in age-specific mortality rate for homicide and suicide among Native Americans: USA, 1959–87.

cent and 7 percent among Alaska Natives, but 19 percent and 14 percent, re-spectively, in the United States nationally (Kettl and Bixler, 1991).

Suicides are not a new phenomenon among Native Americans. Descriptions of the "traditional" pattern of suicide and the cultural beliefs regarding suicide can be found in the ethnographic literature. In some Native American tribes, suicide was used as a means of revenge against an offender, who would then be held responsible for the death of the aggrieved. Other motives for suicide in-cluded grief, sexual deviance, impropriety, shame, jealousy, and marital diffi-culties. In some cultures, suicide victims were believed to be unable to reach the afterworld (Pine, 1981).

Among the Eskimo/Inuit, the image of the noble, but no longer productive, hunter walking out of a snow house into the blizzard to relieve his family's hardship has been a mainstay of Arctic lore. Such suicides, anthropologists have pointed out, occurred mainly among the elderly and infirm. They were carefully considered but nonritualized acts, often carried out after considerable family consultations in response to sickness, suffering, and a feeling of uselessness (Leighton and Hughes, 1955). This is in sharp contrast with the typical pattern among Native American suicides today, committed primarily by adolescents and young adults.

It was possible in Greenland to reconstruct reasonably reliably the suicide rate back to the early twentieth century. Alfred Bertelsen, perhaps Greenland's first epidemiologist, culled church registers and estimated the average annual suicide rate between 1901 and 1930 to be as low as 4/100,000. This compares with the steadily increasing rates of 9 during 1962–66, 17 during 1967–71, 54 during 1972–76, 69 during 1977–81, and 114/100,000 during 1982–86 (Lynge, 1985; Thorslund, 1990).

Suicide mortality represents only the tip of the epidemiological "iceberg." For every successful suicide, there are many more suicide attempts (also called parasuicide). These may or may not result in any contact with the health and social service system, so their true magnitude is difficult to estimate. While many attempts are of the "gestures" variety with minimal health risks, many repeat gestures ultimately succeed.

May (1987) reviewed data from the 1970s and noted that, among various Plains, Plateau, and Northwest Coast tribes, the attempt:suicide ratio ranged from about 9:1 to 17:1. The sex ratio of attempts was usually the reverse of successful suicides, where males predominated.

Data from the Adolescent Health Survey, which involved some 13,500 Native American grade 7–12 students belonging to various Plains, Southeast, and Southwest tribes, revealed that 12 percent of boys and 22 percent of girls had ever attempted suicide, over half of whom tried more than once. The comparison figures for non-Native Minnesota adolescents, among whom a similar survey was administered, were 7 percent in boys and 14 percent in girls (U.S. Congress, 1989; Blum et al., 1992).

Similarly for each homicide, there are usually many more violent assaults resulting in a full spectrum of nonfatal injuries. Data from the justice system (e.g., arrests, convictions) may provide some indication of the extent of the problem, although such statistics should be interpreted with caution. Differential law enforcement standards and judicial practices in a particular locality could explain apparent ethnic differences. Among Alaska Natives, the rate of all arrests during 1977–81 was twice that of whites in the same state, while the rate of arrests for violent felonies was three times higher (Phillips and Inui, 1986). Nationally in the United States the arrest rate for interpersonal conflicts (murders and assaults) in 1970 was five times higher among Indians than whites in urban areas, and three times higher in rural areas. That this could not all be attributed to discrimination against a visible minority group was supported by data from a youth survey in Arizona showing self-reported rates of fights to be 1.3 times and assaults 2.2 times higher among Indians than whites (Jensen et al., 1977). Similarly, data from the Adolescent Health Survey showed that almost 20 percent of respondents had been assaulted by another person to the point of unconsciousness (Blum et al., 1992).

In Canada, data from the Canadian Centre for Justice Statistics indicate that in the country as a whole, Natives accounted for 19 percent of admissions to provincial institutions and 13 percent of admissions to federal custody during 1988–89, even though Natives constituted less than 3 percent of the country's population. In some provinces, particularly those in the Prairies, Natives may account for 30%–65% of admissions to federal and provincial correctional institutions.

One particular form of violence that has received increasing attention in recent years is the abuse and neglect of children. The frequency of such crimes, particularly when they do not result in death, is very difficult to estimate. The increasing incidence of media reports of flagrant cases does not necessarily reflect the true scope of the problem. This is the case in any community, Native or non-Native. In its review of adolescent mental health, the Office of Technology Assessment cited nine studies published from 1969 to 1989 which generated estimates of child abuse and neglect among Native Americans (U.S. Congress, 1989). A variety of methods were used, including participant observation; review of case registries, records of medical care, and social service utilization; and interviews of key informants. Only one, the Adolescent Health Study, involved a large sample survey of adolescent students. It showed that 18 percent of respondents admitted to ever being abused physically, sexually, or both. Among girls, 17 percent had a history of sexual abuse, 19 percent physical abuse, and 9 percent both (Blum et al., 1992).

In his review, Fischler (1985) cited incidence rates from the 1970s of 26, 14, and 6 per 1000 children per year among the Cheyenne, Navajo, and off-reservation Indians in the United States, respectively, compared to a total U.S. average of 4/1000. These were rates of reported cases, which were subject to reporting bias in either direction. Underreporting could occur because of community denial of the problem, suspicion of non-Native social agencies, and inadequate diagnostic and treatment services. Overreporting could also occur because of social class and cultural barriers in the perception and understanding of Native child-rearing practices by non-Native professionals.

In Canada, the proportion of Indian children living in reserves who were "in care" was over 5 percent in 1981, slowly declining to 3 percent by 1987. The national figure, however, was less than 1 percent (Hagey et al., 1989). Although children are taken away from their homes by social welfare agencies for a variety of reasons, a violent and abusive family environment is a major factor.

Etiology and Risk Factors

Opinions abound as to why Native Americans are at such high risk for suicide, homicide, and violence. Depending on the disciplinary orientation of the theorist, explanations have been sought in terms of individual psychopathology, family dynamics, social structure, economic relations, and cultural transition. [Reviews of the large and diverse literature can be found in Shore and Manson (1983), Berlin (1987), and U.S. Congress (1989)]. Some studies have used designs familiar to epidemiologists, several of which are briefly reviewed here.

A small case-control study was conducted by Dizmang and associates (1974) among the Shoshone and Bannock in Idaho during the 1960s. With ten cases and 4 times as many controls matched according to age, sex, and blood quantum, family factors which were significantly associated with suicide included multiple caretakers during childhood, the criminal history of the caretakers, and a history of divorce or desertion. Characteristics of the individual included history of arrest and attending a boarding school. Only univariate analyses were reported.

A somewhat larger case-control study in Alaska [cited in Kettl and Bixler (1991)] analyzed thirty-three suicide victims and their age-sex-matched controls. A history of alcohol abuse and past suicide attempts were the most important risk factors, whereas histories of psychiatric and neurological illnesses were not significantly related. The importance of alcohol in Native suicide was borne out by post-mortem blood alcohol levels in Alaska, which were available from 87 percent of all suicides. Just under 80 percent of Native suicides, compared to 48 percent among whites, had detectable blood alcohol. The proportion with levels greater than 100 mg/dl was 54 percent among Natives and 20 percent among whites (Hlady and Middaugh, 1988).

In a case-control study among Greenland Eskimos, Grove and Lynge (1979) compared successful suicides and suicidal attempts with nonpsychiatric, never-suicidal hospital controls. Among the risk factors identified were a background of disharmonious homes, a family and personal history of alcohol abuse, a personal history of emotional conflict with close contacts, job instability, and criminal convictions.

In a cross-sectional survey of students in one tribally administered boarding school in the Southeast, Manson and colleagues (1989) found that students at greatest risk for suicide were those who reported having either family or friends who had attempted suicide and those who reported on standardized psychological tests as having depressive symptoms, alcohol use, and lack of family support.

The Indian Adolescent Health Survey mentioned earlier also provided information on the risk factors of suicide attempts. Grossman and others (1991) analyzed the Navajo subsample. In a multiple logistic regression where age and all covariates were simultaneously adjusted for, the significant odds ratios for suicide attempts were as follows:

history of treatment for mental problems	3.2
extreme alienation from family/community	3.2
exposure to suicide attempt by friends	2.8
weekly use of hard liquor	2.7
exposure to suicide attempt in family	2.3
poor self-perceived health	2.2
history of child physical abuse	1.9
female sex	1.7
victim of sexual abuse as a child	1.5

Such factors as school performance, and the absence of a biological parent or divorced/deceased parents were not significantly associated with suicide attempts (Grossman et al., 1991).

Compared to suicide, homicide has received far less attention in the medical literature. A pilot study was conducted among inmates incarcerated for criminal homicide in British Columbia in the mid-1970s. It involved extensive record reviews and standardized psychiatric interviews of 22 Natives and a group of whites matched on the basis of sentence, age at first homicide, and IQ (Jilek and Roy, 1976). While Natives were overrepresented in the prison system, manslaughter charges far exceeded capital murders. The typical victim of homicide committed by a Native, if also Native, tended to be female and related to the offender. The non-Native victim of a homicidal Native tended to be male and a stranger. The Native homicide offenders were characterized by limited education, unskilled occupation, and history of alcohol abuse, but were less likely to show evidence of psychiatric illness or sexual deviance. In terms of personality development, a lack of exposure to traditional Indian culture was associated with early onset of antisocial behavior. A positive Native identification, on the other hand, was predictive of benefiting from education and therapy provided in the institutions (Jilek and Roy, 1976).

An analysis of homicide on the Navajo reservation during 1956–65 revealed that the typical offender was a young (age 25–39) *married* man with children, and the victim usually the wife or lover. Marital strife, domestic quarrels and sexual jealousy were the dominant motives. An unusual aspect was that 20 percent of all homicide offenders committed suicide immediately afterwards, a much higher proportion than data from other ethnic groups studied (Levy et al., 1969).

A history of childhood abuse is believed to be a risk factor of later delinquency and criminal or violent behavior, and there is some evidence to support this from longitudinal studies in non-Native populations (e.g., Widom, 1989). While the relative risk may be high, it is important to note that the attributable risk may in fact be quite small; afterall, most abused children do not grow up to become delinquent, criminal, or violent.

The risk factors for committing child abuse itself are complex. Alcoholism is strongly associated: the Navajo Child Abuse Study found that 50 percent of abuse and up to 80 percent of neglect cases were alcohol related (White and Cornely, 1981). Other factors include poor parenting skills, contributed to in part by the former practice of separation of children from their parents for prolonged periods in residential schools, situational stress with ineffective social support and coping mechanisms, and the usual banes of poverty and modernization (Fischler, 1985). Much of this evidence was derived from case series without a non-abused group for comparison.

Oakland and Kane (1973) conducted a case-control study among the Navajos, identifying abuse victims from hospital records and selecting age-matched hospital controls. Their data have been reanalyzed to provide the following odds ratios:

having 1–4 sibs/no sibs	4.0
mother not married/married	3.7
primary education only/secondary or higher	1.3
mother had <5 prenatal clinic visits/ 5+ visits	1.2
mother working/not working	1.1
teenage mother/mother aged 19+	1.0

Such data indicated that single parenthood and multiple sibs were the only factors that showed any strong association with child abuse (Oakland and Kane, 1973).

Prevention and Control Strategies

There are very few formal evaluations of the many suicide-prevention programs in Native American communities, or for that matter, in any population (Streiner and Adam, 1987). Most published studies are program descriptions or uncontrolled observations characterized by small sample size and short duration.

A study on Manitoulin Island, Ontario, five years after a suicide outbreak in the mid-1970s, attributed an apparent decline in suicide, parasuicide, and violent deaths to a multidimensional program consisting of residential alcoholism treatment, family counseling, community feasts, job creation for youths, and self-esteem enhancement in the schools. Native mental health workers were employed to provide crisis intervention as well as liaison with the non-Native professional health and social service sectors (Fox et al., 1984). Shore and others (1972) described the development of a suicide-prevention center in a Pacific Northwest reservation.

It should be noted that the "prevention" label of many programs really refers to crisis intervention and not to primary prevention. In 1989 the Alaska state legislature set aside funds for community-initiated suicide prevention programs. Of 54 projects funded during the first year, about one-third involved improving communications between elders and youth. Other interventions included providing recreational alternatives (both traditional and nontraditional), strengthening support and self-help networks in the community, and cultural projects. This initiative was unusual in that "primary" preventive interventions were in the majority, compared to the more treatment-oriented programs such as crisis response and individual counseling (Berger and Tobeluk, 1991).

It is increasingly recognized that the ultimate solution to the interrelated problems of self-inflicted and interpersonal violence (including child and spouse abuse) lies in a healing process that only the communities themselves can undertake. The reestablishment of individual and community self-esteem requires overcoming the denial of embarrassing and/or painful community problems on the one hand, and emphasizing and enhancing positive traditional values and customs on the other. Significant steps have been taken in scattered locations in Canada and the United States. In the Northwest Coast, spiritual leaders involved their young people in the revived Spirit Dance ceremony, where they find a renewed Native identity and cultural pride (Jilek, 1982). One project, in northern Saskatchewan, set the goal of empowering abused Native women to become independent of violent environments by developing mutual support networks (Dickson, 1989). Various resource guides and training manuals have been developed to assist communities [for example, by the Nechi Institute of Alberta (Martens et al., 1988), and the Quebec Health and Social Service Ministry in collaboration with the Native women's organization, Femmes Autochtones du Québec (Lamoureux, 1991)]. A major international conference with the theme "Healing Our Spirit Worldwide" was held in Edmonton in 1992 and provided a forum for sharing experiences in combating violence and substance abuse by aboriginal groups from around the world.

Alcohol and Substance Abuse

Extent and Magnitude of the Problem

Alcohol and substance abuse can be considered risk factors for a variety of injuries, although they can also be considered health problems, with their own risk factors and control strategies. In this respect, they are analogous to hypertension, obesity, and diabetes, all risk factors for ischemic heart disease and all diseases in their own right.

There is considerable terminological confusion, particularly in distinguishing such terms as "abuse," "dependency," "addiction," "alcoholism," and "problem drinking." A multidisciplinary group of experts have reached some consensus on these definitions (Rinaldi et al., 1988). In the literature on Native American drinking, some definitions of alcoholism emphasize the chronicity and the disruptive effect on social harmony and economic well-being, while the relativist approach would only consider drinking to be a problem when it exceeds community norms or results in loss of control (Brod, 1975). The dominant theoretical framework in public health (as distinct from, say, theology and clinical psychiatry) is the so-called availability theory. Drinking is considered neither a sin nor a disease; rather, alcohol is recognized as a risk factor with many health effects, and the higher the population's overall consumption, the more frequent such health effects occur. The emphasis is thus no longer on "alcoholics" but on all drinkers in a community (Rankin and Ashley, 1992).

An epidemiological assessment of the extent and health impact of alcohol use and abuse based on traditional sources of mortality and morbidity data is likely to be inaccurate. In the ICD-9, only a few codes make direct reference to alcohol—for example, conditions such as alcoholic psychosis (code 291), alcohol dependence (303), and alcohol abuse (305) are grouped under the rubric "mental disorders." Other conditions that can be directly attributed to alcohol use include alcoholic cardiomegaly (code 425.5), alcohol gastritis (535.3), acute alcoholic hepatitis (571.1), and alcoholic cirrhosis of the liver (571.2). Comparisons can be made between Native Americans and the general North American populations in terms of some of these alcohol-related diseases. Since the 1970s, when the excess was over 7 times, the gap has narrowed to about 4 times (Fig. 6.8). In terms of age-sex pattern, an excess over non-Natives occurs among adults in both sexes. Regional variation also exists (Fig. 6.9).

Within specific regions, for example in Oklahoma, a high proportion of alcohol-related deaths among Native Americans (9%) compared to other racial groups (3% in blacks and 2% in whites) can be observed. Within that state, tribal differences can also be demonstrated, with the Cheyenne-Arapaho, Comanche, and Kiowa in the western part of the state more severely affected than the Cherokee, Choctaw, Creek, Seminole, and Pawnee in the east (Christian et al., 1989). In a tri-ethnic community in the Southwest, Native Americans exceeded both Anglos and Hispanics in three survey-based indices: the quantity and frequency of intake, the number of times "drunk," and alcohol-related offenses (Graves, 1967).

In addition to the entire group of injuries and the more directly related medical conditions such as cirrhosis, there are a host of other conditions in which alcohol

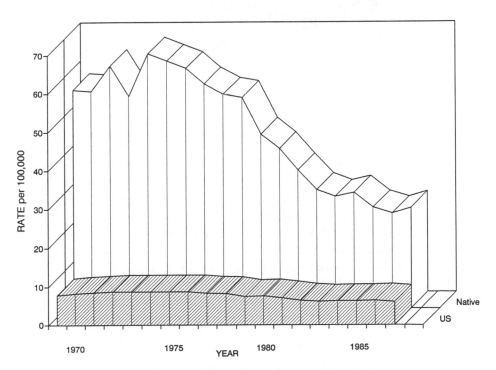

Figure 6.8. Age-standardized mortality rate for alcohol-related diseases: USA, 1969–87, Native American and U.S. all-race populations.

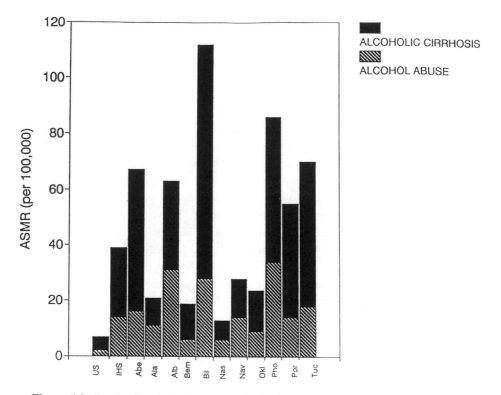

Figure 6.9. Regional variation in age-standardized mortality rate for alcohol-related diseases among Native Americans: USA, 1981–83.

plays some etiologic role (e.g., various gastrointestinal cancers, tuberculosis, and pancreatitis, among others). To obtain a complete picture of the impact of alcohol on the overall mortality pattern, one would need to know the etiologic fraction or population attributable risk for alcohol in these diseases. Such pieces of information are not readily available for the larger North American population and are mostly lacking for Native Americans. The impact of alcohol abuse extends also into the second generation in the form of the fetal alcohol syndrome, although considerable uncertainty exists as to its true extent in Native communities (May et al., 1983; Bray and Anderson, 1989).

   The law enforcement and justice systems provide additional sources of data of the extent and impact of alcohol on the health and social well-being of a community. For example, U.S. crime data for 1970 indicated that alcohol-related offenses (drinking and driving, liquor law violations, public drunkenness) were 22 times higher among Indians than whites in urban areas and seven times higher in rural areas. Note that the urban-rural difference was also significant among

Indians, with the urban rate 10 times higher than the rural rate (Jensen et al., 1977). In Oklahoma tribal variation in alcohol-related arrests correlated with alcohol-related mortality (Stratton et al., 1978).

Westermeyer (1976) advocated the surveillance of alcohol-related health and social problems utilizing a basket of routinely collected data, including mortality, hospital morbidity, admission to chemical dependency units, and arrests and incarceration for public drunkenness and drunk driving. A broad-based approach was necessary to overcome institutional bias, where Native Americans with alcohol problems generally showed up as statistics in "lower-cost problem-maintenance institutions" rather than "higher-cost problem-resolving resources." They were more likely to turn up in morgues, prisons, and foster homes than in treatment facilities.

To assess the extent of alcohol abuse in the community, particularly abuse that does not result in contact with any element of the health, social service, or justice systems, a survey is the only means available. Regional surveys on the prevalence of alcohol use as well as "drinking styles" have been conducted in many tribes [reviewed in May (1982)]. Whittaker (1982) was able to repeat a survey on a Sioux reservation over a span of 20 years and reported a relatively stable prevalence in overall alcohol use but a substantial increase in the proportion of heavy drinkers.

In some Native populations the prevalence of ever-drinkers has been found to be lower than non-Natives. For example, only about 20 percent of adult Cree and Ojibwa in northwestern Ontario, compared to 80 percent in the general population of Ontario, were ever-drinkers. The prevalence declined with age but was highest among those with the most education (Young, 1982). In the Northwest Territories, the 1985 Health Promotion Survey revealed that 34 percent of Inuit and 64 percent of Indian adults reported drinking alcohol at least once per month during the past year, a proportion lower than the 73 percent reported by non-Natives (Imrie and Warren, 1988).

Beauvais and his group conducted six surveys between 1975 and 1987 of Native adolescents age 12–16 attending reservation schools. Each of their national cluster samples covered some 5–6 tribes representative of a variety of geographical locations and cultural affiliations (Beauvais et al., 1989). In terms of lifetime prevalence of alcohol and drug use, there had been an increase between 1975 and 1987. In the latest survey the prevalence of alcohol use was 81 percent and that of marijuana 61 percent. Stimulants, inhalants, cocaine, and hallucinogens (in descending order of importance) were used to a much lesser extent. The sex ratio was about one, which was different from most non-Native populations surveyed, where males predominated. In almost all categories of substances apart from cocaine, the prevalence was higher among Native youths than among non-Natives. The age of onset was also earlier: by the fourth to sixth grade, about one-third of Native youths had tried alcohol, and about 10 percent had been intoxicated.

A survey on illicit drug use has been conducted annually in the United States since 1975 on a nationally representative sample of high school seniors (Bachman et al., 1991). The 1985–89 combined samples were based on over 73,000 students, of whom more than 1,000 were Native Americans. Compared to other ethnic groups, Native students had the highest prevalence of use of illicit drugs. The time trends over the three 5-year periods between 1976 and 1985 showed an overall decline in all ethnic groups but their relative ranking remained except for alcohol. Native Americans had the highest prevalence during 1976–79 but "crossed-over" during 1980–84, when they were overtaken by whites (Bachman et al., 1991).

While survey data often give the veneer of statistical rigor, their validity in the cross-cultural setting is not always assured. Segal (1983) cautioned about the translation of standard research instruments designed for use in non-Native populations into a Native language. Survey questions on frequency and quantity of consumption presume that alcohol consumption occurs in an orderly and controlled manner and that it is available "by the drink" and purchased from liquor stores. In many Native communities, particularly those that are legally "dry," the supply, distribution, and consumption patterns can be very different from those in non-Native communities.

Ethnographic research can provide rich data on drinking behavior and suggest clues to etiology and control that cannot be elicited from survey questionnaires. Some of the earlier literature characterized Native American drinking as a group activity rather than a solitary pastime, often serving a ceremonial or spiritual role (e.g., the seeking of visions). Little social stigma was attached to such drinking, and excesses and misbehaviors did not result in social sanctions. Drinking tended to be periodic and explosive but nonaddictive (Littman, 1970; Brod, 1975). For most North American tribes, alcohol was introduced soon after contact with Europeans. A few tribes, primarily agricultural societies in the Southwest and Mesoamerica, had knowledge in the manufacture and use of alcohol. The Pima and Pagago, for example, made wine from cactus (Price, 1975). However, drinking patterns vary geographically and differ in their historical evolution, so it is difficult to determine if there is a "generic" drinking pattern common to most Native American communities.

While alcohol use may have some antiquity in North America or may have been part of some tribes' cultural repertoire, substance abuse is in all likelihood a "new" problem. Among the substances abused, gasoline sniffing is particularly prevalent among Native children and adolescents in some areas. Gasoline contains a variety of highly toxic hydrocarbons, and it may also contain tetraethyl lead as an antiknock additive. Gasoline sniffers suffer from various acute symptoms of encephalopathy. Severe poisoning may culminate in death from central nervous system depression and respiratory obstruction (Ross, 1982). Long-term inhalers suffer from a chronic organic brain syndrome. Some geneticists have even queried the existence of a fetal gasoline syndrome among the offspring of gasoline sniffers who have grown up to become parents (Hunter et al., 1979).

In some communities in northern Manitoba in the 1970s, between 50 percent and 100 percent of children and adolescents were reputed to be current and recent gasoline sniffers or showed depressed levels of aminolevulinic acid dehydrase, evidence of tetraethyl lead poisoning (Boeckx et al., 1977). In one Indian reserve in northwestern Ontario, 25 percent of children 5–15 years of age, or 10 percent of the total population, were identified as sniffers (Remington and Hoffman, 1984). Cases of toxic encephalopathy have also been reported from the Navajo Reservation. In a survey of high school students in a boarding school, 11 percent reported having tried it "for fun." Sniffers tended to have poor school performance and delinquent behaviors, but few seemed to engage in the activity frequently enough to develop either symptomatic or asymptomatic lead overload (Coulehan et al., 1983).

Etiology and Risk Factors

A substantial literature has developed on the relation between Native Americans and alcohol [see the bibliography by Mail and McDonald (1980)]. Researchers, clinicians, and policy-makers from a variety of disciplines and orientations have tried to understand the problem from diverse approaches. One compendium on alcoholism enumerated eleven theories, which can be grouped into the biological, psychological, and social (Chaudron and Wilkinson, 1988):

Biological: genetic, neurobiological, and neurobehavioral theories

Psychological: psychoanalytic, personality, classical conditioning, and social learning theories

Social: systems, availability, anthropological, and economic theories

The biological approach, particularly genetically determined differences in the rate of alcohol metabolism and physiologic responses, is discussed in more detail in a later section of this chapter.

Some anthropologists and cross-cultural psychiatrists attribute a central role to acculturation or "socio-cultural deprivation" (Dozier, 1966) and the emotional stresses that accompany it. The Native American, caught in the proverbial "no-man's land" between Native and non-Native societies, seeks relief and solace in alcohol. Littman (1970) summarized the prevailing views on "why Indians drink:"

to relieve anxiety from economic insecurities

to release repressed aggression

to relieve pressure from acculturation

to promote group solidarity

Or, as Brod (1975) eloquently summed it up: "Drunkenness can provide short-cut gratification by providing fantasy solutions to culture-bound problems." A fuller discussion of sociocultural theories of alcohol and drug abuse in conjunction with the other social pathologies is provided in a later section.

A more individual-oriented approach, subscribed to by some psychologists and sociologists, tends to emphasize the similarity between Natives and non-Natives and seeks individual psychosocial variables that explain why, given the same social environment (poverty, low education, and unemployment, etc.) certain individuals take up drinking while others do not. An example of this approach is the study by Oetting and colleagues (1988). Comparing nondrinkers and drinkers among 12–16-year-old Native students using a variety of psychological scales, they found little difference in terms of symptoms of emotional problems, feelings of alienation, self-confidence, or social acceptance. However, drinkers were characterized by use of other drugs, social deviance, family dysfunction, poor school adjustment, loss of hope for the future, and most significantly, association with peers who drink. Using path analysis, these researchers hypothesized that all but last of these determinants operate in creating the potential for involvement with peers who have similar problems, which then became the immediate antecedent of drinking.

In another study, this group compared Indian and Anglo youths. Again, peer association was the main determinant, while emotional distress (in the form of depression, anxiety or alienation) was not associated with drinking behavior, with the exception of anger. Among Anglo youths, however, anger led to problem behaviors, whereas among Native youths, anger led to improved self-esteem, which decreased the likelihood of alcohol use (Oetting et al., 1989).

Shoshone and Arapahoe high school students in Wyoming, when compared with their white classmates, tended to have more favorable attitudes towards marijuana and other drug use, were more likely to try them, and tried them at an earlier age. However, having once tried, they did not seem any more prone to continuing the practice (Cockerham et al., 1976). Students who already used one substance such as alcohol were more likely to use another drug (Cockerham, 1977).

In a survey of residents over the age of 5 in an Ojibwa community in eastern Manitoba, it was found that adults and school pupils who participated in hobbies were less likely to use alcohol. Young people who reported good family relationships were also less likely to use alcohol and marijuana (Longclaws et al., 1980).

Among Pueblo school children in New Mexico, Kaufman (1973) was not able to detect any difference in the prevalence of alcoholic families or broken homes between sniffers and non-sniffers, or between different categories of sniffers based on frequency of use.

Barnes, in his review of solvent abuse in a variety of populations, concluded that parental alcohol abuse was the most significant determinant of gasoline sniffing. He proposed a causal model that listed four environmental risk factors—low social assets, acculturative stress, parental drug use, and peer/sibling influence—mediated through a filter of "psychological vulnerability," consisting of learned helplessness and alienation (Barnes, 1979).

Prevention and Control Strategies

The approach to alcohol and drug abuse in most health jurisdictions is one of treatment and rehabilitation of people who have demonstrated a problem, whether residential, outpatient, or "community-based." Government, tribal, and contract agencies responsible for Native health services, in both Canada and the United States, operate a variety of alcohol treatment programs. Both in terms of professional manpower and facilities, the demand far exceeds the supply. In a detailed review of Native American alcoholism, Lamarine (1988) lamented that despite the extensive literature, preventive efforts were conspicuous by their virtual absence. It should be noted that in the non-Native population, education-based prevention programs, whether directed at school students or adults, have not been shown to be effective in terms of such outcome measures as reducing current use and preventing future use (Kinder et al., 1980; Moskowitz, 1989).

In a survey among the Navajos, it was found that the respondents were knowledgeable about the consequences of alcohol abuse, and a majority believed that drinking even a small amount of alcohol was harmful. Despite the relatively low prevalence of drinking in the community, over 90 percent of those questioned believed that "Indians had a problem with alcohol," and most attributed this to a "physical weakness" present among Indians but not other groups. From a policy perspective, it would appear that more knowledge on the adverse consequences of alcohol was not necessary, while correcting inaccuracies and expanding knowledge on policies of intervention and prevention might have more promising results (May and Smith, 1988).

Attempts to prevent and control alcohol problems among Native Americans are not new. Dozier (1966) enumerated various approaches: legal prohibition, nativistic/messianic religious movements, individual education, counseling and psychotherapy, and group-based programs that encouraged Native participation in substitute activities. Such specific interventions can be reduced into three broad categories: (1) controlling the supply of alcoholic beverages; (2) shaping drinking practices; and (3) reducing the physical and social environmental risks (May, 1992).

In response to the onslaught of missionaries and the demoralization of military conquests, various Native "revivalist" religions have sprung up over the past century, such as the Handsome Lake cult among the Iroquois, the Ghost Dance of the Plains tribes, and the Native American Church in the southwest. These had all denounced or prohibited alcohol use. In more recent years, evangelistic Protestant sects, many of which gained wide popularity in many Native communities, adhere to similar views on alcohol. In a somewhat different context, the principles of Alcoholics Anonymous have been transformed into Native revival movements, and meetings have become community-wide social events (Jilek-Aall, 1981).

While prohibition, whether legal or religious, does not eradicate drinking, it does reduce overall consumption and alcohol-related health effects. This was shown in the U.S. experience earlier this century: both per capita consumption and cirrhosis mortality declined when Prohibition was in effect, and they rebounded when it was abandoned. This is also borne out by cross-national comparisons (Rankin and Ashley, 1992).

In the United States federal law prohibited the sale of alcohol to Indians until 1953, after which time individual tribal governments decided if prohibition would continue. In Canada, various amendments to the Indian Act prohibited the possession and use of alcohols by Indians until 1963 (Price, 1975). Some scholars (e.g., Price 1975) considered prohibition to have deleterious social effects, since it:

created an unnecessary class of legal offenses

stimulated conflict with law-enforcement agencies

led to financial exploitation

reinforced the binge drinking patterns

prevented the development of internal controls

A comparison of "dry" with "wet" reservations in Montana and Wyoming during 1959–74 found that mortality from cirrhosis, motor vehicle accidents, suicides, and homicides were reduced after legalization. Also, alcohol-related arrests and overall crime were lower in the "wet" reservations (May, 1986). This was explained on the basis of a change in social value and a shift to social, rather than legal, control of drinking.

The effectiveness of prohibition is difficult to assess in a single, small community using "hard" health outcome measures. Qualitative and ethnographic methods may provide useful data for policy decisions. In a Canadian Inuit community, O'Neil (1985) observed over a 4-year period that alcohol prohibition had contributed to an increase in family integrity and respect between generations, an increase in youthful interest in traditional values and lifestyles, and a decrease in aggressive behaviors and abuse of other substances. Enforcement of the by-laws was through local social pressure without resort to the externally imposed law-enforcement and justice systems. To be sure, clandestine drinking occurred, but it was tolerated as long as it remained private and did not result in disruptive behaviors in public. The difficulty of supply meant that even habitual heavy drinkers had to reduce their consumption substantially (O'Neil, 1985).

Beauvais and LaBoueff (1985) pointed out that the many drug and alcohol programs in reservations across the United States, while reflecting different treatment philosophies and theoretical frameworks, tended to be imposed in a "top-down" fashion by health professionals who were usually non-Native. Community action that began with a core group of stakeholders and community members who had personal experience, around which other community members could coalesce, was seen as a preferable alternative.

Physical training has been identified as a potential means of enhancing Native adolescents' self-image and reducing drug and alcohol abuse. Scott and Myers (1988) reported on a quasi-experimental study in an Algonquin community in northwestern Quebec during which students age 12–18 were assigned to either a 24-week fitness program or regular physical education classes. The fitness program (intervention) was designed to enhance aerobic capacity, flexibility, and strength, while the classes (control) emphasized traditional, competitive sports-specific skills. The impact was modest, perhaps the result of the insufficient duration, intensity, or continuity of the intervention. Alcohol and drug use remained stable in the intervention group but increased among controls. Scores of self-esteem and body image did not change in either group, while physical "self-efficacy" (perceived physical ability and self-confidence) did increase over time in the intervention group (Scott and Myers, 1988).

The IHS launched a strategic plan for alcohol control in 1986 which stressed prevention. Included in the plan were various school-based education programs aimed at improving self-image, values, attitudes, and decision-making. The other major component consisted of providing alternative activities for youths (Rhoades et al., 1988).

A Role for Genes?

The discussion so far has emphasized the overwhelming importance of environmental determinants in injuries among Native Americans. This makes injuries very different from the other two groups of diseases considered, particularly the chronic diseases. Superficially it would seem that genetics would play no role in the causation of injuries. While it would be difficult to conceive of a motor vehicle collision as genetically determined, closer examination reveals that genetic factors do contribute to the susceptibility to, initiation of, and recovery from injuries (Haddon, 1980). While there are rare genetic syndromes of bleeding disorders and brittle bones that cause afflicted individuals to be more susceptible to serious injuries from relatively minor energy transfers, of more public health importance are such genetic conditions as myopia and color-blindness. However, it is clear that nongenetic (such as psychosocial, economic, cultural, and political) factors have far greater impact on the incidence and prevention of injuries.

Whether alcohol abuse or alcoholism has any genetic basis has been the subject of much controversy, particularly its policy implications among Native Americans. A large body of data from twin, half-siblings, adoption, metabolic, and neurophysiologic studies is available (Cloninger, 1987), and there is widespread acceptance among biologically oriented researchers that "susceptibility," "vulnerability," and "predisposition" to the development of alcohol abuse is heritable. The opposition to the biogenetic explanation takes two forms. While some researchers have challenged the strength and quality of the scientific evidence (e.g., Lester 1989), others opposed it on the assumption that a genetic "cause" of alcohol abuse means that the problem is unchangeable and that it precluded application of broad environmental strategies to eliminate socioeconomic determinants of alcohol abuse. Some investigators prefer to attribute alcohol abuse among Native Americans to "relations to the means of production," which have nothing whatsoever to do with peoples' ethnic or racial status (Fisher, 1987).

Reed (1985) enumerated nine categories of alcohol response where ethnic differences have been shown to occur: consumption rate, absorption rate from the digestive tract, metabolism rate, prevalence of variants of the enzyme alcohol dehydrogenase (ADH) and acetaldehyde dehydrogenase (ALDH), alcohol sensitivity, cardiovascular changes, psychological changes, and alcohol abuse. Of these, he concluded that enzyme differences were very probably due to single genes, while rates of absorption and metabolism were likely polygenic.

The speed with which alcohol is absorbed from the stomach can be measured by the time it takes to reach peak blood alcohol concentration (BAC) after a test drink. A clinical study of 17 Oklahoma Indian men showed that they had significantly shorter mean time to peak BAC and higher peak BAC than Caucasian controls (Farris and Jones, 1978).

Once absorbed into the blood stream, alcohol is metabolized in the liver first to acetaldehyde (catalyzed by the enzyme ADH), and ultimately to acetate (catalyzed by the enzyme ALDH). The rate of metabolism can be measured by the rate of disappearance of alcohol from the blood following a test dose, expressed as mg/dl/hr. This rate can be adjusted for body weight (mg/dl/kg/hr).

A study in Alberta (Fenna et al., 1971) compared white volunteers with Inuit and Indian hospital patients and found that when they were given alcohol intravenously, both Native groups had slower rates of disappearance of blood alcohol. This differential response persisted even after stratifying for the history of usual alcohol consumption (categorized as light, moderate, and heavy drinkers). This study lent credence to the impression that Natives take a longer time to "sober up."

The Canadian study, however, was not corroborated by subsequent studies in other Native groups, some of which actually showed the opposite trend. Bennion and Li (1976) found that Indians belonging to several Southwestern tribes had a *faster* rate of disappearance of blood alcohol, which when adjusted for body weight, was not significantly different from whites. These investigators also obtained liver biopsy specimens from patients undergoing gallbladder surgery and tested them for activity of ADH. While there was substantial individual variation, no group differences could be detected. Other studies among the Ojibwa from northwestern Ontario (Reed et al., 1976), various Indian tribes in Oklahoma (Farris and Jones, 1978), and the largely unacculturated Tarahumara Indians of Mexico (Zeiner et al., 1976) all showed that Indians were able to metabolize ethanol quicker than whites.

J. M. Schaefer enumerated the difficulties in interpreting these "first-generation" studies of racial differences in alcohol metabolism: varying ethanol doses, routes of administration, sample sizes, method of ethnic group identification, and inclusion of information on habitual alcohol use, socioeconomic background, and other behavioral and physiological variables (Schaefer, 1981).

Physiological responses to alcohol ingestion, such as facial flushing and unpleasant symptoms such as headaches and tachycardia, also have been found to vary between ethnic groups, particularly their high prevalence in Asiatic populations. Acetaldehyde, a metabolite of ethanol, is believed to be responsible for flushing. Higher activity of ADH would produce more acetaldehyde, while higher activity of ALDH would result in its quicker removal. Native Americans have higher breath acetaldehyde levels than whites (Wolff, 1973). In their comparative study of whites, Chinese, and Ojibwa Indians, Reed et al. (1976) showed that, in tandem with the fastest decline in blood ethanol concentration among the three groups, the Indians also showed the highest levels of acetaldehyde at various times after the ingestion of ethanol.

Studies of alleles of the enzyme ADH among the Navajo, Pueblo, and Sioux showed that they did not have the "atypical" β_2 subunit encoded by the ADH_2 gene, responsible for high ethanol oxidizing activity and very prevalent among Asians. Overall, their pattern of the ADH_2 and ADH_3 alleles were more similar to whites than to Asians (Rex et al., 1985; Bosron et al., 1988).

The other major enzyme involved in alcohol metabolism, ALDH, also exists in multiple forms (isozymes) that are genetically determined. The isozyme ALDH I has been found to be rarely if ever deficient among Europeans and Africans, while it is deficient in a high proportion of Asians (Goedde et al., 1983). Studies among North and South American Indians, however, showed highly variable proportions of subjects who were deficient. Among South American tribes, the proportions ranged from 40–70 percent (Goedde et al., 1983, 1986), 16 percent among Indians in Oklahoma, and 0–5 percent among the Sioux, Navajo, and Pueblo in the Southwest (Rex et al., 1985; Goedde et al., 1986; Bosron et al., 1988).

The sensitivity to alcohol and its metabolic byproducts would appear to be a "protective" mechanism in populations with deficient or abnormal enzymes. Even if this were the case with Native Americans, and the evidence is by no means consistent, it would appear that social and cultural factors could overcome this physiologically based aversion to alcohol such that this group now has higher rates of alcohol use, dependence, and abuse.

The biological basis of suicide and violence has also been investigated, though such studies have not focused on Native Americans. Lower levels of neurotransmitters such as the serotonin precursors 5-hydroxyindoleacetic acid (5-HIAA) and 5-hydroxytryptophan (5-HTP) have been demonstrated in the cerebrospinal fluid of patients with depression, suicidal behavior, and aggression. Genetic studies involving adoption have shown that adoptees who committed suicide were more likely than nonsuicide adoptees to have had biological relatives who committed suicide [see Monk (1987) for a recent review].

A complete understanding of the social pathologies among Native Americans must incorporate both biomedical and sociocultural data. The relative contribution of genetic and environmental factors in disease etiology may differ from the infectious and chronic diseases. While the current state of knowledge is still rudimentary, rapidly developing new techniques and procedures can be expected to shed further light on the genetic basis of complex, multifactorial diseases.

Traditional Culture vs Social Change

In explaining the high incidence of suicide, homicide, accidents, and alcohol abuse (called collectively the social pathologies), cultural anthropologists and sociologists have often invoked concepts such as cultural conflict, "anomie," social disintegration, and acculturation. That the explanation of such a highly individual act as suicide can indeed be sought in terms of broad social factors can be traced to the classic work by the nineteenth century French sociologist Émile Durkheim, whose opus *On Suicide* was only translated into English and published in 1951.

Various researchers have attempted to amplify and clarify the complex relationships involved and offered their explanatory models. Hackenberg and Gallagher (1972), assigned "modernization" scores based on ethnohistorical data to 42 villages in the Papago reservation in southern Arizona. These were grouped into four zones of increasing modernization based on their scores as well as kinship ties and dialect differences. The accidental injury rates in the four zones were positively related to their modernization ranks. The high injury rates among the more "modern" villages could not be attributed to differences in demographic structure or access to treatment facilities, but they were related to the greater proportion of wage labor, higher formal education levels and Protestant religious affiliation, evidence of "an attempt to escape traditionalism" (Hackenberg and Gallagher, 1972).

Further research among the Papagos attempted to demonstrate whether accidental injury rates could distinguish four types of individuals: "modern" individuals in "modern" villages, "traditional" individuals in "modern" villages, "modern" individuals in "traditional" villages, and "traditional" individuals in "traditional" villages (Stull, 1972). The results showed that individuals in traditional villages, regardless of their own personal "modernity" had the lowest injury rates, while modern individuals in modern villages were the worst off. Traditional individuals in modern villages occupied an intermediate position (Stull, 1972).

Levy and Kunitz (1971, 1987) argued against the utility of sweeping "social disintegration" theories to account for observed inter-tribal differences in the rate of social pathologies. They reconstructed homicide rates from 1883–89 in various Southwest, Plains and Plateau tribes and found considerable variation. They observed that tribes that were highly integrated socially and politically had the lowest rate of homicide, whereas the loosely organized band societies had the highest rate (Levy and Kunitz, 1971). They believed that persistent aspects of traditional social structure probably played a larger role than more recent responses to externally imposed modernization/acculturation in the development of social pathologies. Similarly, a general process of acculturation and social disintegration could not satisfactorily explain the consistently low suicide rates among the Navajos, which did not show an increase until the 1970s, or the fact that Hopis in Arizona and the Pueblos in New Mexico showed a similar trend despite the longer history of intense contact, economic change, and outmigration from the reservation. Hopis, when compared to neighboring predominantly non-Native rural counties, also seemed to share similar rates and time trends (Levy and Kunitz, 1987).

When isolated from acculturation pressures, and possibly even prior to their existence, traditional social integration may explain much of the variance in suicide rates (the more socially integrated, the lower the suicide rate). However, as acculturation pressures increase, not only are overall suicide rates elevated but also acculturation interacts with social integration in determining the relative rankings between tribal and cultural groups (Van Winkle and May, 1986).

Graves (1967) contended that acculturation affected both the psychosocial pressures for engaging in deviant behavior and the controls that kept such behavior in check. When traditional cultural strategies for personal satisfaction became inoperative, a reorientation toward a new and more attainable goal occurred as a result of acculturation. Where traditional controls were weak, acculturation also served to promote the development of new controls and prevent disruptive behavior. Acculturation also interacted with other socioeconomic factors. While a low level of acculturation was associated with a high risk of alcohol abuse and deviant behavior, regardless of economic status, a low economic status was also associated with high risk, regardless of acculturation status. [Acculturation was measured based on residence, language, military service, types of friends, and television ownership]. When both acculturation and economic status were high, the risk of alcohol abuse and deviant behavior was lowest.

That some types of injuries can be considered "positive" indicators of social change and modernization is illustrated by data from Greenland. Citing the landmark studies of Bertelsen, Bjerregaard (1990) noted that traditional Eskimo lifestyle was associated with high rates of drowning and boat accidents. With modernization, the mortality rate from such injuries declined as more people took on less hazardous, "modern jobs. [The rate during 1968–85 was 202/100,000, compared to over 500/100,000 during the first three decades of the twentieth century]. There was also geographical variation—the more remote (and thus traditional) the communities, the higher the rate of drowning deaths. Suicides, on the other hand, had the reverse geographical distribution and historical trend. During 1979–82, when there was alcohol prohibition in Greenland, many people reverted to traditional activities such as hunting and fishing, with the result that the rate of non-alcohol-related accidents increased while that of alcohol-related accidents declined.

While theories of social integration within traditional society and cultural change/modernization help explain between-population differences in the frequency of social pathologies, May (1982) proposed a model for individual susceptibility. An individual with strong integration to both traditional and modern societies would have the lowest risk, followed by those who were attached to either one (i.e., derive their identity and self-esteem from job and education achievements, or through adherence to traditional Indian values). Those at highest risk were those integrated into neither.

7

Toward a Biocultural Epidemiology

Native Americans in North America have shown remarkable tenacity in the face of adversity inflicted upon them from the time of contact. From a continental perspective, the population reached its nadir toward the end of the nineteenth century, although substantial regional variation likely existed. From the beginning of the twentieth century, the Native American population has begun to recover, and with it the pattern of health and disease has also changed.

The overall poor health status of Native Americans is well recognized and has been demonstrated in many research studies and official statistics. While there are disparities in health status between the Native and all-race national populations of Canada and the United States, there has also been significant improvement over the past 40 years, particularly in such indicators as life expectancy, infant mortality rate, and the incidence of tuberculosis. The gap continues to narrow; the American Indian infant mortality rate, for example, had converged with that of the U.S. all-race rate by the 1980s.

Like many other populations in the world, Native Americans have undergone "epidemiologic transition," which is characterized by the precipitous decline in the incidence of infectious diseases, followed by the rise of chronic, non-communicable diseases and accidents and violence. Yet infectious diseases, while greatly controlled, have by no means disappeared. Native Americans are still exposed to high risks for such diseases as meningitis, hepatitis, pneumonia, and sexually transmitted diseases.

Many chronic diseases such as diabetes, hypertension, obesity, and cardiovascular disease are the result of the rapid changes in lifestyle, particularly in dietary habits and physical activity levels. The situation with obesity is particu-

216

larly striking. As recently as the 1940s caloric and nutrient deficiency was a real threat in many communities; today, obesity is widespread.

Accidental and violent deaths (including suicide, homicide, and family violence) are primarily social and economic in origin, and reflect the wide gap between Native and non-Native Americans in such socioeconomic indicators as income, housing, social assistance, and children in care.

Throughout this book, when discussing the three groups of health conditions—infectious diseases, chronic diseases, and injuries—the relative contribution of genetic and environmental risk factors has been presented. For the chronic diseases, there is overwhelming evidence that genetic susceptibility plays a major role in etiology, and theories such as the "thrifty gene" (Neel, 1982) and "New World" syndrome (Weiss et al., 1984b) have been proposed to explain the recent emergence of various chronic diseases among Native Americans.

Although the notion that the high burden of infectious diseases was evidence of a "racial" predilection among Native Americans has been abandoned, renewed research in ethnic differences in disease susceptibility and host resistance suggests that genetics does play a role, although probably not as significant a role as in the chronic diseases.

The genetic contribution in injuries is likely to be the least among the three disease categories discussed, although not entirely absent. Genetically determined enzyme differences affecting ethanol metabolism have been demonstrated between Native Americans and other ethnic groups (Reed, 1985), although the causal pathway relating such differences to alcohol abuse, and ultimately to an increased risk of accidents and violence is by no means clear.

A declared objective of this book is to use the health of Native Americans as a case study in "biocultural epidemiology." There are many examples of cultural factors that affect the distribution and natural history of diseases. Infestations with parasites such as trichinosis, for example, are promoted by traditional food sources and methods of food preparation (Margolis et al., 1979). Echinococcosis or hydatid disease may result from the intimate relationship between humans and dogs or farm animals. The northern form, once common in Alaska and northern Canada (Wilson et al., 1968), has almost disappeared with the obsolescence of the dog team as a means of transport. The "European" form, which has become a problem in the Southwest since the mid-1960s, involves the farm sheep and the practice of home-butchering (Schantz et al., 1977). Botulism is almost an exclusively Inuit and Indian disease in Canada and Alaska, attributable to the consumption of traditional delicacies, foods that are raw, partially cooked, or fermented (Hauschild and Gauvreau, 1985).

Cultural influences on disease patterns are not restricted to infectious diseases. Cancers of the salivary glands, nasopharynx, and esophagus are considered traditional among the Inuit/Eskimo population. In fact, a certain histological type of salivary gland tumor has been called "Eskimoma." With cultural change, the declining importance of these cancers relative to the "modern" cancers of the lung, breast, and cervix has been observed (Hildes and Schaefer, 1984). Interestingly, before the large-scale importation and adoption of tobacco smoking, lung cancer was more common among Inuit women, an observation that has led to the hypothesis that hydrocarbons from seal oil lamps, which were tended by women for many hours every day, may have been responsible. Indeed, the lungs of centuries-old female mummies in the Arctic have been found to contain carbonaceous deposits (Zimmerman and Aufderheiden, 1984). In the Southwest, the heavy involvement of Native Americans in some occupations such as uranium miming (Samet et al., 1984) and silver jewelry manufacturing (Driscoll et al., 1988) is associated with specific exposures and their attendant cancer risks.

In the category of injuries such as accidents, suicides, and homicides, there are also "traditional" and "modern" patterns. In Greenland, the traditional Eskimo hunting lifestyle was associated with high mortality from drowning and boating accidents, now supplanted by suicide and alcohol-related violence. During a period of alcohol prohibition, when many Greenlanders reverted to hunting and fishing, a reversal in the accident mortality pattern was observed (Bjerregaard, 1990). In the Southwest, differences in traditional social organization were assigned an important role in explaining the observed historical tribal differences in injury mortality (Levy and Kunitz, 1971).

Contributions of Native American Populations to Epidemiology

Rather than focusing on the general organization and delivery of health care services for Native Americans, this book emphasizes disease-specific prevention and control strategies that either have been shown to be effective or are potentially applicable to Native Americans. Indeed, many advances in public health interventions can be traced back to their initial application in Native American communities. Often the excessive burden of illness in Native American communities, well-defined geographical boundaries, accurately enumerated population, and the existence of a centralized health service system provide methodologically and logistically the optimal conditions for launching disease control programs. The benefits of such demonstration projects accrues to both the Native and non-Native populations.

Tuberculosis has held a central position in the epidemiologic history of almost all Native American groups. Native American populations were important in the evolution of prevention strategies against this disease, which still has a worldwide prevalence. In the 1930s, two early randomized controlled trials of bacille Calmette Guérin (BCG) vaccine were conducted among newborn Indian infants in Saskatchewan (Ferguson and Sime, 1949), and among seven tribes of American Indians in five Western states up to 20 years of age (Aronson et al., 1958). The positive results of these two trials, with protective efficacy in the 80 percent range, whether mortality or incidence of new cases was used as the end-point, contributed to the widespread acceptance of BCG as a major method of disease control. Later trials in other populations, however, were inconsistent in demonstrating efficacy (Clemens et al., 1983).

Where randomized controlled trials are no longer economically feasible, case-control studies have been suggested to evaluate health programs. While such studies have a long tradition in research into disease etiology, their use in evaluating interventions such as vaccines and screening programs is of relatively recent vintage. Of several case-control studies around the world evaluating BCG (Fine, 1988), most of which were indicative of a protective effective, two were conducted in Native American populations, one in Manitoba (Young and Hershfield, 1986) and the other in Alberta (Houston et al., 1990).

The other strategy for the prevention of tuberculosis is mass prophylactic treatment with isoniazid. Again, successful randomized controlled trials were conducted in Native American populations, in this case the Inuit/Eskimo in Alaska (Comstock et al., 1979), Greenland (Horwitz ct al., 1966), and the Northwest Territories (Dorken et al., 1984), demonstrating the safety and efficacy of the intervention.

Hemophilus influenzae type b (Hib), which causes serious morbidity including meningitis and pneumonia, can now be prevented by active immunization. Various generations of vaccines against Hib were successfully field tested among the Navajos (Santosham et al., 1991a), Apaches (Siber et al., 1990), and Alaska Natives (Ward et al., 1990). The effectiveness of a population-based hepatitis B vaccination program has been demonstrated among Alaska Natives (Wainwright et al., 1991). Hepatitis B vaccine can be considered not only a vaccine against a viral infection, but also a vaccine against hepatocellular cancer.

The alarmingly rapid increase in prevalence of diabetes in many Native American populations has prompted the design of community-based intervention programs. The U.S. Indian Health Service has spearheaded model programs. Of these, the Zuni project of weight control and physical exercise has been documented and evaluated in the scientific literature (Heath et al., 1991). Lessons learned from such programs have potential applications beyond the tribe or community.

The enormity of the problem of accidents and violence in Native American communities is well documented. While many prevention programs exist, evidence of their effectiveness is not generally available. An evaluation of community education programs to prevent injuries in 54 Indian Health Service units indicated substantial declines in hospitalization rates for certain injuries, associated with the extent of coverage of training in general safety, recreational safety, and first aid (Robertson, 1986).

In addition to the demonstration and evaluation of disease-control programs, Native American populations have also contributed substantially to the "universal" pool of epidemiological knowledge on the etiology and mechanisms of specific diseases. Investigations of the unique spatial and temporal patterns of health and disease produced by the interaction of biology and culture have yielded important clues, with implications that extend far beyond the local and parochial.

Much of what endocrinologists know about human diabetes today is derived from studies conducted among the Pima in Arizona. In the mid-1960s essentially the entire population of the Gila River Reservation was enrolled into a cohort that underwent detailed biennial examinations (Bennett et al., 1976). The prolific productivity of the research group [see the recent review by Knowler et al. (1990)] over the years increased the understanding of the genetic and metabolic bases of the disease, the role of various risk factors, and the development of complications. The establishment of screening and diagnostic criteria, now accepted universally (World Health Organization, 1985), is also heavily influenced by data originating from the Pima Study.

In cardiovascular diseases, the extensive dietary, metabolic, and hemostatic studies among Greenland Eskimos led to recognition of the importance of marine-based polyunsaturated fatty acids in the prevention of atherosclerosis (Dyerberg, 1989).

In infectious diseases, the epidemics of streptococcal A infection in the Red Lake Reservation in Minnesota in the 1960s and 1970s (Anthony et al., 1976) provided important data on the natural history of the disease, particularly the development of serious sequelae such as acute glomerulonephritis. The name Red Lake has since been associated with a particular nephritogenic strain of streptococci.

Integrating Anthropology and Epidemiology

The biocultural approach to the study of health and disease by necessity must involve the integration of anthropology and epidemiology. The integration of these two sciences is not a new idea. Collaborative efforts in research and public health programs in fact date back to the early days of both disciplines. There have been instances of "anthropology in epidemiology" as well as "epidemiology in anthropology" (Dunn and Janes, 1986), although the former has been predominant. The classic volume by Paul (1955), *Health, Culture and Community,* established the contribution of the social sciences in applied public health programs, especially in international development. The Cornell community health project among the Navajos, which began in the 1950s, provided a unique population laboratory for both epidemiological and anthropological field investigations (Adair et al., revised 1988). The classic studies on the health consequences of sociocultural change in the Appalachians by Cassel (e.g., 1976), have often gone under the rubric of "social epidemiology."

Anthropologists and epidemiologists may study the same subject, but traditionally their methodology differs. One could facetiously refer to an epidemiologist as someone who knows a little about a lot of people, and an anthropologist as someone who knows a lot about a few people. Thus epidemiologists are more likely to be dealing with large databases of survey results, vital statistics, and health care utilization data, while anthropologists, at least in the public's imagination, spend months doing fieldwork in exotic locales, "going native," and finding out what's going on around them. There are also conceptual differences. Epidemiology is more likely to view disease mechanistically and from the Western biomedical perspective, with risk factors and pathogenetic pathways. Anthropology tends to view disease within society as a whole, and is more likely to regard the indigenous culture's medical constructs and perceptions as central to the understanding of disease processes.

The appearance of such works as Rothschild (1981), Janes et al. (1986), Polednak (1989), and Swedlund and Armelagos (1990) is indicative of the growing confluence of the two disciplines. Rothschild's edited volume *Biocultural Aspects of Disease,* had the declared objective to explore the relationship between disease and ethnicity and the relative role of genetics and culture. It had a global perspective, with case studies of specific ethnic groups such as Jews, Chinese, Native Americans, and blacks. This effort was complemented by Polednak's *Racial and Ethnic Differences in Disease,* which catalogued racial and ethnic differences in a wide variety of diseases. Also global in reach, the book was arranged according to disease rather than ethnic group. Swedlund and Armelagos in *Disease in Populations in Transition* focused on those populations undergoing "transition," from modern-day hunter-gatherers in the rainforest to urban dwellers in Oxfordshire.

As the term implies, "biocultural" connotes the interface between biological and cultural factors in studies of human populations. One could ask, why must epidemiology and anthropology be integrated in order to pursue "biocultural" studies of human health and disease? One would have thought that such integration is already inherent within a discipline such as anthropology. Second, what could epidemiology possibly "gain" from such an integration?

Although in name the "study of man" could not be any broader in scope, anthropology in fact has long been fragmented into the two solitudes of physical (or biological) anthropology and cultural (or social) anthropology, leaving aside linguistics and archaeology. The development of the subdiscipline "medical anthropology," by focusing on human health and disease, would ideally achieve a rapprochement (e.g., Alland, 1970). Even in the study of human health and disease, however, the biologically oriented anthropologists emphasize the ecological and evolutionary aspects, while the cultural anthropologists are more concerned with ethnomedical concepts of health and disease and cross-cultural relationships in the clinical setting. "Medical" anthropology has in fact become a branch of cultural anthropology, while biological anthropology (or "human biology") goes its separate way and continues to study disease within the context of human evolution, variation, growth, and adaptability (e.g., Harrison et al., 1988). Thus when Janes, Stall, and Gifford (1986) called for the integration of anthropology and epidemiology, they were concerned exclusively with epidemiology in relation to medical anthropology as a branch of social/cultural anthropology, with very little contribution from biological anthropology.

Johnston and Lowe (1984) coined the term "biomedical anthropology" for a renewed collaboration between medical (i.e., cultural) and physical (biological) anthropology. McElroy (1990) used "biocultural medical anthropology" more or less for the same thing. Polednak (1989) considered that its difference from classical physical anthropology lay in its concern with modern rather than ancient populations.

Although I have used the term "biocultural epidemiology" in the subtitle of this book, it comes very close to the field labeled "human population biology" (e.g., Little and Haas, 1989). As a discipline, human population biology matured during the International Biological Program's human adaptability studies, although its subject matter is concentrated on demography, genetics, physiology, and growth and development, all with a strong evolutionary perspective. Little and Haas in fact called it "transdisciplinary," rather than multi-disciplinary, science. It definitely utilizes epidemiological methods and approaches, in both descriptive and analytical studies. The main distinguishing feature between it and biocultural epidemiology is the latter's inclusion of design, implementation, and evaluation of intervention programs in the public health setting, although there is nothing to stop "pure" scientists such as human biologists from collaborating in such endeavors.

The cultural content of biocultural health research that has been conducted to date varies, ranging from the inclusion of a few sociocultural variables in the research instrument to a model where cultural data are systematically collected and integrated with biological and environmental data (McElroy, 1990).

It may seem astounding that the need exists to emphasize the biological basis of human health in a branch of anthropology. Nevertheless, within medical anthropology there is a school that calls itself "critical medical anthropology," whose denial of biological contribution to health is matched by its conviction that disease is political, both in its causation and its resolution. Thus Baer yearned for the triumph of world socialism—"only when such a time [sic] will we be able to say that humans have bioculturally adapted to their environment" (1990). Certainly, political and economic factors need not be excluded from the basic host-agent-environment paradigm common to epidemiology, human biology, and medical ecology. The "environment" logically includes the political structures and economic relations under which a particular population endures or thrives, as the case may be. Sometimes the political system shields the population from the effects of pathogens, susceptible hosts, and other environmental hazards—as in the case of the welfare state in the liberal democracies. In contrast, sometimes the political system is itself the cause of population ill health, an extreme example of which is the genocides perpetrated by totalitarian regimes of the left and right.

A similar question can be asked of epidemiology: should not cultural diversity be recognized in research design? Afterall, "culture" is very much part of "time, place and person." What more can epidemiology gain by integrating with anthropology? Surprisingly, much of mainstream epidemiology tends to think in terms of a universal man, typified by the good burgher of Framingham, Massachusetts! Such a universal man may smoke, drink, gain weight, and suffer heart attacks, but is otherwise devoid of a culture. What is more, data derived from culturally undifferentiated people are then assumed to be applicable elsewhere unless proved otherwise. Thus, white Americans become the "standard." Blacks, Hispanics, Native Americans and the diverse populations around the world become "special" populations. While there have been migrant studies and in-situ studies of special populations, the aim of epidemiological research is not to understand the pattern of health and its determinants in these populations in their own right, but primarily to derive "universal truths" about etiology and mechanism that are supposed to be applicable to all human beings.

The lack of interest in studying health and disease in its cultural context is reflected in epidemiology's value system. A study of hypertension screening, say, in a group of workers in a North American city would be considered to be of general interest. The same study conducted among the Eskimo/Inuit would be considered parochial and only of interest to a small circle of devotees of Arctic arcana.

Anthropology of course has no such constraint. The study of diverse peoples has been its main concern and is the end in itself, not a means to deciphering mechanisms that might be applicable to the "general" population.

Anthropology, both biological and medical, has benefited from epidemiological methods and concepts. It is not uncommon for graduate programs in biological and medical anthropology to send students to departments of epidemiology in schools of medicine or public health for courses in epidemiology and biostatistics. Fewer epidemiologists, on the other hand, have consciously gone in the other direction.

Even epidemiologists who have studied Native Americans have often done so in a cultural vacuum. There is a prevailing notion of a homogenized Indian. It is not uncommon for reviewers of research proposals or papers on Native American health studies to demand a "nationally representative sample" of Native Americans. Such epidemiologists, of course, never require that their own "non-cultural" studies be done on representative samples of the entire North American population.

In this book regional variation can be demonstrated in almost all diseases, often markedly so, reflecting the differences in genetic makeup, cultural background, ecological habitats, and social circumstances. The term "biocultural epidemiology" is used not so much to suggest a new discipline in the sense of a unified body of knowledge with unique methods and accompanying graduate programs and academic chairs, as to encourage an attitudinal change within an unsplintered "mother" discipline. Much of current mainstream epidemiologic research is concerned with fine-tuning well-worn etiologic relationships. Cassel (1976) distinguished creative epidemiologic studies from "studies which may display considerable rigor in their methods but which are essentially pedestrian," or as Nations (1986) put it, "epidemiology often forsakes the richness of a people's way of living for quantitative rigor," the extreme form of which becomes rigor mortis.

Issues in Native American Health Research

Biocultural epidemiology can only advance if research continues. The examples given in this book suggest that the health of Native Americans is a suitable and exciting field for such research. However, many Native American communities have become wary of research and researchers, which they consider irrelevant to their needs, paternalistic, colonial, inquisitive, and even worse. Often one hears "There is too much research," and perceived and actual cases of unethical experimentation, breach of confidentiality, cultural arrogance, and lack of consultation and feedback are cited. Nevertheless, research is needed as long as there are unanswered questions. The problem lies in how research is done rather than whether it should be done. Good research can lead to good health policy, although by itself it is not sufficient. Good policy cannot be formulated without support from valid research data. Political convictions and passionate rhetoric by themselves are unlikely to achieve the improvement of health among Native Americans.

The issue of community participation is probably the most crucial one in Native American health research. While everyone agrees that it is desirable, there are different forms that it can take. In North America, three basic patterns can be distinguished:

1. *Research on the people.* This is the traditional and predominant model. A project is initiated by the investigator, and the community plays a passive role. Its sole participation is in serving as subjects—a source of information through interviews/surveys or a source of biological specimens and measurements. The investigator recognizes a need—whether based on personal interest or based on an assessment of the health status of the population—and then convinces the community to participate.
2. *Research for the people.* This is a step forward. The research project is community-initiated rather than investigator-initiated. The community recognizes a need, assigns it high priority, seeks and "contracts" out to external experts to design, execute and analyze the research for them. While a partnership exists, it is still an unequal partnership because of the community's lack of specialized knowledge. During research, the community's role is usually one of providing publicity, facilitating access to materials and services, hiring support staff, etc.
3. *Research by the people.* The community initiates and executes projects, having already possessed the necessary skills to manage each project in its entirety, including the design, data collection, analysis, and dissemination of results. Examples of this type of health research are few and far between and will require the nurturing of innovative training programs and partnerships between communities and educational and research institutions.

What types of research are needed? Studies in biocultural epidemiology may be descriptive, analytical, and interventional, dealing respectively with investigations into the extent and magnitude of the disease burden, the risk factors and determinants, and the strategies for the prevention and control of various diseases that have been, or are likely to become, particularly significant among Native Americans.

Properly designed descriptive epidemiological studies are still needed. Continuing surveillance is important, whether for diseases that have declined in importance among Native Americans but are by no means eradicated, such as tuberculosis, gastroenteritis, and other infectious diseases, or more recently emergent problems such as diabetes, HIV/AIDS, and various injuries. New techniques of screening and diagnosis can be tested.

In terms of causation of prevalent diseases, there is a need to confirm among Native Americans genetic and environmental risk factors that have been found to be important in other populations, and to seek risk factors that may be unique to Native Americans. The identification of risk factors, not all of which can be modified, is a prerequisite to the design of prevention and control programs.

Native American communities are particularly interested in action to ameliorate their pressing health problems, and biocultural epidemiologists have a responsibility to ensure that where existing interventions exist, they are rigorously assessed and evaluated; where none exist, new ones should be designed and implemented.

Until recently, typical approaches to health education, disease prevention, and health promotion in Native American communities have ranged from a modification of existing programs to suit local needs, to an imposition of predominantly Eurocentric values and standards. In culturally affected areas such as alcohol abuse, Native communities themselves have achieved some success at control through the development of culturally constituted prevention and treatment programs. Successful strategies need to be adapted to other pressing needs such as diabetes control.

While at one level research can focus on Native Americans nationally and internationally, with their many shared experiences and needs, there is an equally important place for health research at the individual tribe and community level, taking into account the unique historical experience, cultural background, and socioeconomic conditions of each community.

Research on Native American health is necessarily a multidisciplinary effort. In this respect biocultural epidemiology is ideally suited to respond to the task of identification and resolution of community health problems by applying a unique blend of the research methods and traditions of the social and biomedical sciences.

Bibliography

Abott WG, Foley JE (1987) Comparison of body composition, adipocyte size, and glucose and insulin concentration in Pima Indian and Caucasian children. Metabolism 36:576–9.

Abraham S, Miller DC (1959) Serum cholesterol levels in American Indians. Public Health Rep 74:392–8.

Abu-Zeid HA, Maini KK, Choi NW (1978) Ethnic differences in mortality from ischemic heart disease: a study of migrant and native populations. J Chron Dis 31:137–46.

Adair J, Deuschle KW, Barnett CR (1988) The People's Health: Medicine and Anthropology in a Navajo Community. rev. ed. Albuquerque, NM: University of New Mexico Press.

Adamson JD, Moody JP, Peart AF, et al. (1949) Poliomyelitis in the Arctic. Can Med Assoc J 61:339–48.

Alfred BM (1970) Blood pressure changes among male Navajo migrants to an urban environment. Can Rev Sociol Anthropol 7:189–200.

Alland A (1970) Adaptation in Cultural Evolution: An Approach to Medical Anthropology. New York: Columbia University Press.

Alpert JS, Goldberg R, Ockene IS, Taylor P (1991) Heart disease in Native Americans. Cardiology 78:3–12.

Alter MJ, Hadler SC, Margolis HS, et al. (1990) The changing epidemiology of hepatitis B in the United States: need for alternative strategies. JAMA 263:1218–22.

Alward WL, McMahon BJ, Hall DB, et al. (1985) The long-term serological course of asymptomatic hepatitis B virus carriers and the development of primary hepatocellular carcinoma. J Infect Dis 151:604–9.

American Thoracic Society (1986) Treatment of tuberculosis and tuberculous infection in adults and children. Am Rev Respir Dis 134:355–63.

Anthony BF, Kaplan EL, Wannamaker LW, et al. (1969) Attack rates of acute nephritis after type 49 streptococcal infection of the skin and of the respiratory tract. J Clin Invest 48:1697–704

Anthony BF, Kaplan EL, Wannamaker LW, Chapman SS (1976) The dynamics of streptococcal infection in a defined population of children: serotypes associated with skin
and respiratory infections. Am J Epidemiol 104:652–6.

Arch I (1960) Fish tapeworms in Eskimos in Port Harrison area, Canada. Can J Public
Health 51:268–71.

Aronoff SL, Bennett PH, Gorden P, et al. (1977) Unexplained hyperinsulinemia in normal
and prediabetic Pima Indians compared with normal Caucasians: an example of racial
differences in insulin secretion. Diabetes 26:827–40.

Aronson J, Aronson C, Taylor H (1958) A 20-year appraisal of BCG vaccination in the
control of tuberculosis. Arch Intern Med 101:881–93.

Arthaud JB (1970) Causes of death in 339 Alaskan Eskimos as determined by autopsy.
Arch Pathol 90:433–8.

Ashburn PM (1947) The Ranks of Death: A Medical History of the Conquest of the
Americas. New York: Coward-McCann.

Auger F, Jamison PL, Balslev-Jorgensen J, et al. (1980) Anthropometry of circumpolar
populations. In: Milan F, ed. The Human Biology of Circumpolar Populations. Cambridge: Cambridge University Press; 213–55.

Avery ME, Snyder J (1990) Oral therapy for acute diarrhea: the underused simple solution. N Engl J Med 323:891–4.

Ayoub EM, Barrett DJ, Maclaren NK, Krischer JP (1986) Association of class II human histocompatibility leukocyte antigens with rheumatic fever. J Clin Invest 77:
2019–26.

Bachman JG, Wallace JM, O'Malley PM, et al. (1991) Racial/ethnic differences in smoking, drinking, and illicit drug use among American high school seniors. Am J Public
Health 81:372–7.

Baer HA (1990) Biocultural approaches in medical anthropology: a critical medical anthropology commentary. Med Anthropol Q 4:344–8.

Bagley C, Wood M, Khumar H (1990) Suicide and careless death in young males: ecologic study of an aboriginal population in Canada. Can J Comm Mental Health 29:127–
42.

Baikie M, Ratnam S, Bryant DG, Jong M, Bokhout M (1989) Epidemiologic features of
hepatitis B virus infection in northern Labrador. Can Med Assoc J 141:791–5.

Bailey TM, Schantz PM (1990) Trends in the incidence and transmission patterns of
trichinosis in humans in the United States: comparisons of the periods 1975–1981 and
1982–1986. Rev Infect Dis 12:5–11.

Baker PT (1966) Human biological variation as an adaptive response to the environment.
Eugen Q 13:81–9.

Baker PT (1967) The biological race concept as a research tool. Am J Phys Anthropol
27:21–25.

Baker PT, Little MA, eds (1976) Man in the Andes: A Multidisciplinary Study of High
Altitude Quechua. Stroudsburg, PA: Dowden, Hutchison, and Ross.

Baker SP, O'Neill B, Ginsburg MJ, Li G (1992) Injury Fact Book. 2nd ed. New York:
Oxford University Press.

Baker SP, Whitfield RA, O'Neill B (1987) Geographic variations in mortality from motor
vehicle crashes. N Engl J Med 316:1384–7.

Bancroft WH (1992) Hepatitis A vaccine. N Engl J Med 327:488–90.

Bang HO, Dyerberg J, Sinclair HM (1980) The composition of the Eskimo food in northwestern Greenland. Am J Clin Nutr 33:2657–61.

Bang HO, Dyerberg J (1972) Plasma lipids and lipoproteins in Greenlandic west-coast Eskimos. Acta Med Scand 192:85–94.

Barnes GE (1979) Solvent abuse: a review. Int J Addict 14:1–26.

Barrett DH, Burks JM, McMahon B et al. (1977) Epidemiology of hepatitis B in two Alaskan communities. Am J Epidemiol 105:118–22.

Barrett-Connor E (1989) Epidemiology, obesity, and non-insulin-dependent diabetes mellitus. Epidemiol Rev 11:172–81.

Bartha JG, Burch TA, Bennett PH (1973) Hyperglycemia in Washoe and northern Paiute Indians. Diabetes 22:58–62.

Bass MA, Wakefield LM (1974) Nutrient intake and food patterns of Indians on Standing Rock Reservation. J Am Diet Assoc 64:36–41.

Bates C, Van Dam C, Horrobin DF et al. (1985) Plasma essential fatty acids in pure and mixed race American Indians on and off a diet exceptionally rich in salmon. Prostaglandins Leukotrienes Med 17:77–84.

Battista RN, Grover SA (1988) Early detection of cancer: an overview. Annu Rev Public Health 9:21–45.

Beauvais F, LaBoueff S (1985) Drug and alcohol abuse intervention in American Indian communities. Int J Addict 20:139–71.

Beauvais F, Oetting ER, Wolf W, Edwards RW (1989) American Indian youth and drugs, 1976–87: a continuing problem. Am J Public Health 79:634–6.

Becker TM, Wheeler CM, McGough NS, Jordan SW, et al. (1991) Cervical papillomavirus infection and cervical dysplasia in Hispanic, Native American, and non-Hispanic white women in New Mexico. Am J Public Health 81:582–6.

Becker TM, Wiggins CR, Key R, Samet JM (1988) Ischemic heart disease mortality in Hispanics, American Indians, and non-Hispanic whites in New Mexico. Circulation 78:302–9.

Becker TM, Wiggins C, Peek C, et al. (1990) Mortality from infectious diseases among New Mexico's American Indians, Hispanic whites, and other whites, 1958–87. Am J Public Health 80:320–3.

Bender TR, Jones TS, DeWitt WE, et al. (1972) Salmonellosis associated with whale meat in an Eskimo community: serologic and bacteriologic methods as adjuncts to an epidemiologic investigation. Am J Epidemiol 96:153–60.

Bennett PH, Knowler WC, Baird HR, et al. (1984) Diet and development of non-insulin-dependent diabetes mellitus: an epidemiological perspective. In: Pozza G, Micozzi P, Catapano AL, Paoletti R, eds. Diet, Diabetes and Atherosclerosis. New York: Raven Press; 109–19.

Bennett PH, Rushforth NB, Miller M, Lecompte PM (1976) Epidemiological studies of diabetes in the Pima Indians. Recent Prog Horm Res 32:333–76.

Bennion LJ, Knowler WC, Mott DM, et al. (1979) Development of lithogenic bile during puberty in Pima Indians. N Engl J Med 300:873–6.

Bennion LJ, Li TK (1976) Alcohol metabolism in American Indians and whites: lack of racial differences in metabolic rate and liver alcohol dehydrogenase. N Engl J Med 294:9–13.

Berger CJ, Tobeluk HA (1991) Community-based suicide prevention programs in rural Alaska: self-determination as a new approach. In: Postl BD, Gilbert P, Goodwill J, et al., eds. Circumpolar Health 90. Winnipeg: University of Manitoba Press; 291–3.

Berkes F, Farkas CS (1978) Eastern James Bay Cree Indians changing patterns of wild food use and nutrition. Ecol Food Nutr 7:155–72.

Berlin IN (1987) Suicide among American Indian adolescents: an overview. Suicide Life Threat Behav 17:218–32.

Bishop JM (1991) Molecular themes in oncogenesis. Cell 64:235–48.

Bisno AL (1991) Group A streptococcal infections and acute rheumatic fever. N Engl J Med 325:783–93.

Bjerager P, Kromann N, Thygesen K, Harvald B (1982) Blood pressure in Greenland Eskimos. In: Harvald B, Hansen JP, eds. Circumpolar Health 81. Oulu, Finland: Nordic Council for Arctic Medical Research; 317–20.

Bjerregaard P (1983) Housing standards, social group, and respiratory infections in children of Upernavik, Greenland. Scand J Soc Med 11:107–11.

Bjerregaard P (1990) Fatal accidents in Greenland. Arct Med Res 49:132–41.

Bjerregaard P (1991) Disease pattern in Greenland: studies on morbidity in Upernavik 1979–1980 and mortality in Greenland 1968–1985. Arct Med Res 50(Suppl 4):1–62.

Bjerregaard P, Dyerberg J (1988) Mortality from ischemic heart disease and cerebrovascular disease in Greenland. Int J Epidemiol 17:514–9.

Black FL (1975) Infectious diseases in primitive societies. Science 187:515–8.

Black WC, Key CR, Carmany TB, Herman D (1977) Carcinoma of the gallbladder in a population of southwestern American Indians. Cancer 39:1267–79.

Blackburn H (1983) Research and demonstration projects in community cardiovascular disease prevention. J Public Health Policy 4:398–421.

Blacklow NR, Greenberg HB (1991) Viral gastroenteritis. N Engl J Med 325:252–64.

Blackwood L (1981) Alaska Native fertility trends, 1950–1978. Demography 18:173–9.

Blaser MJ, Pollard RA, Feldman RA (1983) Shigella infections in the United States, 1974–1980. J Infect Dis 147:771–75.

Blum RW, Harmon B, Harris L, Bergeisen L, Resnick MD (1992) American Indian-Alaska Native youth health. JAMA 267:1637–44.

Boeckx RL, Postl B, Coodin FJ (1977) Gasoline sniffing and tetraethyl lead poisoning in children. Pediatrics 60:140–5.

Bosron WF, Rex DK, Harden CA, et al. (1988) Alcohol and aldehyde dehydrogenase isoenzymes in Sioux North American Indians. Alcoholism Clin Exp Res 12:454–5.

Boss LP, Lanier AP, Dohan PH, Bender TR (1982) Cancers of the gallbladder and biliary tract in Alaskan Natives: 1970–79. J Natl Cancer Inst 69:1005–7.

Botash AS, Kavey RW, Emm N, Jones D (1991) Cardiovascular risk factors in Native American children. Ann NY Acad Sci 623:416–18.

Bouchard C, Pérusse L (1988) Heredity and body fat. Annu Rev Nutr 8:259–77.

Brant LJ, Bender TR, Marnell RW (1982) Factors affecting streptococcal colonization among children in selected areas of Alaska. Public Health Rep 97:460–64.

Brassard P, Hoey J, Ismail J, Gosselin F (1985) The prevalence of intestinal parasites and enteropathogenic bacteria in James Bay Cree Indians, Quebec. Can J Public Health 76:322–5.

Bray DL, Anderson PD (1989) Appraisal of the epidemiology of fetal alcohol syndrome among Canadian Native peoples. Can J Public Health 80:42–5.

Bray GA (1989) Classification and evaluation of the obesities. Med Clin North Am 73:161–84.

Brenneman G, Silimperi D, Ward J (1987) Recurrent invasive Haemophilus influenzae type b disease in Alaskan Natives. Pediatr Infect Dis J 6:388–92.

Briscoe J (1984) Water supply and health in developing countries: selective primary health care revisited. Am J Public Health 74:1009–13.

Brod T (1975) Alcoholism as a mental health problem of Native Americans. Arch Gen Psychiatry 32:1385–91.

Brody JA (1965) Lower respiratory illness among Alaskan Eskimo children. Arch Environ Health 11:620–3.

Broome CV, Breiman RF (1991) Pneumococcal vaccine—past, present, and future. N Engl J Med 325:1506–8.

Brosseau JD, Eelkema RC, Crawford AC, Abe TA (1979) Diabetes among the Three Affiliated Tribes: correlation with degree of Indian inheritance. Am J Public Health 69:1277–8.

Broudy DW, May PA (1983) Demographic and epidemiologic transition among the Navajo Indians. Soc Biol 30:1–16.

Broussard BA, Johnson A, Himes JH, et al. (1991) Prevalence of obesity in American Indians and Alaska Natives. Am J Clin Nutr 53:1535–42S.

Brown JE, Christensen C (1967) Biliary tract disease among the Navajos. JAMA 202:138–40.

Brown PK, Taylor-Robinson D (1966) Respiratory virus antibodies in sera of persons living in isolated communities. Bull WHO 34:895–900.

Brown RC, Gurunamjappa BS, Hawk RJ, Bitsure D (1970) The epidemiology of accidents among the Navajo Indian. Pub Health Rep 85:881–8.

Buikstra JE, Cook DC (1980) Paleopathology: an American account. Annu Rev Anthropol 9:433–70.

Cadien JD, Mamula PW, Hecht F (1979) Phosphoglycolate phosphatase phenotypes and association with Pima Indian diabetes. Am J Hum Genet 31:40A.

Callegari PR, Alton JD, Shankowski HA, Grace MG (1989) Burn injuries in native Canadians: a 10-year experience. Burns 15:15–19.

Canada, Department of National Health and Welfare (1974) A New Perspective on the Health of Canadians: A Working Document. Ottawa: DNHW.

Canada, Department of National Health and Welfare (1975a) Nutrition Canada: Eskimo Survey Report. Ottawa: DNHW.

Canada, Department of National Health and Welfare (1975b) Nutrition Canada: Food Consumption Patterns Report. Ottawa: DNHW.

Canada, Department of National Health and Welfare (1975c) Nutrition Canada: Indian Survey Report. Ottawa: DNHW.

Canada, Department of National Health and Welfare (1980) Nutrition Canada: Anthropometry Report. Ottawa: DNHW.

Canada, Department of National Health and Welfare (1986) Indians and Inuit of Canada: Health Status Indicators 1974–1983. Ottawa: DNHW, Medical Services Branch.

Canada, Department of National Health and Welfare (1988) Health Indicators Derived from Vital Statistics for Status Indian and Canadian Populations 1978–1986. Ottawa: DNHW, Medical Services Branch.

Canada, Department of National Health and Welfare (1990) Nutrition Recommendations: The Report of the Scientific Review Committee. Ottawa: DNHW.

Carr BA, Lee ES (1978) Navajo tribal mortality: a life table analysis of the leading causes of death. Soc Biol 25:279–87.

Carter J, Horowitz R, Wilson R, Sava S, et al. (1989) Tribal differences in diabetes prevalence among American Indians in New Mexico. Public Health Rep 104:665–9.

Carvalho JM, Baruzzi RG, Howard PF, et al. (1989) Blood pressure in four remote populations in the INTERSALT study. Hypertension 14:238–46.

Cassel JC (1976) The contribution of the social environment to host resistance. Am J Epidemiol 104:107–23.

Cates W, Hinman AR (1991) Sexually transmitted diseases in the 1990s. N Engl J Med 325:1368–70.

Cates W, Wasserheit JN (1991) Genital chlamydial infections: epidemiology and reproductive sequelae. Am J Obstet Gynecol 164:1771–81.

Cavalli-Sforza LL, Piazza A, Menozzi P, Mountain JL (1988) Reconstruction of human evolution: bringing together genetic, archeological and linguistic data. Proc Natl Acad Sci USA 85:6002–6.

Centers for Disease Control (1985) Tuberculosis among American Indians and Alaskan Natives—United States, 1985. MMWR 36:493–5.

Centers for Disease Control (1989) Pneumococcal polysaccharide vaccine: recommendations of the Immunization Practices Advisory Committee. MMWR 38:64–76.

Centers for Disease Control (1989) Motor vehicle crashes and injuries in an Indian community—Arizona. MMWR 38:589–91.

Centers for Disease Control (1989) The Surgeon General's 1989 Report on Reducing the Health Consequences of Smoking: 25 Years of Progress (Executive Summary). MMWR 38(No S-2):1–32.

Centers for Disease Control (1989) A strategic plan for the elimination of tuberculosis in the United States. MMWR 38(No S-3):1–25.

Centers for Disease Control (1989) 1989 sexually transmitted diseases treatment guidelines. MMWR 38(No S-8):1–43.

Centers for Disease Control (1990) Diabetes Surveillance, 1980–1987. Atlanta, GA: USDHSS/PHS/ CDC/Division of Diabetes Translation.

Centers for Disease Control (1990) Prevention and control of influenza: recommendations of the Immunization Practices Advisory Committee (ACIP). MMWR 39(No RR-7):1–15.

Centers for Disease Control (1990) The Surgeon General's 1990 Report on the Health Benefits of Smoking Cessation (Executive Summary). MMWR 39(No RR-12): 1–12.

Centers for Disease Control (1991) Haemophilus b conjugate vaccine for prevention of Haemophilus influenzae type b disease among infants and children two months of age and older: recommendations of the Immunization Practices Advisory Committee (ACIP). MMWR 40(No RR-1):1–7.

Centers for Disease Control (1991) Hepatitis B virus—a comprehensive strategy for eliminating transmission in the United States through universal childhood vaccination: recommendations of the Immunization Practices Advisory Committee (ACIP). MMWR 40(No RR-13):1–25.

Chakraborty R, Szathmary EJ, eds. (1985) Diseases of Complex Etiology in Small Populations: Ethnic Differences and Research Approaches. New York: Alan R. Liss.

Chaudron CD, Wilkinson DA, eds. (1988) Theories on Alcoholism. Toronto: Addiction Research Foundation.

Chin J, Mann JM (1990) HIV infection and AIDS in the 1990s. Annu Rev Public Health 11:127–42.

Christian CM, Dufour M, Bertolucci D (1989) Differential alcohol-related mortality among American Indian tribes in Oklahoma, 1968–1978. Soc Sci Med 28:275–84.

Ciba Foundation Symposium (1977) Health and Disease in Tribal Societies. Amsterdam: Excerpta Medica.

Clark GA, Kelley MA, Grange JM, Hill MC (1987) The evolution of mycobacterial disease in human populations. Curr Anthropol 28:45–62.

Clausen J (1974) An epidemiological and demographic study of coronary heart deaths in Denmark, the Faroes and Greenland. Arct Med Res 11:13–28.

Clemens JD, Chuong JJ, Feinstein AR (1983) The BCG controversy: a methodological and statistical reappraisal. JAMA 249:2362–69.

Clements F (1931) Racial differences in mortality and morbidity. Hum Biol 3:397–419.

Clifford NJ, Kelly JJ, Leo TF, Eder HA (1963) Coronary heart disease and hypertension in the White Mountain Apache tribe. Circulation 28:926–31.

Cloninger CR (1987) Neurogenetic adaptive mechanisms in alcoholism. Science 236:410–16.

Cockburn TA (1971) Infectious diseases in ancient populations. Curr Anthropol 12:45–62.

Cockerham WC (1977) Pattern of alcohol and multiple drug use among rural white and American Indian adolescents. Int J Addict 12:271–85.

Cockerham WC, Forslund MA, Raboin RM (1976) Drug use among white and American Indian high school youth. Int J Addict 11:209–20.

Cohen MM, Young TK, Hammarstrand KM (1989) Ethnic variation in cholecystectomy rates and outcomes, Manitoba, Canada, 1972–1984. Am J Public Health 79:751–55.

Colbert MJ, Mann GV, Hursh LM (1978) Nutrition studies: clinical observations on nutritional health. In: Jamison PL, Zegura SL, Milan FA, eds. Eskimos of Northwestern Alaska. Stroudsburg, PA: Dowden; 162–73.

Cole SA, Szathmary EJ, Ferrell RE (1989) Gene and gene-product variation in the apolipoprotein A-I/C-III/A-IV cluster in the Dogrib Indians of the Northwest Territories. Am J Hum Genet 44:835–43.

Comess LJ, Bennett PH, Burch TA (1967) Clinical gallbladder disease in Pima Indians: its high prevalence in contrast to Framingham, Massachusetts. N Engl J Med 277:894–8.

Comstock GW (1975) Frost revisited: the modern epidemiology of tuberculosis. Am J Epidemiol 101:363–82.

Comstock GW, Baum C, Snider DE (1979) Isoniazid prophylaxis among Alaskan Eskimos: a final report of the Bethel isoniazid studies. Am Rev Respir Dis 119:827–30.

Connop PJ (1983) A Canadian Indian health status index. Med Care 21:67–81.

Cooper R (1985) A note on the biological concept of race and its application in epidemiological research. Am Heart J 108:715–23.

Corcoran AC, Rabinowitch IM (1937) A study of the blood lipids and blood proteins in Canadian Eastern Arctic Eskimos. Biochem J 31:343–8.

Coulehan JL, Baacke G, Welty T, Goldtooth NL (1982) Cost-benefit of a streptococcal surveillance program among Navajo Indians. Public Health Rep 97:73–7.

Coulehan JL, Hallowell C, Michaels, et al. (1983a) Immunogenicity of a Haemophilus influenzae type b vaccine in combination with diphtheria-pertussis-tetanus vaccine in infants. J Infect Dis 148:530–4.

Coulehan JL, Hirsch W, Brillman J, et al. (1983) Gasoline sniffing and lead toxicity in Navajo adolescents. Pediatrics 71:113–7.

Coulehan JL, Michaels RH, Hallowell C, et al. (1984) Epidemiology of Haemophilus influenzae type b disease among Navajo Indians. Public Health Rep 99:404–9.

Coulehan JL, Lerner G, Helzlsouer K, et al. (1986) Acute myocardial infarction among Navajo Indians, 1976–83. Am J Public Health 76:412–4.

Coulehan JL, Michaels RH, Williams KE, et al. (1976) Bacterial meningitis in Navajo Indians. Public Health Rep 91:464–8.

Coulehan JL, Topper MD, Arena V, Welty T (1990) Determinants of blood pressure in Navajo adolescents. Am Ind Alaska Native Ment Health Res 3(3):27–36.

Creagan ET, Fraumeni JF (1973) Cancer mortality among American Indians, 1950–67. J Natl Cancer Inst 49:959–67.

Crosby AW (1972) The Columbian Exchange: Biological and Cultural Consequences of 1492. Westport, CT: Greenwood Press.

Crosby AW (1976) Virgin soil epidemics as a factor in aboriginal depopulation in America. William and Mary Q 33:289–99.

Curtis MA, Byland G (1991) Diphyllobothriasis: fish tapeworm disease in the circumpolar North. Arct Med Res 50:18–25.

Darby WJ, Salsbury CG, McGaninty WJ, et al. (1956) A study of the dietary background and nutriture of the Navajo Indians. J Nutr 60(Suppl 2):1–85.

Davidson M, Schraer CD, Parkinson AJ, et al. (1989) Invasive pneumococcal disease in an Alaska Native population, 1980 through 1986. JAMA 261:715–18.

Davis S, Kunitz SJ (1978) Hospital utilization and elective surgery on the Navajo Indian reservation. Soc Sci Med 12B:263–72.

De Zoysa I, Feachem RG (1985) Interventions for the control of diarrhoeal diseases among young children: chemoprophylaxis. Bull WHO 63:295–315.

Dean HJ, Carson J (1989) Insulin-dependent diabetes mellitus in an Inuit child. Can Med Assoc J 140:527–8.

Dean HJ, Mundy RL, Moffatt M (1992) Non-insulin-dependent diabetes mellitus in Indian children in Manitoba. Can Med Assoc J 147:52–7.

DeFronzo RA, Bonadonna RC, Ferrannini E (1992) Pathogenesis of NIDDM. Diabetes Care 15:318–68.

DeFronzo RA, Ferrannini E (1991) Insulin resistance: a multifaceted syndrome responsible for NIDDM, obesity, hypertension, dyslipidemia, and atherosclerotic cardiovascular disease. Diabetes Care 14:173–94.

Deprez RD, Miller E, Hart SK (1985) Hypertension prevalence among Penobscot Indians of Indian Island, Maine. Am J Public Health 75:653–4.

Desai ID, Lee M (1971) Nutritional status of British Columbia Indians. III: Biochemical studies at Ahousat and Anaham Reserves. Can J Public Health 62:526–36.

Desai ID, Lee M (1974) Nutritional status of Canadian Indians. I: Biochemical studies at Upper Liard and Ross River, the Yukon Territory. Can J Public Health 65:369–74.

Desrochers F, Curtis MA (1987) The occurrence of gastrointestinal helminths in dogs from Kuujjuaq (Fort Chimo), Quebec, Canada. Can J Public Health 78:403–6.

DeStefano F, Coulehan JL, Wiant MK (1979) Blood pressure survey on the Navajo Indian Reservation. Am J Epidemiol 109:335–45.

Dickson G (1989) Iskwew: empowering victims of wife abuse. Native Studies Rev 5:115–35.

Diehl AK (1991) Epidemiology and natural history of gallstone disease. Gastroenterol Clin North Am 20:1–19.

Diehl AK, Haffner SM, Hazuda HP, Stern MP (1987) Coronary risk factors and clinical gallbladder disease: an approach to the prevention of gallstones? Am J Public Health 77:841–5.

Dillehay TD, Meltzer DJ (1991) The First Americans: Search and Research. Boca Raton, FL: CRC Press.

Dippe SE, Bennett PH, Dippe DW, et al. (1976) Glucose tolerance among Aleuts on the Pribilof Islands. In: Shephard RJ, Itoh S, eds. Circumpolar Health: Proceedings of the 3rd International Symposium. Toronto: University of Toronto Press; 156.

Dizmang LH, Watson J, May PA, Bopp J (1974) Adolescent suicide at an Indian reservation. Am J Orthopsychiat 44:43–9.

Dobyns HF (1966) Estimating aboriginal American population. I. An appraisal of techniques with a new hemispheric estimate. Curr Anthropol 7:395–416.

Dobyns HF (1983) Their Number Become Thinned: Native American Population Dynamics in Eastern North America. Knoxville, TN: University of Tennessee Press.

Doeblin TD, Evans K, Ingall GB, et al. (1969) Diabetes and hyperglycemia in Seneca Indians. Hum Hered 19:613–27.

Dohrenwend BP, Levav I, Shrout PE, et al. (1992) Socioeconomic status and psychiatric disorders: the causation-selection issue. Science 255:946–52.

Doll R, Peto R (1981) The Causes of Cancer: Quantitative Estimates of Avoidable Risks of Cancer in the United States Today. New York: Oxford University Press.

Dorken E, Grzybowski S, Enarson DA (1984) Ten year evaluation of a trial of chemoprophylaxis against tuberculosis in Frobisher Bay, Canada. Tubercle 65:93–9.

Dozier EP (1966) Problem drinking among American Indians: the role of sociocultural deprivation. Q J Stud Alcohol 27:72–87.

Draper HH (1976) A review of recent nutritional research in the Arctic. In: Shephard RJ, Itoh S, eds. Circumpolar Health: Proceedings of the Third International Symposium. Toronto: University of Toronto Press; 120–9.

Draper HH (1977) The aboriginal Eskimo diet in modern perspective. Am Anthropologist 79:309–16.

Dressler WW (1984) Social and cultural influences in cardiovascular disease: a review. Transcult Psychiat Res Rev 21:5–41.

Driscoll RJ, Mulligan WJ, Schultz D, Candelaria A (1988) Malignant mesothelioma: a cluster in a Native American pueblo. N Engl J Med 318:1437–8.

Driver HE (1969) Indians of North America. 2nd rev. ed. Chicago: University of Chicago Press.

Duncan MH, Wiggins CL, Samet JM, Key CR (1986) Childhood cancer epidemiology in New Mexico's American Indians, Hispanic whites, and non-Hispanic whites, 1970–82. J Natl Cancer Inst 76:1013–8.

Dunn FL (1968) Epidemiological factors: health and disease in hunter-gatherers. In: Lee RL, DeVore I, eds. Man The Hunter. Chicago: Aldine Press; 221–8.

Dunn FL, Janes CR (1986) Introduction: medical anthropology and epidemiology. In: Janes CR, Stall R, Gifford SM, eds. Anthropology and Epidemiology: Interdisciplinary Approaches to the Study of Health and Disease. Dordrecht, the Netherlands: D. Reidel; 3–34.

Dyerberg J (1989) Coronary heart disease in Greenland Inuit: a paradox. Arct Med Res 48:47–54.

Dyerberg J, Bang HO (1975) Hemostatic function and platelet polyunsaturated fatty acids in Eskimos. Lancet 2:433–5.

Dyerberg J, Bang HO, Hjorne N (1975) Fatty acid composition of the plasma lipids in Greenland Eskimos. Am J Clin Nutr 28:958–66.

Dyerberg J, Bang HO, Hjorne N (1977) Plasma cholesterol concentration in Caucasian Danes and Greenland west coast Eskimos. Dan Med Bull 24:52–5.

Eaton RD (1968) Amebiasis in northern Saskatchewan: epidemiological considerations. Can Med Assoc J 99:706–11.

Eaton SB, Konner M (1985) Paleolithic nutrition: a consideration of its nature and current implications. N Engl J Med 312:283–9.

Ehrstrom MC (1951) Medical studies in north Greenland 1948–1949. VI: Blood pressure, hypertension and atherosclerosis in relation to food and mode of living. Acta Med Scand 140:416–22.

El-Najjar MY (1979) Human treponematosis and tuberculosis: evidence from the New World. Am J Phys Anthropol 51:599–618.

Ellestad-Sayed J, Coodin FH, Dilling LA, Haworth JC (1979) Breast-feeding protects against infection in Indian infants. Can Med Assoc J 120:295–8.

Elsea WR, Partridge RA, Neter E (1967) Epidemiologic and microbiological study of a Shigella flexneri outbreak. Public Health Rep 82:347–52.

Elston RC, Namboodiri KK, Nino HV, Pollitzer WS (1974) Studies on blood and urine glucose in Seminole Indians: indications for segregation of a major gene. Am J Hum Genet 26:13–34.

Enarson DA, Grzybowski S (1986) Incidence of active tuberculosis in the Native population of Canada. Can Med Assoc J 134:1149–52.

Engleberg NC, Holburt EN, Barrett TJ, et al. (1982) Epidemiology of diarrhea due to rotavirus on an Indian reservation: risk factors in the home environment. J Infect Dis 145:894–8.

Esrey SA, Habicht JP (1986) Epidemiologic evidence for health benefits from improved water and sanitation in developing countries. Epidemiol Rev 8:117–28.

Evers S, McCracken E, Antone I, Deagle G (1987) Prevalence of diabetes in Indians and Caucasians living in southwestern Ontario. Can J Public Health 78:240–3.

Evers SE, McCracken E, Deagle G (1989) Body fat distribution and non-insulin dependent diabetes mellitus in North American Indians. Nutr Res 9:977–87.

Evers S, Orchard J, McCracken E (1985) Lower respiratory disease in Indian and non-Indian infants. Can J Public Health 76:195–8.

Evers SE, Rand CG (1982) Morbidity in Canadian Indian and non-Indian children in the first year of life. Can Med Assoc J 126:249–52.

Evers SE, Rand CG (1983) Morbidity in Canadian Indian and non-Indian children in the second year of life. Can J Public Health 74:191–4.

Fagan BM (1987) The Great Journey: The Peopling of Ancient America. New York: Thames and Hudson.

Farris JJ, Jones BM (1978) Ethanol metabolism and memory impairment in American Indian and white women social drinkers. J Stud Alcohol 39:1975–9.

Farris JJ, Jones BM (1978) Ethanol metabolism in male American Indians and whites. Alcoholism Clin Exp Res 2:77–81.

Feachem RG (1983) Interventions for the control of diarrhoeal diseases among young children: supplementary feeding programmes. Bull WHO 61:967–79.

Feachem RG, Hogan RC, Merson MH (1983) Diarrhoeal disease control: reviews of potential interventions. Bull WHO 61:637–40.

Feachem RG, Koblinsky MA (1984) Interventions for the control of diarrhoeal diseases among young children: promotion of breast-feeding. Bull WHO 62:271–91.

Feldman SA, Ho K, Lewis LA, et al. (1972) Lipid and cholesterol metabolism in Alaskan Arctic Eskimos. Arch Pathol 94:42–58.

Fenna D, Mix L, Schaefer O, Gilbert JA (1971) Ethanol metabolism in various racial groups. Can Med Assoc J 105:472–5.

Ferebee SH (1970) Controlled chemoprophylaxis trials in tuberculosis: a general review. Adv Tuberc Res 17:28–106.

Ferguson RG (1955) Studies in Tuberculosis. Toronto: University of Toronto Press.

Ferguson RG, Sime AB (1949) BCG vaccination of Indian infants in Saskatchewan. Tubercle 30:5–11.

Fine PE (1988) BCG vaccination against tuberculosis and leprosy. Br Med Bull 44:691–703.

Fischler RS (1985) Child abuse and neglect in American Indian communities. Child Abuse Negl 9:95–106.

Fisher AD (1987) Alcoholism and race: the misapplication of both concepts to North American Indians. Can Rev Sociol Anthropol 24:81–98.

Fleshman JK, Wilson JF, Cohen JJ (1968) Bronchiectasis in Alaska Native Children. Arch Environ Health 17:517–23.

Forman MR, Graubard BI, Hoffman HJ, et al. (1984a) The Pima Infant Feeding Study: breast feeding and gastroenteritis in the first year of life. Am J Epidemiol 119:335–49.

Forman MR, Graubard BI, Hoffman HJ, et al. (1984b) The Pima Infant Feeding Study: breast feeding and respiratory infections during the first year of life. Int J Epidemiol 13:447–53.

Fortuine R (1989) Chills and Fever: Health and Disease in the Early History of Alaska. Fairbanks, AK: University of Alaska Press.

Fournelle HJ, Rader V, Allen C (1966) A survey of enteric infections among Alaskan Indians. Public Health Rep 81:797–803.

Fox J, Manitowabi D, Ward JA (1984) An Indian community with a high suicide rate— 5 years after. Can J Psychiat 29:425–7.

Franco EL (1991) Viral etiology of cervical cancer: a critique of the evidence. Rev Infect Dis 13:1195–206.

Fraser G (1986) Preventive Cardiology. New York: Oxford University Press.

Freeman RS, Jamison J (1976) Parasites of Eskimos at Igloolik and Hall Beach, N.W.T. In: Shephard RJ, Itoh S, eds. Circumpolar Health: Proceedings of the Third International Symposium, Yellowknife, NWT. Toronto: University of Toronto Press; 306–15.

Freeman WL, Hosey GM, Diehr P, Gohdes D (1989) Diabetes in American Indians of Washington, Oregon and Idaho. Diabetes Care 12:282–8.

French JG (1967) Relationship of morbidity to the feeding patterns of Navajo children from birth through twenty-four months. Am J Clin Nutr 20:375–85.

Friesen B (1985) Haddon's strategy for prevention: application to Native house fires. In: Fortuine R, editor. Circumpolar Health 84. Seattle, WA: University of Washington Press; 105–9.

Frohman LA, Doeblin TD, Emerling FG (1969) Diabetes in the Seneca Indians. Diabetes 18:38–43.

Frost F, Taylor V, Fries E (1992) Racial misclassification of Native Americans in a Surveillance, Epidemiology, and End Results Cancer Registry. J Nat Cancer Inst 84:957–62.

Fulmer HS, Roberts RW (1963) Coronary heart disease among the Navajo Indians. Ann Intern Med 59:740–64.

Gallagher RP, Elwood JM (1979) Cancer mortality among Chinese, Japanese, and Indians in British Columbia, 1964–73. Natl Cancer Inst Monogr 53:89–94.

Gallaher MM, Fleming DW, Berger LR, Sewell CM (1992) Pedestrian and hypothermia deaths among Native Americans in New Mexico: between bar and home. JAMA 267:1345–8.

Gardner LI, Stern MP, Haffner SM, et al. (1984) Prevalence of diabetes in Mexican Americans: relationship to percent of gene pool derived from Native American sources. Diabetes 33:86–92.

Garnick MB, Bennett PH, Langer T (1979) Low density lipoprotein metabolism and lipoprotein cholesterol content in southwestern American Indians. J Lipid Res 20: 31–9.

Garro LC (1988) Explaining high blood pressure: variation in knowledge about illness. Am Ethnologist 15:98–119.

Garro LC (1988) Suicides by status Indians in Manitoba. In: Linderholm H, Backman C, Broadbent N, Joelsson I, eds. Circumpolar Health 87: Proceedings of the 7th International Congress on Circumpolar Health. Oulu, Finland: Nordic Council for Arctic Medical Research; 590–2.

Garro LC, Lang GC (1993) Explanation of diabetes: Anishinaabe and Dakota deliberate upon a new illness. In: Joe JR, Young RS, eds. Culture Change, Diabetes, and Native Americans. Berlin: Mouton Press; 394–444.

Gaudette LA, Dufour R, Freitag S, Miller AB (1991) Cancer patterns in the Inuit population of Canada, 1970–1984. In: Postl BD, Gilbert P, et al., eds. Circumpolar Health 90: Proceedings of the 8th International Congress on Circumpolar Health. Winnipeg: University of Manitoba Press; 443–6.

Gerber A, King L, Dunleavy G, Novik L (1989) An outbreak of syphilis on an Indian reservation: descriptive epidemiology and disease-control measures. Am J Public Health 79:83–5.

Gibson RS (1990) Principles of Nutritional Assessment. New York: Oxford University Press.

Gillis DC, Irvine J, Tan L, et al. (1991) Cancer incidence and survival of Saskatchewan northerners and registered Indians, 1967–1986. In: Postl BD, Gilbert P, et al., eds. Circumpolar Health 90: Proceedings of the 8th International Congress on Circumpolar Health. Winnipeg: University of Manitoba Press; 447–51.

Gillum RF (1988) Ischemic heart disease mortality in American Indians, United States, 1969–1971 and 1979–1981. Am Heart J 115:1141–4.

Gillum RF, Gillum B, Smith N (1984) Cardiovascular risk factors in urban American Indians. Am Heart J 107:765–6.

Gillum RF, Prineas RJ, Palta M, Horibe H (1980) Blood pressure of urban Native American school children. Hypertension 2:744–9.

Gilsdorf JR (1977) Bacterial meningitis in southwestern Alaska. Am J Epidemiol 1977:388–91.

Goedde W, Agarwal DP, Harada S, et al. (1983) Population genetic studies on aldehyde dehydrogenase isozyme deficiency and alcohol sensitivity. Am J Hum Genet 35:769–72.

Goedde HW, Agarwal DP, Harada S, et al. (1986) Aldehyde dehydrogenase polymorphism in North American, South American, and Mexican Indian populations. Am J Hum Genet 38:395–9.

Gohdes DM (1986) Diabetes in American Indians: a growing problem. Diabetes Care 9:609–13.

Graham NM (1990) The epidemiology of acute respiratory infections in children and adults: a global perspective. Epidemiol Rev 12:149–78.

Granner DK, O'Brien RM (1992) Molecular physiology and genetics of NIDDM. Diabetes Care 15:369–95.

Graves TD (1967) Acculturation, stress, and alcohol in a tri-ethnic community. Am Anthropologist 69:306–21.

Greenberg JH, Ruhlen M (1992) Linguistic origins of Native Americans. Sci Am 267(5):60–5.

Greenberg JH, Turner CG, Zegura SL (1986) The settlement of the Americas: a comparison of the linguistic, dental and genetic evidence. Curr Anthropol 27:447–97.

Griffin PM, Tauxe RV, Redd SC, et al. (1989) Emergence of highly trimethoprim-sulfamethoxazole-resistant Shigella in a Native American population: an epidemiological study. Am J Epidemiol 129:1042–51.

Grossman DC, Milligan C, Deyo RA (1991) Risk factors for suicide attempts among Navajo adolescents. Am J Public Health 81:870–4.

Grove O, Lynge I (1979) Suicide and attempted suicide in Greenland. Acta Psychiatr Scand 60:375–91.

Grundy SM, Metzger AL, Adler RD (1972) Mechanisms of lithogenic bile formation in American Indian women with cholesterol gallstones. J Clin Invest 51:3026–43.

Grzybowski S, Dunaj Z (1959) Tuberculin survey of the population of Manitoulin Island. Can Med Assoc J 81:366–9.

Grzybowski S, Styblo K, Dorken E (1976) Tuberculosis in Eskimos. Tubercle 57(Suppl 4):S1–S58.

Hackenberg RA, Gallagher MM (1972) The costs of cultural change: accidental injury and modernization among the Papago Indians. Hum Organization 31:211–26.

Haddon W (1980) Advances in the epidemiology of injuries as a basis for public policy. Public Health Rep 95:411–21.

Haffner SM, Stern MP, Hazuda HP, Pugh JA, Patterson JK (1986) Hyperinsulinemia in a population at high risk for non-insulin-dependent diabetes mellitus. N Engl J Med 315:220–4.

Haffner SM, Diehl AK, Mitchell BD, Stern MP, Hazuda HP (1990) Increased prevalence of clinical gallbladder disease in subjects with non-insulin-dependent diabetes mellitus. Am J Epidemiol 132:327–35.

Haffner SM, Stern MP, Hazuda HP, Pugh J, Patterson JK (1987) Do upper-body and centralized adiposity measure different aspects of regional body-fat distribution? Relationship to non-insulin-dependent diabetes mellitus, lipids, and lipoproteins. Diabetes 36:43–51.

Hagey NJ, Larocque G, McBride C (1989) Highlights of Aboriginal Conditions 1981–2001: Part I—Demographic Trends; Part II—Social Conditions; Part III—Economic Conditions. Ottawa: Department of Indian Affairs and Northern Development.

Hagey R (1984) The phenomenon, the explanations and the responses: metaphors surrounding diabetes in urban Canadian Indians. Soc Sci Med 18:265–72.

Hall DB, Lum MK, Knutson LR, Heyward WL, Ward JI (1987) Pharyngeal carriage and acquisition of anticapsular antibody to Haemophilus influenzae type b in a high risk population in southwestern Alaska. Am J Epidemiol 126:1190–7.

Hall RL, Wilder D, Bodenroeder P, Hess M (1990) Assessment of AIDS knowledge, attitudes, behaviors, and risk level of northwestern American Indians. Am J Public Health 80:875–7.

Hall TR, Hickey ME, Young TB (1991) The relationship of body fat distribution to non-insulin-dependent diabetes mellitus in a Navajo community. Am J Hum Biol 3:119–26.

Hamby C, Beach DA, Pinder N (1988) Snowmobile injuries in northern Newfoundland and Labrador, 1985–86 winter season. In: Linderholm H, Backman C, Broadbent N, Joelsson I, eds. Circumpolar Health 87: Proceedings of the 7th International Congress on Circumpolar Health. Oulu, Finland: Nordic Council for Arctic Medical Research; 406–8.

Hamer J, Steinbring J, eds (1980) Alcohol and Native Peoples of the North. Washington, DC: University Press of America.

Hamilton MK (1990) The Health and Activity Limitation Survey: disabled aboriginal persons in Canada. Statistics Canada Health Reports 2:279–87.

Hammond GW, Rutherford BE, Malazdrewicz R, et al. (1988) Haemophilus influenzae meningitis in Manitoba and the Keewatin District, NWT: potential for mass vaccination. Can Med Assoc J 139:743–7.

Hanis CL, Chakraborty R, Ferrell RE, Schull WJ (1986) Individual admixture estimates: disease associations and individual risk of diabetes and gallbladder disease among Mexican-Americans in Starr County, Texas. Am J Phys Anthropol 70:433–41.

Hanis CL, Ferrell RE, Tulloch BR, et al. (1985) Gallbladder disease epidemiology in Mexican Americans in Starr County, Texas. Am J Epidemiol 122:820–9.

Hanna JM (1970) Responses of native and migrant desert residents to arid heat. Am J Phys Anthropol 32:187–96.

Hansen JP, Hancke S, Moller-Petersen J (1990) Atherosclerosis in Native Greenlanders: an ultrasonographic investigation. Arct Med Res 49:151–6.

Hansen JP, Meldgaard J, Nordqvist J (1985) The mummies of Qilakitsoq. Natl Geographic 167:191–207.

Harris MI, Hadden WC, Knowler WC, Bennett PH (1987) Prevalence of diabetes and impaired glucose tolerance and plasma glucose level in U.S. population aged 20–74 years. Diabetes 36:523–34.

Harrison GA, Tanner JM, Pilbeam DR, Baker PT (1988) Human Biology: An Introduction to Human Evolution, Variation, Growth, and Adaptability. Oxford: Oxford University Press; 1988.

Harrison H, Boyce W, Haffner W, et al. (1983) The prevalence of genital Chlamydia trachomatis and Mycoplasma infections during pregnancy in an American Indian population. Sex Transm Dis 10:184–6.

Hauschild AH, Gauvreau L (1985) Food-borne botulism in Canada, 1971–84. Can Med Assoc J 133:1141–6.

Havlik RJ, Feinleib M (1982) Epidemiology and genetics of hypertension. Hypertension 4(Suppls III):121–7.

Heath GW, Wilson RH, Smith J, Leonard BE (1991) Community-based exercise and weight control: diabetes risk reduction and glycemic control in Zuni Indians. Am J Clin Nutr 53:1642S–6S.

Helm J (1980) Female infanticide, European diseases, and population levels among the MacKenzie Dene. Am Ethnologist 7:259–85.

Helmrich SP, Ragland DR, Leung RW, Paffenbarger RS (1991) Physical activity and reduced occurrence of non-insulin-dependent diabetes mellitus. N Engl J Med 325:147–52.

Henry RE, Burch TA, Bennett PH, Miller M (1969) Diabetes in the Cocopah Indians. Diabetes 18:33–7.

Herbert FA, Mahon WA, Wilkinson D, et al. (1967) Pneumonia in Indian and Eskimo infants and children. Part I: a clinical study. Can Med Assoc J 96:257–65.

Herbert FA, Wilkinson D, Burchak E, Morgante O (1977) Adenovirus type 3 pneumonia causing lung damage in childhood. Can Med Assoc J 116:274–6.

Heyward WL, Bender TR, McMahon BJ, Hall DB, et al. (1985) The control of hepatitis B virus infection with vaccine in Yupik Eskimos: demonstration of safety, immunogenicity, and efficacy under field conditions. Am J Epidemiol 121:914–23.

Heyward WL, Lanier AP, Bender TR, McMahon BJ, et al. (1983) Early detection of primary hepatocellular carcinoma by screening for alpha-fetoprotein in high risk families. Lancet 2:1161–2.

Hildes JA, Schaefer O (1973) Health of Igloolik Eskimos and change with urbanization. J Hum Biol 2:241–6.

Hildes JA, Schaefer O (1984) The changing picture of neoplastic disease in the western and central Canadian Arctic (1950–1980). Can Med Assoc J 130:25–33.

Hill CA, Spector MI (1971) Natality and mortality of American Indians compared to US whites and non-whites. HSMHA Health Reports 86:229–49.

Hislop TG, Deschamps M, Band PR, Smith JM, Clarke HF (1992) Participation in the British Columbia cervical cytology screening program by Native Indian women. Can J Public Health 83:344–5.

Hislop TG, Threlfall WJ, Gallagher RP, Band PR (1987) Accidental and intentional violent deaths among British Columbia Native Indians. Can J Public Health 78:271–4.

Hlady WG, Middaugh JP (1988) Suicides in Alaska: firearms and alcohol. Am J Public Health 78:179–80.

Hoffer J, Ruedy J, Verdier P (1981) Nutritional status of Quebec Indians. Am J Clin Nutr 34:2784–9.

Horrobin DF (1987) Low prevalence of coronary heart disease (CHD), psoriasis, asthma and rheumatoid arthritis in Eskimos: are they caused by high dietary intake of eicosapentaenoic acid (EPA), a genetic variation of essential fatty acid (EFA) metabolism or a combination of both? Med Hypotheses 22:421–8.

Horsburgh CR, Douglas JM, LaForce FM (1987) Preventive strategies in sexually transmitted diseases for the primary care physician. JAMA 258:814–21.

Horwitz O, Payne PG, Wilbek E (1966) Epidemiological basis of tuberculosis eradication. 4: the isoniazid trial in Greenland. Bull WHO 35:509–23.

House JS, Landis KR, Umberson D (1988) Social relationships and health. Science 241:540–5.

Houston CS, Weiler RL, Habbick BF (1979) Severity of lung disease in Indian children. Can Med Assoc J 120:1116–21.

Houston S, Fanning A, Soskolne CL, Fraser N (1990) The effectiveness of Bacillus Calmette-Guérin (BCG) vaccination against tuberculosis. Am J Epidemiol 131:340–8.

Howard BV, Bogardus C, Ravussin E, Foley JE, et al. (1991) Studies of the etiology of obesity in Pima Indians. Am J Clin Nutr 53:1577S–85S.

Howard BV, Davis MP, Pettitt DJ, et al. (1983) Plasma and lipoprotein cholesterol and triglyceride concentrations in the Pima Indians: distribution differing from those of Caucasians. Circulation 68:714–24.

Howland J, Hingson R (1987) Alcohol as a risk factor for injuries or death due to fires and burns: review of the literature. Public Health Rep 102:475–83.

Hrabovsky SL, Welty TK, Coulehan JL (1989) Acute myocardial infarction and sudden death in Sioux Indians. West J Med 150:420–22.

Hrdlička A (1908) Physiological and Medical Observations among the Indians of Southwestern United States and Mexico. Washington, DC: Smithsonian Institution; Bureau of American Ethnology Bulletin No. 34.

Hsu JS, Williams SD (1991) Injury prevention awareness in an urban Native American population. Am J Public Health 81:1466–8.

Hull J (1984) 1981 Census coverage of the Native population in Manitoba and Saskatchewan. Can J Native Stud 4:147–56.

Hunter AG, Thompson D, Evans JA (1979) Is there a fetal gasoline syndrome? Teratology 20:75–9.

Hurlich MD, Steegman AT (1979) Contrasting laboratory response to cold in two Subarctic Algonkian villages: an admixture effect? Hum Biol 51:255–78.

Imrie R, Warren R (1988) Health promotion survey in the Northwest Territories. Can J Public Health 79:16–24.

Ingelfinger JA, Bennett PH, Liebow IM, Miller M (1976) Coronary heart disease in Pima Indians: electrocardiographic findings and postmortem evidence of myocardial infarctions in a population with a high prevalence of diabetes mellitus. Diabetes 25:561–5.

Inhorn MC, Brown PJ (1990) The anthropology of infectious diseases. Annu Rev Anthropol 19:89–117.

Innis SM, Kuhnlein HV (1987) The fatty acid composition of northern Canadian marine and terrestrial mammals. Acta Med Scand 222:105–9.

Innis SM, Kuhnlein HV, Kinloch D (1988) The composition of red cell membrane phospholipids in Canadian Inuit consuming a diet high in marine mammals. Lipids 23:1064–8.

Ireland B, Lanier AP, Knutson L, Clift SE, Harpster A (1988) Increased risk of cancer in siblings of Alaskan Native patients with nasopharyngeal carcinoma. Int J Epidemiol 17:509–11.

Irvine J, Gillis DC, Tan L, et al. (1991) Lung, breast, and cervical cancer incidence and survival in Saskatchewan northerners and registered Indians (1967–86). In: Postl BD, Gilbert P, et al., eds. Circumpolar Health 90: Proceedings of the 8th International Congress on Circumpolar Health. Winnipeg: University of Manitoba Press; 452–6.

Jackson MY, Proulx JM, Pelican S (1991) Obesity prevention. Am J Clin Nutr 53:1625S–30S.

Janes CR, Stall R, Gifford SM, eds. (1986) Anthropology and Epidemiology. Dordrecht, the Netherlands: D. Reidel.

Jarrett RJ (1989) Epidemiology and public health aspects of non-insulin-dependent diabetes mellitus. Epidemiol Rev 11:151–71.

Jarvis GK, Boldt M (1982) Death styles among Canada's Indians. Soc Sci Med 16:1345–52.

Jenkins D (1977) Tuberculosis: the Native Indian viewpoint on its prevention, diagnosis, and treatment. Prev Med 6:545–55.

Jensen GF, Strauss JH, Harris VW (1977) Crime, delinquency, and the American Indian. Hum Organization 36:252–7.

Jilek WG (1982) Indian Healing: Shamanic ceremonialism in the Pacific Northwest Today. Surrey, BC: Hancock House.

Jilek W, Roy C (1976) Homicide committed by Canadian Indians and non-Indians. Int J Offender Therapy Comp Criminol 20:201–16.

Jilek-Aall L (1981) Acculturation, alcoholism and Indian-style Alcoholics Anonymous. J Stud Alcohol (Suppl 9):143–58.

Johansson SR (1982) The demographic history of the Native Peoples of North America: a selective bibliography. Yearbk Phys Anthropol 25:133–52.

Johnson A, Taylor A (1991) Prevalence of chronic diseases: a summary of data from the Survey of American Indians and Alaska Natives. Rockville, MD: USDHHS/PHS/ Agency for Health Care Policy and Research; 1991. National Medical Expenditure Survey Data Summary 3, ACHPR Pub No 91-0031.

Johnson IL, Thomson M, Manfreda J, Hershfield ES (1985) Risk factors for reactivation of tuberculosis in Manitoba. Can Med Assoc J 133:1221–4.

Johnson JE, Jr, McNutt CW (1964) Diabetes mellitus in an American Indian population isolate. Texas Rep Biol Med 22:110–25.

Johnston FE (1985) Health implications of childhood obesity. Ann Intern Med 103:1068–72.

Johnston FE, Low SM (1984) Biomedical anthropology: an emerging synthesis in anthropology. Yearbk Phys Anthropol 27:215–27.

Johnston FE, McKigney JI, Hopwood S, Smelker J (1978) Physical growth and development of urban Native Americans: a study in urbanization and its implications for nutritional status. Am J Clin Nutr 31:1017–27.

Johnston JL, Williams CN, Weldon KL (1977) Nutrient intake and meal patterns of Micmac Indian and Caucasian women in Shubenacadie, NS. Can Med Assoc J 116: 1356–9.

Joint National Committee on Detection, Evaluation and Treatment of High Blood Pressure. (1988) The 1988 Report. Arch Intern Med 148:1023–38.

Joossens JV, Geboers J (1987) Dietary salt and risks to health. Am J Clin Nutr 45:1277–88.

Jordan SW, Key CR (1981) Carcinoma of the cervix in southwestern American Indians: result of a cytologic detection program. Cancer 47:2523–32.

Kaplan GJ, Bender TR, Clark PS, et al. (1972) Echovirus type 4 meningitis and related febrile illness: epidemiologic study of an outbreak in two Eskimo communities in 1970. Am J Epidemiol 96:74–85.

Kaplan GJ, Fraser RI, Comstock GW (1972b) Tuberculosis in Alaska 1970: the continued decline of the tuberculosis epidemic. Am Rev Respir Dis 105:920–6.

Kaufman A (1973) Gasoline sniffing among children in a Pueblo Indian village. Pediatrics 51:1060–4.

Kelso DR, Attneave CL, eds (1981) Bibliography of North American Indian Mental Health. Westport, CT: Greenwood Press.

Kettl PA, Bixler EO (1991) Suicide in Alaska Natives, 1979–1984. Psychiatry 54:55–63.

Key CR (1981) Cancer incidence and mortality in New Mexico, 1973–1977. Natl Cancer Inst Monogr 57:489–595.

Kinder BN, Pape NE, Walfish S (1980) Drug and alcohol education programs: a review of outcome studies. Int J Addict 15:1035–54.

King H, Dowd JE (1990) Primary prevention of type 2 (non-insulin-dependent) diabetes mellitus. Diabetologia 33:3–8.

Kirk R, Szathmary EJ, eds. (1985) Out of Asia: Peopling the Americas and the Pacific. Canberra: Journal of Pacific History Special Publication.

Kjaer SK, De Villiers EM, Haugaard BJ, et al. (1988) Human papillomavirus, herpes simplex virus and cervical cancer incidence in Greenland and Denmark: a population-based cross-sectional study. Int J Cancer 41:518–24.

Kjaer SK, Engholm G, Teisen C, et al. (1990) Risk factors for cervical human papillomavirus and herpes simplex virus infections in Greenland and Denmark: a population-based study. Am J Epidemiol 131:669–82.

Kjaer SK, Teisen C, Haugaard BJ, et al. (1989) Risk factors for cervical cancer in Greenland and Denmark: a population-based cross-sectional study. Int J Cancer 44:40–7.

Klain M, Coulehan JL, Arena VC, Janett R (1988) More frequent diagnosis of acute myocardial infarction among Navajo Indians. Am J Public Health 78:1351–2.

Knowler WC, Bennett PH, Hamman RF, Miller M (1978) Diabetes incidence and prevalence in Pima Indians: a 19-fold greater incidence than in Rochester, Minnesota. Am J Epidemiol 108:497–505.

Knowler WC, Bennett PH, Bottazzo GF, Doniach D (1979) Islet cell antibodies and diabetes mellitus in Pima Indians. Diabetologia 17:161–4.

Knowler WC, Pettit DJ, Bennett PH, Williams RC (1983) Diabetes mellitus in the Pima Indians: genetic and evolutionary considerations. Am J Phys Anthropol 62:107–14.

Knowler WC, Pettitt DJ, Saad MF, Bennett PH (1990) Diabetes mellitus in the Pima Indians: incidence, risk factors and pathogenesis. Diabetes Metab Rev 6:1–27.

Knowler WC, Pettitt DJ, Saad MF, Charles MA, et al. (1991) Obesity in the Pima Indians: its magnitude and relationship with diabetes. Am J Clin Nutr 53:1543S–51S.

Knowler WC, Pettit DJ, Savage PJ, Bennett PH (1981) Diabetes incidence in Pima Indians: contributions of obesity and parental diabetes. Am J Epidemiol 113:144–56.

Knowler WC, Pettitt DJ, Vasquez B, et al. (1984) Polymorphism in the 5' flanking region of the human insulin gene: relationship with non-insulin-dependent diabetes mellitus, glucose and insulin concentrations, and diabetes treatment in the Pima Indian. J Clin Invest 74:2129–35.

Knowler WC, Williams RC, Pettitt DJ, Steinberg AG (1988) Gm[3;5,13,14] and type 2 diabetes mellitus: an association in American Indians with genetic admixture. Am J Hum Genet 43:520–6.

Kordova N, Wilt JC, Selka L, et al. (1983) High prevalence of antibodies to Chlamydia trachomatis in a northern Canadian community. Can J Public Health 74:246–9.

Kositchek RJ, Wurm M, Strauss R (1961) Biochemical studies in full-blooded Navajo Indians: II. Lipids and lipoproteins. Circulation 23:219–24.

Kralt J (1990) Ethnic origins in the Canadian Census, 1871–1986. In: Halli SS, Trovato F, Driedger L. Ethnic Demography: Canadian Immigrant, Racial and Cultural Variations. Ottawa: Carleton University Press; 13–29.

Kraus RF, Buffler PA (1979) Sociocultural stress and the American Native in Alaska: an analysis of changing patterns of psychiatric illness and alcohol abuse among Alaska Natives. Cult Med Psychiatry 3:111–51.

Krech S (1978) Disease, starvation, and northern Athapaskan social organization. Am Ethnologist 5:710–32.

Krishnamurthy S, Lanier AP, Dohan P, Lanier JF, Henle W (1987) Salivary gland cancer in Alaskan Natives, 1966–1980. Hum Pathol 18:986–96.

Kriska AM, Knowler WC, Laporte RE, et al. (1990) Development of a questionnaire to examine relationship of physical activity and diabetes in Pima Indians. Diabetes Care 13:401–11.

Kroman N, Green A (1980) Epidemiological studies in the Upernavik District: incidence of some chronic diseases, 1950–1974. Acta Med Scand 208:401–6.

Kuhnlein HV (1984) Traditional and contemporary Nuxalk foods. Nutr Res 4:789–809.

Kuhnlein HV, Calloway DH (1977) Contemporary Hopi food intake patterns. Ecol Food Nutr 6:159–73.

Kunitz SJ (1976) Fertility, mortality and social organization. Hum Biol 48:361–77.

Kunitz SJ (1983) Disease Change and the Role of Medicine: The Najavo Experience. Berkeley: University of California Press.

Kunitz SJ, Levy J (1986) The prevalence of hypertension among elderly Navajos: a test of the acculturative stress hypothesis. Cult Med Psychiatry 10:97–121.

Kunzelman CL, Knowler WC, Pettitt DJ, Bennett PH (1989) Incidence of proteinuria in type 2 diabetes mellitus in the Pima Indians. Kidney Int 35:681–7.

Kushigemachi M, Schneiderman LJ, Barrett-Connor E (1984) Racial differences in susceptibility to tuberculosis: risk of disease after infection. J Chron Dis 37:853–62.

Labarthe DR, Elissa M, Varas C (1991) Childhood precursors of high blood pressure and elevated cholesterol. Annu Rev Public Health 12:519–41.

Lamarine RJ (1988) Alcohol abuse among Native Americans. J Comm Health 13:143–55.

Lamoureux M, ed (1991) Domestic Violence in Aboriginal Communities: Reference Manual. Quebec: Ministère de la Santé et des Services sociaux.

Lang GC (1985) Diabetes and health care in a Sioux community. Hum Organization 44:251–60.

Lanier AP, Bender TR, Blot WJ, Fraumeni JF (1982) Cancer in Alaskan Natives: 1974–78. Natl Cancer Inst Monogr 62:79–81.

Lanier AP, Bender T, Talbot M, et al. (1980a) Nasopharyngeal carcinoma in Alaskan Eskimos, Indians, and Aleuts: a review of cases and study of Epstein-Barr virus, HLA, and environmental risk factors. Cancer 46:2100–6.

Lanier AP, Blot WJ, Bender TR, Fraumeni JF (1980b) Cancer in Alaskan Indians, Eskimos, and Aleuts. JNCI 65:1157–9.

Lanier AP, Bornkamm GW, Henle W, et al. (1981) Association of Epstein-Barr virus with nasopharyngeal carcinoma in Alaskan Native patients: serum antibodies and tissue EBNA and DNA. Int J Cancer 28:301–5.

Lanier AP, Bulkow LR, Ireland B (1989) Cancer in Alaskan Indians, Eskimos, and Aleuts, 1969–83: implications for etiology and control. Public Health Rep 104:658–64.

Lanier AP, McMahon BJ, Alberts SR, Popper H, Heyward WL (1987) Primary liver cancer in Alaskan Natives, 1980–1985. Cancer 60:1915–20.

Larke RB, Froese GJ, Devine RD, Petruk MW (1987) Extension of the epidemiology of hepatitis B in circumpolar regions through a comprehensive serologic study in the Northwest Territories of Canada. J Med Virol 22:269–76.

La Rosa JC, Hunninghake D, Bush D, et al. (1990) The cholesterol facts: a summary of the evidence relating dietary fats, serum cholesterol and coronary heart disease. Circulation 81:1721–33.

Laughlin WS, Harper AB, eds. (1979) The First Americans: Origins, Affinities, and Adaptations. New York: Gustav Fischer.

Leacock EB, Lurie NO, eds. (1971) North American Indians in Historical Perspective. New York: Random House.

Leacy FH, ed. (1983) Historical Statistics of Canada. Ottawa: Statistics Canada.

Lederman JM, Wallace AC, Hildes JA (1962) Arteriosclerosis and neoplasms in Canadian Eskimos. In: Biological Aspect of Aging: Proceedings of the Fifth International Congress on Gerontology. New York: Columbia University Press; 201–7.

Lee CC, Brunham RC, Sherman E, Harding GK (1987) Epidemiology of an outbreak of infectious syphilis in Manitoba. Am J Epidemiol 125:277–83.

Lee ET, Anderson PS, Jr, Bryan J, et al, (1985) Diabetes, prenatal diabetes and obesity in Oklahoma Indians. Diabetes Care 8:107–13.

Lee ET, Welty TK, Fabsitz R, et al. (1990) The Strong Heart Study: a study of cardiovascular disease in American Indians: design and methods. Am J Epidemiol 132:1141–55.

Lee M, Reyburn R, Carrow A (1971) Nutritional status of British Columbia Indians. 1. Dietary studies at Ahousat and Anaham reserves. Can J Public Health 62:285–96.

Lefkowitz D, Underwood C (1991) Personal health practices: findings from the Survey of American Indians and Alaska Natives. Rockville, MD: USDHHS/PHS/Agency for Health Care Policy and Research (ACHPR Pub No 91-0034).

Leighton AH, Hughes CC (1955) Notes on Eskimo patterns of suicide. Southwest J Anthropol 11:327–8.

Lemon SM (1985) Type A viral hepatitis: new developments in an old disease. N Engl J Med 313:1059–67.

Lester D (1989) The heritability of alcoholism: science and social policy. Drugs Society 3:29–68.

Letson GW, Santosham M, Reid R, et al. (1988) Comparison of active and combined passive/active immunization of Navajo children against Haemophilus influenzae type b. Pediatr Infect Dis J 7:747–52.

Levy JE, Kunitz SJ (1971) Indian reservations, anomie, and social pathologies. Southwest J Anthropol 27:97–128.

Levy JE, Kunitz SJ (1987) A suicide prevention program for Hopi youth. Soc Sci Med 25:931–40.

Levy JE, Kunitz SJ, Everett M (1969) Navajo criminal homicide. Southwest J Anthropol 25:124–52.

Liberatos P, Link BG, Kelsey JL (1988) The measurement of social class in epidemiology. Epidemiol Rev 10:87–121.

Lillioja S, Mott DM, Zawadzki JK, et al. (1987) In vivo insulin action is familial characteristic in nondiabetic Pima Indians. Diabetes 36:1329–35.

Little MA, Haas JD, eds. (1989) Human Population Biology: A Transdisciplinary Science. New York: Oxford University Press.

Littman G (1970) Alcoholism, illness, and social pathology among American Indians in transition. Am J Public Health 60:1769–78.

Long TP (1978) The prevalence of clinically treated diabetes among Zuni reservation residents. Am J Public Health 68:901–3.

Longclaws L, Barnes GE, Grieve L, Dumoff R (1980) Alcohol and drug use among the Brokenhead Ojibwa. J Stud Alcohol 41:21–36.

Longstaffe S, Postl B, Kao H, Nicolle L, Ferguson CA (1982) Rheumatic fever in native children in Manitoba. Can Med Assoc J 127:497–8.

Losonsky GA, Santosham M, Sehgal VM, et al. (1984) Haemophilus influenzae disease in the White Mountain Apaches: molecular epidemiology of a high risk population. Pediatr Infect Dis 3:539–47.

Lowenfels AB, Walker AM, Althaus DP, et al. (1989) Gallstone growth, size, and risk of gallbladder cancer: an interracial study. Int J Epidemiol 18:50–4.

Lynch HT, Drouhard TJ, Scheulke GS, et al. (1985) Hereditary nonpolyposis colorectal cancer in a Navajo family. Cancer Genet Cytogenet 15:209–13.

Lynge I (1985) Suicide in Greenland. Arct Med Res 40:53–60.

Macaulay AC, Hanusaik N (1988) Diabetic education program in the Mohawk community of Kahnawake, Quebec. Can Fam Physician 34:1591–3.

Macaulay AC, Moutour LT, Adelson N (1988) Prevalence of diabetic and atherosclerotic complications among Mohawk Indians of Kahnawake, PQ. Can Med Assoc J 139: 221–4.

MacWilliams L, Mao Y, Nicholls E, Wigle D (1987) Fatal accidental childhood injuries in Canada. Can J Public Health 78:129–35.

Mahoney MC (1991) Fatal motor vehicle traffic accidents among Native Americans. Am J Prev Med 7:112–6.

Mahoney MC, Michalek AM (1991) A meta-analysis of cancer incidence in United States and Canadian Native population. Int J Epideminol 20:323–7.

Mahoney MC, Michalek AM, Cummings KM, et al. (1989a) Years of potential life lost among a Native American population. Public Health Rep 104:279–85.

Mahoney MC, Michalek AM, Cummings KM, et al. (1989b) Cancer mortality in a northeastern Native American population. Cancer 64:187–90.

Mahoney MC, Michalek AM, Cummings KM, et al. (1989c) Cancer surveillance in a northeastern Native American population. Cancer 64:191–5.

Mahoney MC, Michalek AM, Cummings KM, et al. (1989d) Mortality in a northeastern Native American cohort 1955–1984. Am J Epidemiol 129(816–26):

Mail PD, McDonald DR, eds. (1980) Tulapai to Tokay: A Bibliography of Alcohol Use and Abuse among Native Americans of North America. New Haven, CT: HRAF Press.

Mann GV, Scott EM, Hursh LM, et al. (1962) The health and nutritional status of Alaskan Eskimos: a survey of the Interdepartmental Committee on Nutrition for National Defence—1958. Am J Clin Nutr 11:31–75.

Manson JE, Tosteson H, Ridker PM, et al. (1992) The primary prevention of myocardial infarction. N Engl J Med 326:1406–16.

Manson SM, Beals J, Dick RW, Duclos C (1989) Risk factors for suicide among Indian adolescents at a boarding school. Public Health Rep 104:609–14.

Mao Y, Morrison H, Semenciw R, Wigle D (1986) Mortality on Canadian Indian reserves 1976–1983. Can J Public Health 77:263–8.

Marchand JF (1943) Tribal epidemics in the Yukon. JAMA 123:1019–20.

Margolis HS, Lum MK, Bender TR, et al. (1980) Acute glomerulonephritis and streptococcal skin lesions in Eskimo children. Am J Dis Child 134:681–5.

Margolis HS, Middaugh JP, Burgess RD (1979) Arctic trichinosis: two Alaskan outbreaks from walrus meat. J Infect Dis 139:102–3.

Marmot MG, Kogevinas M, Elston MA (1987) Social/economic status and disease. Annu Rev Public Health 8:111–35.

Martens T, Daily B, Hodgson M (1988) Characteristics and Dynamics of Incest and Child Sexual Abuse, with a Native Perspective. Edmonton: Nechi Institute.

May PA (1982) Substance abuse and American Indians: prevalence and susceptibility. Int J Addict 17:1185–209.

May PA (1986) Alcohol and drug misuse prevention programs for Amerian Indians: needs and opportunities. J Stud Alcohol 47:187–95.

May PA (1987) Suicide and self-destuction among American Indian youths. Am Ind Alaska Native Ment Health Res 1:52–69.

May PA (1992) Alcohol policy considerations for Indian reservations and bordertown communities. Am Ind Alaska Nat Mental Health Res 4:5–59.

May PA, Hymbaugh KJ, Aase JM, Samet JM (1983) Epidemiology of fetal alcohol syndrome among American Indians of the Southwest. Soc Biol 30:374–87.

May PA, Smith MB (1988) Some Navajo Indian opinions about alcohol abuse and prohibition: a survey and recommendations for policy. J Stud Alcohol 49:324–34.

Mayberry RH, Lindeman RD (1963) A survey of chronic disease and diet in Seminole Indians in Oklahoma. Am J Clin Nutr 13:127–34.

Maynard JE (1976) Coronary heart disease risk factors in relation to urbanization in Alaskan Eskimo men. In: Shephard RJ, Itoh S, eds. Circumpolar Health. Toronto: University of Toronto Press; 294.

Maynard JE, Hammes LM, Kester FE (1967) Morality due to heart disease among Alaska Natives, 1955–65. Public Health Rep 82:714–20.

McElroy A (1990) Biocultural models in studies of human health and adaptation. Med Anthropol Q 4:243–65.

McIntyre L, Shah CP. (1986) Prevalence of hypertension, obesity and smoking in three Indian communities in northwestern Ontario. Can Med Assoc J 134:345–9.

McKeown T. (1988) The Origins of Human Disease. Oxford: Basil Blackwell.

McKinnon AL, Gartrell JW, Derksen LA, Jarvis GK. (1991) Health knowledge of Native Indian youth in central Alberta. Can J Public Health 82:429–33.

McMahon BJ, Albert SR, Wainwright RB, Bulkow L, Lanier AP. (1990a) Hepatitis B-related seuqelae: prospective study in 1400 hepatitis B surface antigen-positive Alaska Native carriers. Arch Intern Med 150:1051–4.

McMahon BJ, Alward WL, Hall DB, Heyward WL et al (1985) Acute hepatitis B virus infection: relation of age to the clinical expression of disease and subsequent development of the carrier state. J Infect Dis 151:599–603.

McMahon BJ, Rhoades ER, Heyward WL, et al. (1987) A comprehensive programme to reduce the incidence of hepatitis B virus infection and its sequelae in Alaskan Natives. Lancet 2:1134–6.

McMahon BJ, Wainwright K, Bulkow L, et al. (1990b) Response to hepatitis B vaccine in Alaska Natives with chronic alcoholism compared with non-alcoholic control subjects. Am J Med 88:460–4.

McMurtry MP, Cerqueira MT, Connor SL, Connor WE (1991) Changes in lipid and lipoprotein levels and body weight in Tarahumara Indians after consumption of an affluent diet. N Engl J Med 325:1704–8.

Meerovitch E, Eaton RD (1965) Outbreak of amebiasis among Indians in northwestern Saskatchewan, Canada. Am J Trop Med Hyg 14:719–23.

Megill DM, Hoy WE, Woodruff SD (1988) Rates and causes of end-stage renal disease in Navajo Indians, 1971–1985. West J Med 149:178–82.

Meister CW (1976) Demographic consequences of Euro-American contact on selected American Indian populations and their relationship to the demographic transition. Ethnohistory 23:161–72.

Melbye M, Ebbesen P, Levine PH, Bennike T (1984a) Early primary infection and high Epstein-Barr virus antibody titers in Greenland Eskimos at high risk for nasopharyngeal carcinoma. Int J Cancer 34:619–23.

Melbye M, Skinhøj P, Nielsen NH, et al. (1984b) Virus-associated cancers in Greenland:

frequent hepatitis B virus infection but low primary hepatocellular carcinoma incidence. J Natl Cancer Inst. 73:1267–72.

Meltzer DJ (1989) Why don't we know when the first people came to North America? Am Antiquity 54:471–90.

Meltzer H, Kovacs L, Orford T, Matas M (1956) Echinococcosis in North American Indians and Eskimos. Can Med Assoc J 75:121–8.

Menon S, Santosham M, Reid R, et al. (1990) Rotavirus diarrhea in Apache children: a case-control study. Int J Epidemiol 19:715–21.

Metler R, Conway GA, Stehr-Green J (1991) AIDS surveillance among American Indians and Alaska Natives. Am J Public Health 81:1469–71.

Middaugh JP (1990) Cardiovascular deaths among Alaskan Natives, 1980–86. Am J Public Health 80:282–5.

Mikkelson MK, Snoke T, Sharp C, Westley T, Vall-Spinosa A (1973) Ambulatory tuberculosis chemotherapy on an Indian reservation. Chest 64:570–3.

Millar WJ (1982) Mortality patterns in a Canadian Indian population. Can Stud Pop 9:17–31.

Millar WJ (1990) Smoking prevalence in the Canadian Arctic. Arctic Med Res 49(Suppl 2):23–28.

Millar WJ (1992) Place of birth and ethnic status: factors associated with smoking prevalence among Canadians. Statistics Canada Health Reports 4:7–24.

Miller AB, Anderson G, Brisson J, et al. (1991) Report of a national workshop on screening for cancer of the cervix. Can Med Assoc J 145:1301–25.

Minuk GY, Ling N, Postl B, Waggoner JG, et al. (1985) The changing epidemiology of hepatitis B virus infection in the Canadian North. Am J Epidemiol 121:598–604.

Minuk GY, Nicolle LE, Postl B, Waggoner JG, Hoofnagle JH (1982b) Hepatitis virus infection in an isolated Canadian Inuit (Eskimo) population. J Med Virol 10:255–64.

Minuk GY, Nicolle LE, Gauthier T, Brunha J (1991) The prevalence of antibody to hepatitis C virus in an isolated Canadian Inuit settlement. Can J Infect Dis 2:71–3.

Minuk GY, Waggoner JG, Jernigan R, Nicolle LE, et al. (1982a) Prevalence of antibody to hepatitis A virus in a Canadian Inuit community. Can Med Assoc J 127:850–2.

Moffatt MEK, Law B, Tenenbein M (1991) Low relative risk of epiglottitis in Manitoba Indians. In: Postl B, Gilbert P, Goodwill J et al., eds. Circumpolar Health 90: Proceedings of the 8th International Congress on Circumpolar Health. Winnipeg: University of Manitoba Press, 394–5.

Moller DE, Yokota A, Flier JS (1989) Normal insulin-receptor cDNA sequence in Pima Indians with NIDDM. Diabetes 34:1496–500.

Monk M (1987) Epidemiology of suicide. Epidemiol Rev 9:51–69.

Montour LT, Macaulay AC, Adelson N (1989) Diabetes mellitus in Mohawks of Kahnawake, PQ: a clinical and epidemiologic description. Can Med Assoc J 141:549–52.

Montour LT, Macaulay AC (1985) High prevalence rates of diabetes mellitus and hypertension in a North American Indian reservation (letter). Can Med Assoc J 132:1112.

Moore PE, Kruse HD, Tisdall FF, Corrigan RS (1946) Medical survey of nutrition among the northern Manitoba Indian. Can Med Assoc J 54:223–33.

Moorman LJ (1949) Health of the Navajo-Hopi Indians: general report of the American Medical Association. JAMA 139:370–6.

Moran EF (1981) Human adaptation to Arctic zones. Annu Rev Anthropol 10:1025.

Morris K, Morganlander M, Coulehan JL, et al. (1990) Wood-burning stoves and lower respiratory tract infection in American Indian children. Am J Dis Child 144:105–8.

Morrison HI, Semenciw RM, Mao Y, Wigle D (1986) Infant mortality on Canadian Indian reserves, 1976–1983. Can J Public Health 77:269–73.

Moskowitz JM (1989) The primary prevention of alcohol problems: a critical review of the research literature. J Stud Alcohol 50:54–88.

Motulsky AG (1987) Human genetic variation and nutrition. Am J Clin Nutr 45:1108–13.

Mouratoff GJ, Carroll NV, Scott EM (1967) Diabetes mellitus in Eskimos. JAMA 199:107–12.

Mouratoff GJ, Carroll NV, Scott EM (1969) Diabetes mellitus in Athapaskan Indians in Alaska. Diabetes 18:29–31.

Mouratoff GJ, Scott EM (1973) Diabetes mellitus in Eskimos after a decade. JAMA 266:1345–6.

Nagulesparan M, Savage PJ, Knowler WC, Johnson GC, Bennett PH (1982) Increased in vivo insulin resistance in nondiabetic Pima Indians compared with Caucasians. Diabetes 31:952–6.

National Institutes of Health Consensus Development Panel (1985) Health implications of obesity. Ann Intern Med 103:1073–7.

Nations MK (1986) Epidemiological research on infectious disease: quantitative rigor or rigor mortis? Insights from ethnomedicine. In: Janes CR, Stall R, Gifford SM, eds. Anthropology and Epidemiology. Dordrecht, the Netherlands: D. Reidel; 97–123.

Navarro V (1989) Race vs class, or race and class. Int J Health Services 19:311–4.

Naylor CD, Basinski A, Frank JW, Rachlis MM (1990) Asymptomatic hypercholesterolemia: a clinical policy review. J Clin Epidemiol 43:1029–121.

Neel JV (1968) Opening statement. In: Biomedical Challenges Presented by the American Indian. Sci Publ No 165. Washington, DC: Pan American Health Organization, 1968.

Neel JV (1982) The thrifty gene revisited. In: Kobberling J, Tattersall R, eds. The Genetics of Diabetes Mellitus. New York: Academic Press; 283–93.

Nelson RG, Gohdes DM, Everhart JE, et al. (1988) Lower-extremity amputation in NIDDM: 12-year follow-up study in Pima Indians. Diabetes Care 11:8–16.

Nelson RG, Newman JM, Knowler WC, et al. (1988) Incidence of end-stage renal disease in type 2 (non-insulin-dependent) diabetes mellitus in Pima Indians. Diabetologia 31:730–6.

Nelson RG, Wolfe JA, Horton MB, et al. (1989) Proliferative retinopathy in NIDDM. Diabetes 38:435–40.

Newman JM, Marfin AA, Eggers PW, Helgerson SD (1990) End state renal disease among Native Americans, 1983–86. Am J Public Health 80:318–9.

Nicolle LE, Minuk GY, Postl B, et al. (1986) Cross-sectional seroepidemiologic study of the prevalence of cytomegalovirus and herpes simplex virus infection in a Canadian Inuit (Eskimo) community. Scand J Infect Dis 18:19–23.

Nicolle LE, Postl B, Kotelewetz E, et al. (1982a) Chemoprophylaxis for *Neisseria meningitidis* in an isolated Arctic community. J Infect Dis 145:103–9.

Nicolle LE, Postl B, Kotelewetz E, et al. (1982b) Emergence of rifampin-resistant Haemophilus influenzae. Antimicrob Agents Chemother 21:498–500.

Nicolle LE, Postl B, Urias B, et al. (1990a) Group A streptococcal pharyngeal carriage, pharyngitis, and impetigo in two northern Canadian Native communities. Clin Invest Med 13:99–106.

Nicolle LE, Postl B, Urias B, et al. (1990b) Outcome following therapy of group A streptococcal infection in schoolchildren in isolated northern communities. Can J Public Health 81:468–70.

Nielsen NH (1986) Cancer Incidence in Greenland. Oulu, Finland: Nordic Council for Arctic Medical Research; Arctic Medical Research Reports No 43 (Suppl).

Nielsen NH, Jensen H, Hansen PK (1988) Cervical cytology in Greenland and occurrence of cervical carcinoma, carcinoma in situ, and dysplasia: extent and impact of uncoordinated screening activity 1976–1985. Arct Med Res 47:179–88.

Norris MJ (1990) The demography of aboriginal people in Canada. In: Halli SS, Trovato F, Driedger L, eds. Ethnic Demography: Canadian Immigrant, Racial and Cultural Variations. Ottawa: Carleton University Press; 33–59.

Norsted TL, White E (1989) Cancer incidence among Native Americans of western Washington. Int J Epidemiol 18:22–7.

Nutting PA, Strotz CT, Short GI, Berg LE (1975) Reduction of gastroenteritis morbidity in high-risk infants. Pediatrics 55:354–8.

Oakland L, Kane R (1973) The working mother and child: neglect on the Navajo Reservation. Pediatrics 51:849–53.

Oetting ER, Beauvais F, Edwards RW (1988) Alcohol and Indian youth: social and psychological correlates and prevention. J Drug Issues 18:87–101.

Oetting ER, Swaim RC, Edwards RW, Beauvais F (1989) Indian and Anglo adolescent alcohol use and emotional distress: path models. Am J Alcohol Drug Abuse 15:153–72.

Olson LM, Becker TM, Wiggins CL, Key CR, Samet JM (1990) Injury mortality in American Indian, Hispanic, and non-Hispanic white children in New Mexico, 1958–1982. Soc Sci Med 30:479–86.

Omran AR (1971) The epidemiological transition: a theory of the epidemiology of population change. Milbank Mem Fund Q 49:509–38.

O'Malley MS, Fletcher SW (1987) Screening for breast cancer with breast self-examination. JAMA 257:2196–203.

O'Neil JD (1985) Community control over health problems: alcohol prohibition in a Canadian Inuit village. In: Fortuine R, ed. Circumpolar Health 84: Proceedings of the 6th International Symposium on Circumpolar Health. Seattle, WA: University of Washington Press; 340–3.

O'Neil JD (1986) The politics of health in the Fourth World: a northern Canadian example. Hum Organization 45:119–28.

O'Nell TD (1989) Psychiatric investigations among American Indians and Alaska Natives: a critical review. Cult Med Psychiatry 13:51–87.

O'Rahilly SO, Wainscoat JS, Turner RC (1988) Type 2 (non-insulin-dependent) diabetes mellitus: new genetics for old nightmares. Diabetologia 31:407–14.

Oseasohn R, Skipper BE, Tempest B (1978) Pneumonia in a Navajo community. Am Rev Respir Dis 117:1003–9.

Ostergaard Kristensen M (1983) Increased incidence of bleeding intracranial aneurysms in Greenland Eskimos. Acta Neurochir (Wien) 67:37–43.

Ostfield AM, Wilk E (1990) Epidemiology of stroke, 1980–1990: a progress report. Epidemiol Rev 12:253–6.

Overfield T, Klauber MR (1980) Prevalence of tuberculosis in Eskimos having blood group B gene. Hum Biol 52:87–92.

Pabst HF, Godel JC, Spady DW, McKechnie J, Grace M (1989a) Prospective trial of timing of Bacillus Calmette-Guérin vaccination in Canadian Cree infants. Am Rev Respir Dis 140:1007–11.

Pabst HF, Grace M, Godel J, Spady DW (1989b) Effect of breast-feeding on immune response to BCG vaccination. Lancet 1:295–7.

Page IH, Lewis LA, Gilbert J (1956) Plasma lipids and proteins and their relationship to coronary heart disease in the Navajo Indians. Circulation 13:675–9.

Pappaioanou M, Schwabe CW, Sard DM (1977) An evolving pattern of human hydatid disease transmission in the United States. Am J Trop Med Hyg 26:732–42.

Parish KL, Chapman WC, Williams LF, Richards WO (1991) Are new treatment methods of gallbladder stones the death-knell for gallstone surgery? Am Surgeon 57:634–41.

Passel JS (1976) Provisional evaluation of the 1970 Census count of American Indians. Demography 13:397–409.

Paul BD, ed. (1955) Health, Culture and Community. New York: Russell Sage.

Paulsen HJ (1987) Tuberculosis in the Native American: indigenous or introduced? Rev Infect Dis 9:1180–6.

Peart AF, Nagler FP (1954) Measles in the Canadian Arctic, 1952. Can J Public Health 45:146–57.

Perlman LV, Herdman RC, Kleinman H, Vernier RL (1965) Post-streptococcal glomerulonephritis: a ten-year follow-up of an epidemic. JAMA 194:175–82.

Petersen GM, Silimperi DR, Rotter JI, et al. (1987) Genetic factors in Haemophilus influenzae type b disease susceptibility and antibody acquisition. J Pediatr 110:228–33.

Petersen GM, Silimperi DR, Scott EM, et al. (1985) Uridine monophosphate kinase 3: a genetic marker for susceptibility to Haemophilus influenzae type b disease. Lancet 2:417–9.

Peterson NJ, Barrett DH, Bond WW, Berquist KR, et al. (1976) Hepatitis B surface antigen in saliva, impetiginous lesions, and the environment in two remote Alaskan villages. Appl Environ Microbiol 32:572–4.

Pettitt DJ, Aleck KA, Baird HR, Carraher MJ, et al. (1988) Congenital susceptibility to NIDDM: role of intrauterine environment. Diabetes 37:622–28.

Pettitt DJ, Knowler WC, Bennett PH, Aleck KA, Baird HR (1987) Obesity in offspring of diabetic Pima Indian women despite normal birth weight. Diabetes Care 10:76–80.

Pettitt DJ, Lisse JR, Knowler WC, Bennett PH (1982) Mortality as a function of obesity and diabetes mellitus. Am J Epidemiol 115:359–66.

Pfeiffer S (1984) Paleopathology in an Iroquoian ossuary, with special reference to tuberculosis. Am J Phys Anthropol 65:181–9.

Phillips MR, Inui TS (1986) The interaction of mental illness, criminal behavior and culture: native Alaskan mentally ill criminal offenders. Cult Med Psychiatry 10:123–49.

Piché V, George MV (1973) Estimates of vital rates for the Canadian Indians, 1960–1970. Demography 10:367–82.

Pine C (1981) Suicide in American Indian and Alaskan Native tradition. White Cloud J 2:3–8.

Pinkerton RE, Badke FR (1974) Coronary heart disease: an epidemiologic study of Crow and Northern Cheyenne Indians. Rocky Mt Med J 71:577–83.

Poirier S, Ohshima H, De-The G, et al. (1987) Volatile nitrosamine levels in common foods from Tunisia, south China, and Greenland, high-risk areas for nasopharyngeal carcinoma (NPC). Int J Cancer 39:293–6.

Polednak AP (1989) Racial and Ethnic Differences in Disease. New York: Oxford University Press.

Postl BD, Carson JB, Schaefer O (1985) Northwest Territories Perinatal and Infant Morbidity and Mortality Study: follow-up 1982, I. Utilization, morbidity and mortality. In: Fortuine R, ed. Circumpolar Health 84. Seattle: University of Washington Press; 125–8.

Postl B, Moffatt M, Sarsfield P (1987) Epidemiology and intervention for Native Canadians. Can J Public Health 78:219.

Postl BD, Moffatt ME, Black GB, Cameron CB (1987) Injuries and deaths associated with off-road recreational vehicles among children in Manitoba. Can Med Assoc J 137:297–300.

Prener A, Nielsen NH, Hansen JP, Jensen OM (1987) Cancer pattern among Greenlandic Inuit migrants in Denmark, 1968–1982. Br J Cancer 56:679–84.

Prener A, Nielsen NH, Storm HH, Hansen JP, Jensen OM (1991) Cancer in Greenland, 1953–1985. Acta Pathol Microbiol Immunol Scand 99(Suppl 20):7–79.

Price JA (1975) An applied analysis of North American Indian drinking patterns. Hum Organization 34:17–26.

Prosnitz LR, Mandell GL (1967) Diabetes among Navajo and Hopi Indians: the lack of vascular complications. Am J Med Sci 253:700–5.

Proulx JF (1988) Meningitis in Hudson's Bay, northern Quebec, Canada. Arctic Med Res 47(Suppl 1):686–7.

Rankin JG, Ashley MJ (1992) Alcohol-related health problems. In: Last JM, Wallace RB, eds. Maxcy-Rosenau-Last Public Health and Preventive Medicine. Norwalk, CT: Appleton and Lange; 741–67.

Ransohoff DF, Gracie WA, Wolfenson LB, Neuhauser D (1983) Prophylactic cholecystectomy or expectant management for silent gallstones: a decision analysis to assess survival. Ann Intern Med 99:199–204.

Rate RG, Knowler WC, Morse HG, et al. (1983) Diabetes mellitus in Hopis and Navajo Indians: prevalence of microvascular complications. Diabetes 32:894–9.

Rausch RL (1992) Hydatid disease. In: Last JM, Wallace RB, eds. Maxcy-Rosenau-Last Public Health and Preventive Medicine. Norwalk, CT: Appleton and Lange; 275–8.

Rausch RL, Scott EM, Rausch VR (1967) Helminths in Eskimos in western Alaska, with particular reference to Diphyllobothrium infection and anemia. Trans R Soc Trop Med Hyg 61:351–7.

Ravussin E, Lillioja S, Knowler WC, et al. (1988) Reduced rate of energy expenditure as a risk factor for body weight gain. N Engl J Med 318:467–72.

Redfield R, Linton R, Herskovitz M (1936) Memorandum for the study of acculturation. Am Anthropologist 69:661–9.

Reed TE (1985) Ethnic differences in alcohol use, abuse, and sensitivity: a review with genetic interpretation. Soc Biol 32:195–209.

Reed TE, Kalant H, Gibbins RJ, Kapur BM, Rankin JG (1976) Alcohol and acetaldehyde metabolism in Caucasians, Chinese and Amerinds. Can Med Assoc J 115:851–5.

Reeder BA, Shah CP, Williams DA (1988) Serum lipid distributions in Canadian Indians of northwestern Ontario. Can Fam Phys 34:1535–9.

Reeves WC, Rawls WE, Brinton LA (1989) Epidemiology of genital papillomaviruses and cervical cancer. Rev Infect Dis 11:426–39.

Reid JM, Fullmer SD, Pettigrew KD et al (1971) Nutrient intake of Pima Indian women: relationships to diabetes mellitus and gallbladder disease. Am J Clin Nutr 24:1281–9.

Remington G, Hoffman BF (1984) Gas sniffing as a form of substance abuse. Can J Psychiatry 29:31–5.

Rex DK, Bosron WF, Smialek JE, Li TK (1985) Alcohol and aldehyde dehydrogenase isoenzymes in North American Indians. Alcoholism Clin Exp Res 9:147–52.

Rhoades ER (1990) The major respiratory diseases of American Indians. Am Rev Respir Dis 141:595–600.

Rhoades ER, Hammond J, Welty TK, Handler AO, Amler RW (1987) The Indian burden of illness and future health interventions. Public Health Rep 102:361–8.

Rhoades ER, Mason RD, Eddy P, Smith EM, Burns TR (1988) The Indian Health Service approach to alcoholism among American Indians and Alaska Natives. Public Health Rep 103:621–7.

Rice RJ, Roberts PL, Handsfield HH, Holmes KK (1991) Sociodemographic distribution of gonorrhea incidence: implications for prevention and behavioral research. Am J Public Health 81:1252–8.

Rieder HL (1989) Tuberculosis among American Indians of the contiguous United States. Public Health Rep 104:653–7.

Rieder HL, Cauthen GM, Comstock GW, Snider DE (1989) Epidemiology of tuberculosis in the United States. Epidemiol Rev 11:79–98.

Rifkin SB, Walt G (1986) Why health improves: defining the issues concerning "comprehensive primary health care" and "selective primary health care." Soc Sci Med 23:559–66.

Rinaldi RC, Steindles MS, Wilford BB, et al. (1988) Classification and standardization of substance abuse terminology. JAMA 259:555–7.

Ritenbaugh C, Goodby C (1989) Beyond the Thrifty Gene: metabolic implications of prehistoric migration into the New World. Med Anthropol 11:227–36.

Robertson LS (1986) Community injury control programs of the Indian Health Service: an early assessment. Public Health Rep 101:632–7.

Robinson E (1985) Mortality among the James Bay Cree. In: Fortuine R, ed. Circumpolar Health 84. Seattle: University of Washington Press; 166–9.

Robinson E (1988) The health of the James Bay Cree. Can Fam Physician 34:1606–13.

Robinson EJ, Moffatt ME (1985) Outbreak of rotavirus gastroenteritis in a James Bay Cree community. Can J Public Health 76:21–4.

Robitaille N, Choinière R (1985) An Overview of Demographic and Socio-economic Conditions of the Inuit in Canada. Ottawa: Research Branch, Corporate Policy, Indian and Northern Affairs Canada.

Rolf RT, Nakashima AK (1990) Epidemiology of primary and secondary syphilis in the United States, 1981 through 1989. JAMA 264:1432–7.

Romaniuk A (1974) Modernization and fertility: the case of the James Bay Indians. Can Rev Sociol Anthropol 11:344–59.

Romaniuk A (1981) Increase in natural fertility during the early stages of modernization: Canadian Indians case study. Demography 18:157–72.

Rose G (1985) Sick individuals and sick populations. Int J Epidemiol 14:32–8.

Ross CA (1982) Gasoline sniffing and lead encephalopathy. Can Med Assoc J 127:1195–7.

Ross CA, Davis B (1986) Suicide and parasuicide in a northern Canadian native community. Can J Psychiatry 31:331–4.

Ross SA, Fick GH (1990) Vascular complications in diabetic Native Canadians. Diabetes 39(Suppl 1):125A.

Ross SA, Fick GH (1991) Insulin as a risk factor for diabetes complications. Diabetes 40(Suppl 1):333A.

Rothschild HR, ed (1981) Biocultural Aspects of Disease. Orlando, FL: Academic Press.

Roychoudhury AK (1978) Genetic distance between the American Indians and the three major races of man. Hum Hered 28:380–5.

Rubenstein A, Boyle J, Odoroff CL, et al. (1969) Effect of improved sanitary facilities on infant diarrhea in a Hopi village. Public Health Rep 84:1093–7.

Runyan CW, Gerken EA (1989) Epidemiology and prevention of adolescent injury: a review and research agenda. JAMA 262:2273–9.

Rush AG, comp. (1992) HIV Prevention in Native American Communities: A Manual for Native American Health and Human Service Providers. Oakland, CA: National Native American AIDS Prevention Center.

Saad MF, Knowler WC, Pettitt DJ, et al. (1988) The natural history of impaired glucose tolerance in the Pima Indian. N Engl J Med 319:1500–6.

Saad MF, Knowler WC, Pettitt DJ, et al. (1989) Sequential changes in serum insulin concentration during development of non-insulin-dependent diabetes. Lancet 1:1356–9.

Saad MF, Knowler WC, Pettitt DJ, et al. (1991a) A two-step model for development of non-insulin-dependent diabetes. Am J Med 90:229–35.

Saad MF, Lillioja S, Nyomba B, et al. (1991b) Racial differences in the relation between blood pressure and insulin resistance. N Engl J Med 324:733–9.

Saemundsen AK, Albeck H, Hansen JP, et al. (1982) Epstein-Barr virus in nasopharyngeal and salivary gland carcinoma of Greenland Eskimos. Br J Cancer 46:721–8.

Sagild U, Littauer J, Jespersen CS, Andersen S (1966) Epidemiological studies in Greenland 1962–1964. I. Diabetes mellitus in Eskimos. Acta Med Scand 179:29–39.

Saiki JH, Rimoin DL (1968) Diabetes mellitus among the Navajo. I. Clinical features. Arch Intern Med 122:1–5.

Samet JM, Coultas DB, Howard CA (1988) Diabetes, gallbladder disease, obesity, and hypertension among Hispanics in New Mexico. Am J Epidemiol 128:1302–11.

Samet JM, Key CR, Hunt WC, Goodwin JS (1987) Survival of American Indian and Hispanic cancer patients in New Mexico and Arizona, 1969–82. J Natl Cancer Inst 79:457–63.

Samet JM, Kutvirt DM, Waxweiler RJ, Key CR (1984) Uranium mining and lung cancer in Navajo men. N Engl J Med 310:1481–4.

Sampliner RE, Bennett PH, Comess LJ, et al. (1970) Gallbladder disease in Pima Indians: demonstration of high prevalence and early onset by cholecystography. N Engl J Med 283:1358–64.

Santosham M, Hill J, Wolff M, et al. (1991a) Safety and immunogenicity of a Haemophilus influenzae type b conjugate vaccine in a high risk American Indian population. Pediatr Infect Dis J 10:113–7.

Santosham M, Letson GW, Wolff M, et al. (1991b) A field study of the safety and efficacy of two candidate rotavirus vaccines in a Native American population. J Infect Dis 163:483–7.

Santosham M, Reid R, Ambrosino DM, et al. (1987) Prevention of Haemophilus influenzae type b infections in high-risk infants treated with bacterial polysaccharide immune globulin. N Engl J Med 317:923–9.

Santosham M, Wolff M, Reid R, et al. (1991c) The efficacy in Navajo infants of a conjugate vaccine consisting of Haemophilus influenzae type b polysaccharide and

Neisseria meningitidis outer-membrane protein complex. N Engl J Med 324: 1767–72.

Santosham M, Yolken R, Wyatt R, et al. (1985) Epidemiology of rotavirus diarrhea in a prospectively monitored American Indian population. J Infect Dis 152:778–83.

Saracci R (1987) The interactions of tobacco smoking and other agents in cancer etiology. Epidemiol Rev 9:175–93.

Sauberlich HE, Goad W, Herman YF, et al. (1972) Biochemical assessment of the nutritional status of the Eskimos of Wainwright, Alaska. Am J Clin Nutr 25:437–45.

Savage PJ, Hamman RF, Bartha G, et al. (1976) Serum cholesterol levels in American (Pima) Indian children and adolscents. Pediatrics 58:274–82.

Schacht RM (1981) Estimating past population trends. Annu Rev Anthropol 10:119–40.

Schaefer C, Harrison HR, Boyce WT, Lewis M (1985) Illnesses in infants born to women with Chlamydia trachomatis infection. Am J Dis Child 139:127–33.

Schaefer JM (1981) Firewater myths revisited: review of findings and some new directions. J Stud Alcohol 42(Suppl 9):99–117.

Schaefer O (1968) Glycosuria and diabetes mellitus in Canadian Eskimos. Can Med Assoc J 99:201–6.

Schaefer O (1968) Glucose tolerance testing in Canadian Eskimos: a preliminary report and hypothesis. Can Med Assoc J 99:252–62.

Schaefer O (1977) Are Eskimos more or less obese than other Canadians? A comparison of skinfold thickness and ponderal index in Canadian Eskimos. Am J Clin Nutr 30:1623–8.

Schaefer O (1982) Ethnology, demography and medicine in the Arctic. In Harvald B, Hansen JPH, eds. Circumpolar Health 81. Oulu, Finland: Nordic Council for Arctic Medical Research; 187–93.

Schaefer O, Crockford PM, Romanowski B (1972) Normalization effect of preceding protein meals on "diabetic" oral glucose tolerance in Eskimos. Can Med Assoc J 107:733–8.

Schaefer O, Eaton RD, Timmermans FJ, Hildes JA (1980a) Respiratory function impairment and cardiopulmonary consequences in long-time residents of the Canadian Arctic. Can Med Assoc J 123:997–1004.

Schaefer O, Hildes JA, Greidanus P, Leung D (1974) Regional sweating in Eskimos compared to Caucasians. Can J Physiol Pharmacol 52:960–5.

Schaefer O, Hildes JA, Medd LM, Cameron DG (1975) The changing pattern of neoplastic disease in Canadian Eskimos. Can Med Assoc J 112:1399–404.

Schaefer O, Timmermans JF, Eaton RD, Mathews AR (1980b) General and nutritional health in two Eskimo populations at different stages of acculturation. Can J Public Health 71:397–405.

Schanfield MS, Crawford MH, Dossetor JB, Gershowitz H (1990) Immunoglobulin allotypes in several North American Eskimo populations. Hum Biol 62:773–89.

Schantz PM, Von Reye CF, Welty T, et al. (1977) Epidemiologic investigation of echinococcosis in American Indians living in Arizona and New Mexico. Am J Trop Med Hyg 26:121–6.

Schlech WF, Ward JJ, Band JD, et al. (1985) Bacterial meningitis in the United States, 1978 through 1981. JAMA 253:1749–54.

Schmitt N, Hole LW, Barclay WS (1966) Accidental deaths among British Columbia Indians. Can Med Assoc J 94:228–34.

Schraer CD, Lanier AP, Boyko EJ, et al. (1988) Prevalence of diabetes mellitus in Alaskan Eskimos, Indians, and Aleuts, Diabetes Care 11:693–700.

Schreeder MT, Bender TR, McMahon BJ, Moser MR, et al. (1983) Prevalence of hepatitis B in selected Alaskan Eskimo villages. Am J Epidemiol 118:543–9.

Scott EM, Griffith IV (1957) Diabetes mellitus in Eskimos. Metabolism 6:320–5.

Scott EM, Griffith IV, Hoskins DD, Whaley RD (1958) Serum cholesterol levels and blood pressure of Alaskan Eskimo men. Lancet 2:667–8.

Scott KA, Myers AM (1988) Impact of fitness training on Native adolescents' self-evaluations and substance use. Can J Public Health 79:424–9.

Segal B (1983) Alcohol and alcoholism in Alaska: research in a multicultural and transitional society. Int J Addict 18:379–92.

Sewell CM, Becker TM, Wiggins CL et al (1989) Injury mortality in New Mexico's American Indians, Hispanics, and non-Hispanic whites, 1958 to 1982. West J Med 150:708–13.

Shaffer N, Wainwright RB, Middaugh JP, Tauxe RV (1990) Botulism among Alaska Natives: the role of changing food preparation and consumption practices. West J Med 153:390–3.

Shapiro ED, Ward JI (1991) The epidemiology and prevention of disease caused by Haemophilus influenzae type b. Epidemiol Rev 13:113–42.

Shaw FE, Shapiro CN, Welty TK, et al. (1990) Hepatitis transmission among the Sioux Indians of South Dakota. Am J Public Health 80:1091–4.

Shephard RJ (1980) Work physiology and activity patterns. in: Milan FA, ed. Human Biology of Circumpolar Populations. Cambridge: Cambridge University Press; 305–38.

Shephard RJ (1991) Body Composition in Biological Anthropology. Cambridge: Cambridge University Press.

Shore JH (1975) American Indian suicide: fact and fantasy. Psychiatry 38:86–91.

Shore JH, Bopp JE, Waller JR, et al. (1972) A suicide prevention center on an Indian reservation. Am J Psychiatry 128:1086–91.

Shore JH, Manson SM (1983) American Indian psychiatric and social problems. Transcult Psychiatr Res Rev 20:159–80.

Siber GR, Santosham M, Reid R, Thompson C, et al. (1990) Impaired antibody response to Haemophilus influenzae type b polysaccharide and low IgG2 and IgG4 concentrations in Apache children. N Engl J Med 323:1387–92.

Sievers ML (1966) Disease patterns among southwestern Indians. Public Health Rep 81:1075–83.

Sievers ML (1967) Myocardial infarction among southwestern American Indians. Ann Intern Med 67:800–7.

Sievers ML (1968a) Cigarette and alcohol usage by southwestern American Indians. Am J Public Health 58:71–82.

Sievers ML (1968b) Serum cholesterol levels in southwestern American Indians. J Chron Dis 21:107–15.

Sievers ML (1977) Historical overview of hypertension among American Indians and Alaskan Natives. Ariz Med 34:607–10.

Sievers ML, Fisher JR (1979) Increasing rate of acute myocardial infarction in southwestern American Indians. Ariz Med 36:739–42.

Sievers ML, Fisher JR (1981) Diseases of North American Indians. In: Rothschild H, ed. Biocultural Aspects of Disease. New York: Academic Press; 191–252.

Sievers ML, Fisher JR (1985) Diabetes in North American Indians. In: National Diabetes Data Group. Diabetes in America: Diabetes Data Compiled 1984. Bethesda, MD: U.S. Department of Health and Human Services; Chapter XI:1–20. NIH Publication No. 85-1468.

Sievers ML, Marquis JR (1962) The southwestern American Indians' burden: biliary disease. JAMA 182:570–2.

Sievers ML, Nelson RG, Bennett PH (1990) Adverse mortality experience of a southwestern American Indian community: oveall death rates and underlying causes of death in Pima Indians. J Clin Epidemiol 43:1231–42.

Simpson SG, Reid R, Baker SP et al (1983) Injuries among the Hopi Indians. A population-based survey. JAMA 249:1873–6.

Singer DE, Samet JH, Coley CM, Nathan DM (1988) Screening for diabetes mellitus. Ann Intern Med 109:639–49.

Singer M (1989) The limitations of medical ecology: the concepts of adaptation in the context of social stratification and social transformation. Med Anthropol 10:223–34.

Skamene E (1989) Genetic control of susceptibility to mycobacterial infections. Rev Infect Dis 11(Suppl 2):S394–S399.

Skinhøj P (1977) Hepatitis and hepatitis B antigen in Greenland. II. Occurrence and interrelation of hepatitis B associated surface, core and "e" antigen-antibody systems in a highly endemic area. Am J Epidemiol 105:99–106.

Skinhøj P, Mikklesen F, Hollinger FB (1977) Hepatitis A in Greenland: importance of specific antibody testing in epidemiologic surveillance. Am J Epidemiol 105:140–7.

Smith RL (1957) Cardiovascular-renal and diabetes deaths among the Navajos. Public Health Rep 72:33–8.

Smith RL (1957) Recorded and expected mortality among the Indians of the United States with special reference to cancer. J Natl Cancer Inst. 18:385–96.

Smith RJ (1988) IHS fellows program aimed at lowering injuries, deaths of Indians, Alaska Natives. Public Health Rep 103:204.

Smith SM, Colwell LS, Sniezek JE (1990) An evaluation of external cause-of-injury codes using hospital records from the Indian Health Service, 1985. Am J Public Health 80:279–81.

So JK (1980) Human biological adaptation to Arctic and Subarctic zones. Annu Rev Anthropol 9:63–82.

Sole TD, Croll N (1980) Intestinal parasites in man in Labrador, Canada. Am J Trop Med Hyg 29:364–8.

Sorem KA (1985) Cancer incidence in the Zuni Indians of New Mexico. Yale J Biol Med 58:489–96.

Spicer EH, ed. (1961) Perspectives in American Indian Culture Change. Chicago: University of Chicago Press.

Spuhler JN (1979) Genetic distances, trees, and maps of North American Indians. In: Laughlin WS, Harper AB, eds. The First Americans: Origins, Affinities, and Adaptations. New York: Gustav Fischer; 135–83.

Statistics Canada (1984) Canada's Native People: 1981 Census of Canada. Ottawa: Statistics Canada.

Statistics Canada (1989) A Data Book on Canada's Aboriginal Population from the 1986 Census of Canada. Ottawa: Statistics Canada, Aboriginal Peoples Output Program.

Stead WW, Senner JW, Reddick WT, Lofgren JP (1990) Racial differences in susceptibility to infection by Mycobacterium tuberculosis. N Engl J Med 322:422–7.

Steegman AT, Hurlich MG, Winterhalder B (1983) Coping with cold and other challenges of the boreal forest: an overview. In: Steegman TA, ed. Boreal Forest Adaptations: The Northern Algonkians. New York: Plenum Press; 317–51.

Stein JH, West KM, Robey JM, et al. (1965) The high prevalence of abnormal glucose tolerance in the Cherokee Indians of North Carolina. Arch Intern Med 116:842–5.

Stern MP (1991) Primary prevention of type II diabetes mellitus. Diabetes Care 14:399–410.

Stern MP, Ferrell RE, Rosenthal M, et al. (1986) Association between NIDDM, Rh blood group, and haptoglobin phenotype. Diabetes 35:387–91.

Stern MP, Haffner SM (1986) Body fat distribution and hyperinsulinemia as risk factors for diabetes and cardiovascular diseases. Arteriosclerosis 6:123–30.

Stich HF, Hornby AP (1985) Endogenous and exogenous sources of nitrate/nitrite and nitrosamines in Canadian Inuit with a traditional or Western lifestyle. In: Fortuine R, ed. Circumpolar Health 84. Seattle, WA: University of Washington Press; 92–5.

Stich HF, Hornby AP, Dunn BP (1985) A pilot beta-carotene intervention trial with Inuit using smokeless tobacco. Int J Cancer 36:321–7.

Story M, Tompkin RA, Bass MA, Wakefield LM (1986) Anthropometric measurements and dietary intakes of Cherokee Indian teenagers in North Carolina. J Am Diet Assoc 86:1555–60.

Stratton R, Zeiner A, Paredes A (1978) Tribal affiliation and prevalence of alcohol problems. J Stud Alcohol 39:1166–77.

Streeper RB, Massey RU, Liu G, et al. (1960) An electrocardiographic and autopsy study of coronary heart disease in the Navajos. Dis Chest 38:305–12.

Streiner DL, Adam K (1987) Evaluation of the effectiveness of suicide prevention programs: a methodological perspective. Suicide Life Threat Behav 17:93–106.

Stull DD (1972) Victims of modernization: accident rates and Papago Indian adjustment. Hum Organization 31:227–40.

Sturtevant WC, ed. (1978–1990) Handbook of North American Indians. Washington, DC: Smithsonian Institution [20 vols projected, 9 already published].

Stutzman CD, Nelson DM, Lanier AP (1986) Estimates of cancer incidence in Alaskan Natives due to exposure to global radioactive fallout from atmospheric nuclear weapons testing. Alaska Med 28:67–77.

Sugarman JR, Gilbert TJ, Weiss NS (1992) Prevalence of diabetes and impaired glucose tolerance among Navajo Indians. Diabetes Care 15:114–20.

Sugarman JR, Hickey M, Hall T, Gohdes D (1990a) The changing epidemiology of diabetes mellitus among Navajo Indians. West J Med 153:140–5.

Sugarman JR, Percy C (1989) Prevalence of diabetes in a Navajo Indian community. Am J Public Health 79:511–3.

Sugarman JR, White LL, Gilbert TJ (1990b) Evidence for a secular change in obesity, height, and weight among Navajo Indian school children. Am J Clin Nutr 52:960–6.

Sutherland I (1976) Recent studies in the epidemiology of tuberculosis, based on the risk of being infected with tubercle bacilli. Adv Tuberc Res 19:1–63.

Sutherland I (1981) The epidemiology of tuberculosis: is prevention better than cure? Bull Int Union Tuberc 56:127–34.

Swedlund AC, Armelagos GJ, eds (1990) Disease in Populations in Transition: Anthropological and Epidemiological Perspectives. New York: Bergin and Garvey.

Szathmary EJ (1984) Peopling of northern North America: clues from genetic studies. Acta Anthropogenet 8:79–110.

Szathmary EJ (1985) The search for genetic factors controlling plasma glucose levels in Dogrib Indians. In: Chakraborty R, Szathmary EJ, eds. Diseases of Complex Etiology in Small Populations. New York: Alan R Liss; 199–226.

Szathmary EJ (1987) The effect of Gc genotype on fasting insulin level in Dogrib Indians. Hum Genet 75:368–72.

Szathmary EJ (1989) The impact of low carbohydrate consumption on glucose tolerance, insulin concentration and insulin response to glucose challenge in Dogrib Indians. Med Anthropol 11:329–50.

Szathmary EJ (1990) Diabetes in Amerindian populations: the Dogrib studies. In: Armelagos G, Swedlung A, eds. Health and Disease of Populations in Transition. New York: Bergin and Garvey; 75–103.

Szathmary EJ, Ferrell RE (1990) Glucose level, acculturation, and glycosylated hemoglobin: an example of biocultural interaction. Med Anthropol Q 4:315–41.

Szathmary EJ, Holt N (1983) Hyperglycemia in Dogrib Indians of the NWT, Canada: association with age and a centripetal distribution of body fat. Hum Biol 55:493–515.

Szathmary EJ, Ritenbaugh C, Goodby CS (1987) Dietary change and plasma glucose levels in an Amerindian population undergoing cultural transition. Soc Sci Med 24:791–804.

Tanner CE, Staudt M, Adamowski R, et al. (1987) Seroepidemiological study for five different zoonotic parasites in northern Quebec. Can J Public Health 78:262–6.

Terry RD, Bass MA (1984) Obesity among Eastern Cherokee Indian women: prevalence, self perceptions, and experience. Ecol Foods Nutr 14:117–27.

Thacker SB (1986) The persistence of influenza A in human populations. Epidemiol Rev 8:129–42.

Thistle JL, Eckhart KL, Nensel RE et al (1971) Prevalence of gallbladder disease among Chippewa Indians. Mayo Clin Proc 46:603–8.

Thistle JL, Schoenfield LJ (1971) Lithogenic bile among young Indian women: lithogenic potential decreased with chenodeoxycholic acid. N Engl J Med 284:177–81.

Thomas DB (1979) Epidemiologic studies of cancer in minority groups in the western United States. Nat Cancer Inst Monogr 53:103–13.

Thomson G (1988) HLA disease associations in models for insulin dependent diabetes mellitus and the study of complex human genetic disorders. Annu Rev Genet 22:31–50.

Thomson M, Philion J (1991) Children's respiratory hospitalizations and air pollution. Can J Public Health 82:203–4.

Thorne AG, Wolpoff MH (1992) The multiregional evolution of humans. Sci Am 266(4):76–83.

Thornton R (1987) American Indian Holocaust and Survival: A Population History Since 1492. Norman, OK: University of Oklahoma Press.

Thorslund J (1990) Inuit suicides in Greenland. Arct Med Res 49:25–33.

Toomey KE, Oberschelp AG, Greenspan JR (1989) Sexually transmitted diseases and Native Americans: trends in reported gonorrhea and syphilis morbidity, 1984–88. Public Health Rep 104:566–72.

Toomey KE, Rafferty MP, Stamm WE (1987) Unrecognized high prevalence of Chlamydia trachomatis cervical infection in an isolated Alaskan Eskimo population. JAMA 258:53–6.

Torrey EF, Reiff FW, Noble GR (1979) Hypertension among Aleuts. Am J Epidemiol 110:7–14.

Torroni A, Schurr TG, Yang C, Szathmary EJ, et al. (1992) Native American mitochondrial DNA analysis indicates that the Amerind and the NaDene populations were founded by two independent migrations. Genetics 130:153–62.

Trott L, Barnes G, Dumoff R (1981) Ethnicity and other demographic characteristics as predictors of sudden drug-related deaths. J Stud Alcohol 42:564–78.

Trovato F (1988) Mortality differentials in Canada, 1951–1971: French, British, and Indians. Cult Med Psychiatry 12:459–77.

Trowell HC, Burkitt DP, eds. (1981) Western Diseases: Their Emergence and Prevention. Cambridge, MA: Harvard University Press.

U.S. Congress, Office of Technology Assessment (1986) Indian Health Care. Washington, DC: U.S. Government Printing Office (OTA-H-290).

U.S. Congress, Office of Technology Assessment (1989) Indian Adolescent Mental Health. Washington, DC: U.S. Government Printing Office (OTA-H-446).

U.S. Department of Health, Education, and Welfare (1978a) Illness among Indians and Alaska Natives, 1970 to 1978. Rockville, MD: U.S. DHEW/PHS/HSA/IHS/Office of Program Statistics; DHEW Pub No (HSA 79-12040).

U.S. Department of Health, Education and Welfare (1978b) Indian Health Trends and Services. Rockville, MD: U.S. DHEW/PHS/HSA/IHS/Office of Program Statistics; DHEW Pub No (HSA 78-12009).

U.S. Department of Health and Human Services (1988) Indian Health Service Chart Series Book. Rockville, MD: U.S. DHHS/PHS/IHS/Division of Program Statistics.

U.S. Department of Health and Human Services (1988) The Surgeon General's Report on Nutrition and Health. Washington, D.C.: U.S. Government Printing Office; DHHS(PHS) Pub. No. 88-50210.

U.S. Department of Health and Human Services (1990a) Indian Health Conditions. Rockville, MD: U.S. DHHS/PHS/Indian Health Service.

U.S. Department of Health and Human Services (1990b) Trends in Indian Health 1990. Rockville, MD: U.S. DHHS/PHS/IHS/Division of Program Statistics.

Ubelaker DH (1976) Prehistoric New World population size: historical review and current appraisal of North American estimates. Am J Phys Anthropol 45:661–5.

Upadhyay YN, Gerrard JW (1969) Recurrent pneumonia in Indian children. Ann Allergy 27:218–24.

Van Winkle NW, May PA (1986) Native American suicide in New Mexico, 1957–1979: A comparative study. Hum Organization 45:296–309.

Verdier PC, Eaton RD, Cooper B (1987) A study of the nutritional status of an Inuit population in the Canadian high Arctic. Part 1: Biochemical evaluation. Can J Public Health 78:229–35.

Vivian RP, McMillan C, Moore PE, et al. (1948) The nutrition and health of the James Bay Indian. Can Med Assoc J 59:505–18.

Wainwright RB, McMahon BJ, Bulkow LR, et al. (1989) Duration of immunogenicity and efficacy of hepatitis B vaccine in a Yupik Eskimo population. JAMA 261: 2362–6.

Wainwright RB, McMahon BJ, Bulkow LR, et al. (1991) Protection provided by hepatitis B vaccine in a Yupik Eskimo population: seven-year results. Arch Intern Med 151:1634–6.

Waldram JB (1985) Hydroelectric development and dietary delocalization in northern Manitoba, Canada. Hum Organization 44:41–9.

Waller AE, Baker SP, Szocka A (1989) Childhood injury deaths: national analysis and geographical variations. Am J Public Health 79:310–5.

Walsh JA, Warren KS (1979) Selective primary health care: an interim strategy for disease control in developing countries. N Engl J Med 301:967–74.

Ward JA, Fox J (1977) A suicide epidemic on an Indian reserve. Can Psychiatr Assoc J 22:423–6.

Ward JI, Brenneman G, Lepow M et al (1988) Haemophilus influenzae type b anticapsular antibody responses to PRP-Pertusis and PRP-D vaccines in Alaska Native infants. J Infect Dis 158:719–23.

Ward JI, Brenneman G, Letson GW, Heyward WL et al (1990) Limited efficacy of a Haemophilus influenzae type b conjugate vaccine in Alaska Native infants. N Engl J Med 323:1393–401.

Ward JI, Lum MK, Hall DB, Silimperi DR, Bender TR (1986) Invasive Haemophilus influenzae type b disease in Alaska: background epidemiology for a vaccine efficacy trial. J Infect Dis 153:17–26.

Ward JI, Margolis HS, Lum MK, Fraser DW, Bender TR (1981) Haemophilus influenzae disease in Alaskan Eskimos: characteristics of a population with an unusual incidence of invasive disease. Lancet 1:1281–4.

Warwick OH, Phillips AJ (1954) Cancer among Canadian Indians. Br J Cancer 8:223–30.

Watson TG, Freeman RS, Staszak M (1979) Parasites in native peoples of the Sioux Lookout Zone, northwestern Ontario. Can J Public Health 70:179–82.

Wein EE, Sabry JH, Evers FT (1991a) Food consumption patterns and use of country foods by Native Canadians near Wood Buffalo National Park, Canada. Arctic 44:196–205.

Wein EE, Sabry JH, Evers FT (1991b) Nutrient intakes of Native Canadians near Wood Buffalo National Park. Nutr Res 11:5–13.

Weiss KM, Ferrell RE, Hanis CL, Styne PN (1984a) Genetics and epidemiology of gallbladder disease in New World Native Peoples. Am J Hum Genet 36:1259–78.

Weiss KM, Ferrell RE, Hanis CL (1984b) A New World syndrome of metabolic diseases with a genetic and evolutionary basis. Yearbk Phys Anthropol 27:153–78.

Welty TK, Freni-Titulaer L, Zack MM, et al. (1986) Effects of exposure to salty drinking water in an Arizona community: cardiovascular mortality, hypertension prevalence, and relationships between blood pressure and sodium intake. JAMA 255:622–6.

Welty TK, Tanaka ES, Leonard B, Rhoades ER, Hurlburt WB (1987) Indian Health Service facilities become smoke-free. MMWR 36:348–50.

Wendorf M, Goldfine ID (1991) Archaeology of NIDDM: excavation of the "thrifty" genotype. Diabetes 40:161–5.

West KM (1974) Diabetes in American Indians and other native populations of the New World. Diabetes 23:841–55.

West KM (1978) Epidemiology of Diabetes and Its Vascular Lesions. New York: Elsevier.

West KM, Erdreich LJ, Stober JA (1980) A detailed study of risk factors for retinopathy and nephropathy in diabetes. Diabetes 29:501–8.

Westermeyer J (1976) Use of a social indicator system to assess alcoholism among Indian people in Minnesota. Am J Drug Alcohol Abuse 3:447–56.

Westfall DN, Rosenbloom AL (1971) Diabetes mellitus among the Florida Seminoles. HSMHA Health Rep 86:1037–41.

Wherrett GJ (1977) The Miracle of the Empty Beds: A History of Tuberculosis in Canada. Toronto: University of Toronto Press.

White R, Cornely D (1981) Navajo child abuse and neglect study: A comparison group examination of abuse and neglect of Navajo children. Child Abuse and Neglect 5:9–17.

Whittaker JO (1982) Alcohol and the Standing Rock Sioux tribe: a twenty-year follow-up study. J Stud Alcohol 43:191–200.

Widom CS (1989) The cycle of violence. Science 244:160–6.

Wilber CG, Levine VE (1950) Fat metabolism in Alaskan Eskimos. Exp Med Surg 8: 422–5.

Wilkinson D, King G (1987) Conceptual and methodological issues in the use of race as a variable: policy implications. Milbank Q 65(suppl 1):56–71.

Willctt WC (1990) Nutritional Epidemiology. New York: Oxford University Press.

Williams CN, Johnston JL, Weldon KL (1977) Prevalence of gallstones and gallbladder disease in Canadian Micmac Indian women. Can Med Assoc J 117:758:60.

Williams R (1986) Prevalence of hepatitis A virus antibody among Navajo school children. Am J Public Health 76:282–3.

Williams RC, Knowler WC, Butler WJ, et al. (1981) HLA-A2 and type 2 (insulin-dependent) diabetes mellitus in Pima Indians: an association of allele frequency with age. Diabetologia 21:460–3.

Williams RC, Steinberg AG, Gershowitz H, et al. (1985) Gm allotypes in Native Americans: evidence for three distinct migrations across the Bering land bridge. Am J Phys Anthropol 66:1–19.

Wilson AC, Cann RL (1992) The recent African genesis of humans. Sci Am 266(4):68–73.

Wilson JF, Diddams AC, Rausch RL (1968) Cystic hydatid disease in Alaska: a review of 101 autochthonous cases of Echinococcus granulosus infection. Am Rev Respir Dis 98:1–15.

Wilson LG (1990) The historical decline of tuberculosis in Europe and America: its causes and significance. J Hist Med 45:366–96.

Wilt J, Wilt P, Kordova N, Martin C (1976) The human placenta as a possible reservoir of chlamydial infection in northern Canada. Can J Public Health 67:114–6.

Winawer SJ, Schottenfield D, Flehinger BJ (1991) Colorectal cancer screening. J Natl Cancer Inst 83:243–53.

Winterhalder B (1983) Boreal foraging strategies. In: Steegman AT, ed. Boreal Forest Adaptations: The Northern Algonkians. New York: Plenum Press; 201–41.

Wirsing RL (1985) The health of traditional societies and the effects of acculturation. Curr Anthropol 26:303–22.

Wolff P (1973) Vasomotor sensitivity to alcohol in diverse Mongoloid populations. Am J Hum Genet 25:193–9.

Wolfgang RW (1954) Indian and Eskimo diphyllobothriasis. Can Med Assoc J 70: 536–9.

Wood JW, Milner GR, Harpending HC, Weiss KM (1992) The osteological paradox: problems of inferring prehistoric health from skeletal samples. Curr Anthropol 33:343–70.

Woodward WE, Hirschhorn N, Sack RB, et al. (1974) Acute diarrhea on an Apache Indian reservation. Am J Epidemiol 99:281–90.

World Health Organization (1982) Tuberculosis Control: Report of a Joint IUAT/WHO Study Group. Tech Rep Ser No 671. Geneva: WHO.

World Health Organization (1985) Diabetes Mellitus: Report of a WHO Study Group. Tech Rep Ser; No 727. Geneva: WHO.

World Health Organization (1990) Prevention in Childhood and Youth of Adult Cardio-vascular Diseases: Time for Action. Tech Rep Ser No 792. Geneva: WHO.

Wotton KA, Stiver HG, Hildes JA (1981) Meningitis in the Central Arctic: a 4-year experience. Can Med Assoc J 124:887–90.

Yamashita T, Mackay W, Rushforth NB, Bennett P, Houser H (1984) Pedigree anlayses of non-insulin dependent diabetes mellitus (NIDDM) in the Pima Indians suggests au-tosomal dominant mode of inheritance. Am J Hum Genet 36:183–S.

Yolken R, Leister F, Almeido-Hill J, et al. (1989) Infantile gastroenteritis associated with excretion of pestivirus antigens. Lancet 1:517–9.

Yost GC, Kaplan AM, Bustamante R, et al. (1986) Bacterial meningitis in Arizona Amer-ican Indian children. Am J Dis Child 140:943–6.

Young JL, Ries LG, Pollock ES (1984) Cancer patient survival among ethnic groups in the United States. J Natl Cancer Inst 73:341–52.

Young TK (1982) Self-perceived and clinically assessed health status of Indians in north-western Ontario: analysis of a health survey. Can J Public Health 73:272–7.

Young TK (1983) Mortality pattern of isolated Indians in northwestern Ontario: a 10-year review. Public Health Rep 98:467–75.

Young TK (1985) BCG vaccination among Canadian Indians and Inuit: the epidemiolog-ical bases for policy decision. Can J Public Health 76:124–9.

Young TK (1988a) Are Subarctic Indians undergoing the epidemiologic transition? Soc Sci Med 26:659–71.

Young TK (1988b) Health Care and Cultural Change: the Indian Experience in the Central Subarctic. Toronto: University of Toronto Press.

Young TK (1991) Prevalence and correlates of hypertension in a subarctic Indian popu-lation. Prev Med 20:474–85.

Young TK, Bruce L, Elias J, O'Neil JD, Yassi A (1991) The Health Effects of Housing and Community Infrastructure on Canadian Indian Reserves. Ottawa: Department of Indian Affairs and Northern Development.

Young TK, Casson I (1988) The decline and persistence of tuberculosis in a Canadian Indian population: implications for control. Can J Public Health 79:302–6.

Young TK, Choi NW (1985) Cancer risks among residents of Manitoba Indian reserves, 1970–79. Can Med Assoc J 132:1269–72.

Young TK, Frank JW (1983) Cancer surveillance in a remote Indian population in north-western Ontario. Am J Public Health 73:515–20.

Young TK, Hershfield ES (1986) A case-control study to evaluate the effectiveness of mass BCG vaccination among Canadian Indians. Am J Public Health 76:783–6.

Young TK, Kaufert JM, McKenzie JK, Hawkins A, O'Neil JD (1989) Excess burden of end-stage renal disease among Canadians Indians: a national survey. Am J Public Health 79:756–8.

Young TK, McIntyre LL, Dooley J, Rodriguez J (1985) Epidemiologic features of dia-betes mellitus among Indians in northwestern Ontario and northeastern Manitoba. Can Med Assoc J 132:793–7.

Young TK, Roche BA (1990) Factors associated with clinical gallbladder disease in a Canadian Indian population. Clin Invest Med 13:55–9.

Young TK, Schraer CD, Shubnikoff EV, Szathmary EJ, Nikitin YP (1992) Prevalence of diagnosed diabetes in circumpolar indigenous populations. Int J Epidemiol 21:730–6.

Young TK, Sevenhuysen G (1989) Obesity in northern Canadian Indians: patterns, determinants, and consequences. Am J Clin Nutr 49:786–93.

Young TK, Sevenhuysen G, Ling N, Moffatt MEK (1990a) Determinants of plasma glucose levels and diabetes in a northern Canadian Indian population. Can Med Assoc J 142:821–30.

Young TK, Szathmary EJ, Evers S, Wheatley B (1990b) Geographical distribution of diabetes among the Native population of Canada: a national survey. Soc Sci Med 31:129–39.

Zeiner AR, Giradot JM, Nichols N, Jones-Saumty D (1984) ALDHI isozyme deficiency among North American Indians. Alcoholism Clin Exp Res 8:129.

Zeiner AR, Parades A, Cowden L (1976) Physiologic response to ethanol among the Tarahumara Indians. Ann NY Acad Sci 273:151–8.

Zimmerman MR, Aufderheiden AC (1984) The frozen family of Utriagvik: the autopsy findings. Arct Anthropol 21:53–64.

Zimmet PZ (1992) Challenges in diabetes epidemiology—from West to the rest. Diabetes Care 15:232–52.

Zimmet P, Dowse G, Finch C, Serjeantson S, King H (1990) The epidemiology and natural history of NIDDM—lessons from the South Pacific. Diabetes Metab Rev 6:91–124.

Zur Hausen H (1989) Papillomaviruses in anogenital cancer as a model to understand the role of viruses in human cancer. Cancer Res 49:4677–81.

Geographical and Tribal Index

Includes names of tribes, language families, culture areas, geographical place names

267

Subject Index

Fires, 46, 179, 181–89
Fish, 48, 91, 108
Folate, 50–51
Food hygiene, 93
Framingham Study, 130, 133, 223

Gallbladder disease, 101, 103, 108, 139,
    168–71, 174
Gasoline sniffing, 204–5; *see also* Substance
    abuse
Gastroenteritis. *See* Diarrhea
Gene effect, 161
Gene frequencies, 21
Gene pool, 22
Genetic
    admixture, 160, 168
    counseling, 168
    distance, 7
    factors in disease, 56, 125, 135, 157, 217,
        220–24, 226
    markers, 8, 62, 67–68, 90, 105, 160–61,
        173
    origins and diversity of Native Americans,
        3, 7–10
    polymorphism, 8
    susceptibility, 7, 62, 106, 108, 146, 164,
        210–15
    theory of alcoholism, 205
Genocide, 15, 28
Geographical distribution, 16–21
Ghost Dance, 208
Giardiasis (*Giardia lamblia*), 70, 92
Glomerulonephritis, 88–90, 220
Gonorrhea, gonococcus, 84–86
Gm allotype. *See* Serum proteins.

Hair color and texture, 8
Habitats, ecological, 10–11
Handsome Lake cult, 208
Health
    definition of, 23–25
    field concept, 23
    indicators, 23
    insurance claims databases, 44, 96
    policy, 224
    status, 12, 216
Health care services, 23–24, 138, 194, 218
Health education, 74, 87, 93, 109, 136, 145,
    167, 188, 207–9, 220, 226
Heart disease, ischemic, 21, 94, 113–23,
    129, 135–37, 139, 165–66, 200
Helminths, 90–93
Hemophilus influenzae, 65–69, 75–76, 79,
    219
Hepatitis, 79–84, 107, 110, 112, 216, 219
Herpes simplex, 84–85, 106–7
Historical development, 12–15
Homicide, 176–77, 182, 189–98, 217
Horticulture, 14

Hospitalizations, 43, 70, 77, 96, 114–18,
    176, 203
Human biology, 23, 24, 222
Human immunodeficiency virus (HIV), 61,
    84, 86–88, 225
Human leukocyte antigen (HLA), 8, 62, 67,
    90, 105, 161
Human papillomavirus, 84, 106–7
Hunter-gatherer, 26, 221
Hydatid disease. *See* Echinococcosis.
Hydroelectric development, 49
Hypertension, 94, 121, 123–29, 135–37,
    139, 163, 166, 171–73, 200, 216, 223

Immunizations, 55, 62–64, 68–69, 74–75,
    79, 83, 110, 112, 219
Immune globulins (immunoglobulins), 69,
    82–83
Impaired glucose tolerance (IGT), 164, 172;
    see also Diabetes
Impetigo, 89
Indian Health Service (IHS), 29, 31, 44, 52–
    53, 57, 62, 83, 87, 155–56, 167, 180,
    188, 219–20
Infant mortality rate, 37–41, 65, 216
Infectious diseases, 3, 4, 24–26, 42, 43–44,
    52–94, 216–17, 220, 225
Infertility, 85
Influenza and parainfluenza, 75–76, 79
Injuries, 3, 4, 24, 41–44, 53, 94, 176–215,
    216–20, 225
Insulin resistance, 125, 160, 164, 171–74
International Biological Program, 125, 143,
    222
International Classification of Diseases
    (ICD), 41–42, 56, 176, 200
INTERSALT Study, 125
Intestinal tract, infections of. *See* Diarrhea.
Intrauterine growth retardation, 46
Iron, 50–51
Isoniazid (INH), 62, 64

Km allotype. *See* Serum proteins

Languages, 8–10, 12–14, 129, 157, 204, 214
Life expectancy, 37–38, 216
Lifestyles, 23, 24, 46, 93, 113, 145, 209,
    216
Lipids, 94, 121, 123, 125, 128–37, 162, 166,
    169–73

Mammogram, 110–12
Measles, 53, 55–56
Medical Services Branch, 29–31
Meningitis. *See* Nervous system.
Meningococcus, 65–69
Mental disorders, 42, 189, 200
Metabolic bone disease, 26
Migration, 7–8, 105